MAKE INFORMED CHOICES ABOUT YOUR HEALTH . . .
BY KNOWING THE FACTS.

1. Which everyday foods can help restore your body's estrogen?
2. Which glands most strongly influence your postmenopausal health?
3. What is the most significant factor in preventing osteoporosis?
4. What is gamma-oryzynol?
5. True or false: Deep breathing can reduce hot flashes.
6. Is there any specific treatment for night sweats?

1. Soy products, apples, figs, dates, apricots, alfalfa, garlic, sprouted green peas, fennel and anise seeds, parsley, celery, nuts and legumes, whole grains
2. Your *adrenal* glands
3. Exercise
4. A component of rice bran oil shown to be effective in treating hot flashes, chills, heart palpitations, dizziness, insomnia, fatigue, and digestive problems
5. True. One study showed it helped 50 percent of women.
6. Oat straw, motherwort, and garden sage are helpful, and the homeopathic remedy sepia

FEELING BETTER . . . NATURALLY

The MEND Clinic Guide to
Natural Medicine for Menopause and Beyond

**Paula Maas, D.O., M.D. (H),
Susan E. Brown, Ph.D.,
and Nancy Bruning**

A Lynn Sonberg Book

A Dell Trade Paperback

A DELL TRADE PAPERBACK

Published by
Dell Publishing
a division of
Bantam Doubleday Dell Publishing Group, Inc.
1540 Broadway
New York, New York 10036

Copyright © 1997 by Lynn Sonberg Book Associates

Neither this nor any other book should be used as a substitute for professional medical care or treatment. It is advisable to seek the guidance of a physician or other qualified health practitioner before implementing any of the approaches to health suggested in this book. Also, please note that research about menopause and aging is ongoing and subject to interpretation. Although all reasonable efforts have been made to include the most up-to-date and accurate information in this book, there can be no guarantee that what we know about this complex subject won't change with time. It is essential that any reader who has any reason to suspect that she has an illness or health problem should check with her health practitioner before using any of the methods described in this book.

Library of Congress Cataloging in Publication Data
Maas, Paula.
The MEND clinic guide to natural medicine for menopause and beyond /
by Paula Maas, Susan E. Brown, and Nancy Bruning.
p.   cm.
"A Lynn Sonberg book."
ISBN 0-440-50703-0
1. Menopause—Popular works.   2. Menopause—Complications—
Alternative treatment.   3. Middle aged women—Health and hygiene.
I. Brown, Susan E., Ph.D.   II. Bruning, Nancy.   III. Title.
RG186.M22   1997
618.1'75—dc20   96-5709
CIP

Published by arrangement with:
Lynn Sonberg Book Associates
10 West 86 Street
New York, NY 10024

Printed in the United States of America
Published simultaneously in Canada

March 1997

10   9   8   7   6   5   4   3   2   1

BVG

Contents

Appendixes

Acknowledgments from Dr. Paula Maas:

Appreciation to my mother, who suffered with monthly migraines as a result of prescription estrogen, and the many other unique and strong women who sought to understand and doctor their own bodies and taught me from their experience. Special appreciation to those great healing physicians Robert Fulford, Lyn Patrick, Jesse Stoff, Reggie Stout, Andrew Weil; Dharma Singh Khalsa; the teaching of Elias at DiagnosTechs; Wally at Women's International Pharmacy and the many others who create excellent products and develop laboratory means of helping women through the "pause." For the support team leaders: Martin, Jeff, Lisa, Donna and Pattie; coauthors Susan Brown and Nancy Bruning and packager Lynn Sonberg for their patience with my meticulousness; and to Mary at the Complementary Medical Association.

Introduction

Not so long ago menopause was talked about in hushed tones, if at all. Going through menopause meant that you were getting old, and that your life was practically over. But that is changing. Today, a new generation of health-conscious American women is not shy about asking questions. About 1.25 million American women are becoming menopausal each year. Instead of looking back, today's women are looking forward. We invite you to join them. Perhaps you are one of them already.

If so, you have picked up this book because you want to know what happens during menopause and what you can do to feel better as you undergo this major change. What can you expect during menopause? Why do some women have such a bumpy ride while others sail through it smoothly, even joyfully? Is there sex after menopause—and how satisfying is it? What about other signs of aging (such as wrinkles) and the serious diseases (such as heart disease and breast cancer) that occur more frequently during and after the menopause years? We wrote this book to provide you with answers to such questions and to guide you in making informed decisions about your health care at this important time in your life.

Menopause can be a time of physical, spiritual, and emotional growth for women. At the same time, however, the characteristic hormonal fluctuations can cause troublesome symptoms in up to 80 percent of all American women. Hot flashes are the most notorious of these, but many women are also bothered by fatigue, depression, vaginal dryness, insomnia, urinary problems, heavy or irregular bleeding, breast tenderness, mood swings, and problems with sexual desire and arousal.

The good news is that these unpleasant symptoms are not an inevitable part of menopause. The natural approach—a healthy, balanced lifestyle and natural medicine—offers a safe, gentle alternative or complement to traditional medicine, including hormone replacement therapy, in treating many of these problems. The natural approach can not only help you deal with current menopausal problems, but also help reduce your risk of future serious age-related diseases such as cardiovascular disease, breast cancer, osteoporosis, and diabetes.

The two expert authors of this book are health professionals who are committed to improving women's health. One of us, Paula Maas, D.O., M.D. (H) is a physician board certified in Family Practice as well as Homeopathy. For over twenty years she has worked in the healing arts, integrating the most effective therapies from her eclectic study and practice. In 1988 she founded and directed the MEND Clinic in Tucson, Arizona. The MEND Clinic multidisciplinary approach has included experts in osteopathy, naturopathy, psychotherapy, acupuncture, herbal therapy, homeopathy, and a variety of manual medicine disciplines. Dr. Maas has found that although many women respond adequately to the common menopause prescription, women thrive and obtain optimal wellness when their needs are addressed as individuals. Beginning with the Balanced Life Plan guidelines presented in this book, she encourages every woman to discover her own body's needs and the natural choices available to meet them. The other author is Susan E. Brown, Ph.D., a medical anthropologist and certified clinical nutritionist. She directs the Nutrition Education and Consulting Service, in Syracuse, New York, which develops health maximization programs specifically tailored to the needs of each client. She also heads the Osteoporosis Education Project, specializing in the development of natural programs for regeneration of bone health. We have teamed up with a veteran health writer who has authored or co-authored fifteen books on a variety of subjects including nutritional supplements, homeopathy, swimming, and chemotherapy.

We have found there are some general books about natural medicine for women and books about a single type of alternative treatment. However, there was no book available that covered the major natural therapies for women who were concerned about menopause and age-related diseases, and that provided the information in easy-to-use A-to-Z format.

To fill that gap, we have written *The MEND Clinic Guide to Natural Medicine for Menopause and Beyond,* an easy-to-understand yet comprehensive look at menopause and the years that follow. We talk about the hormonal changes that occur, and we separate the facts from the myths associated with this period of transition and transformation in women's lives. Most of all, we want you to know that today you have choices—you don't have to turn automatically to prescription hormones such as estrogen. There are many alternatives that can complement and enhance traditional medical treatment.

Although you may find it tempting to turn directly to the A-to-Z section (Chapter 5), we hope you'll begin at the beginning of the book because it lays the foundation for all that follows. Chapter 1 opens up the door to a whole new way of thinking about menopause and aging that differs from the one that has become prevalent in the United States. It explains why menopause happens, and what you can expect from menopause and aging. Did you know that most women in many other parts of the world don't experience as many unpleasant physical and psychological problems as we do? It's true: They suffer less from both minor annoyances like hot flashes and insomnia, and from serious disease such as cardiovascular disease and osteoporosis. We explain why this is so. We discuss the underlying causes of menopause problems and aging disorders and how our attitudes toward aging and our modern lifestyles contribute toward less-than-perfect health. What you got away with in your younger years no longer works. Bad habits such as poor diet, little or no exercise, and coffee drinking combine with stress to throw your hormonal system out of kilter, making menopause more difficult than nature intended it to be. Such lifestyles increase our risk of such major killers as cardiovascular disease, breast cancer, osteoporosis, and diabetes. But it's never too late to begin to turn your life and your health around, using our three-part natural approach to menopause and aging disorders.

In Chapter 2, we give you the *Balanced Life Plan.* This is the most important component of the plan because it acts as a foundation. This program—consisting of a balanced, whole-food eating pattern, exercise, relaxation and stress management, and establishing a partnership with your doctor—may be all you need.

In Chapter 3, we explain how you can use *natural therapies for the common conditions of menopause and aging.* These include nutritional supplements, herbal therapy, bodywork, homeopathy, acupressure and traditional Chinese medicine, aromatherapy, and relaxation therapies. This is the next step to add if the Balanced Life Plan doesn't solve your problems or if you are at higher-than-average risk for serious age-related diseases. Through self-care or working with a professional natural health care practitioner, we explain how these therapies can address specific symptoms and/or reduce the risk of disease.

In Chapter 4, you learn about the various options for *replacing your dwindling hormones.* Although this may be the riskiest step to take, sometimes you may need to go beyond natural therapies if they don't help enough or if you are at very high risk for certain age-related diseases. We provide the kind of straightforward information you need to help you decide whether to undergo prescription hormone replacement therapy (HRT), or to rely on hormonelike substances found in plants. The important thing is to take charge of your life, and to keep your body and mind healthy through the midlife years and beyond.

Chapter 5 provides an *A-to-Z guide to the natural remedies for common conditions of menopause and aging.* We provide a short description of the condition, why it occurs, and then supply specific suggestions for natural therapies that you can use yourself to help prevent, alleviate, and eliminate the physical and psychological problems that might occur during the second half of your life. From hot flashes to fatigue and from mood swings to insomnia—you'll find safe, practical, natural steps to take that have helped many other women.

Serious diseases are covered in Chapter 6. You'll find easy-to-use questionnaires to fill out that show you if you are at higher-than-average risk for the four major diseases associated with aging in women: cardiovascular disease, breast cancer, osteoporosis, and diabetes. Then, we give you the latest information about how to reduce your risk through natural therapies or hormone replacement.

We save the best—sex—for last. In Chapter 7, we discuss ways to *enjoy your sexuality beyond menopause.* We provide natural alternatives to hormone replacement therapy that will help you continue to be sexually active—and perhaps to discover and more fully take advantage of a newfound sexuality.

Finally, in the appendixes, we provide a *glossary* of terms you may be unfamiliar with, a method for *testing food allergies,* lists of *resources* for more information about specific alternative therapies and products, and a bibliography of books and articles.

No longer dismissed as ineffective or too far out, alternative therapies are now entering mainstream medicine. The National Institutes of Health has established its groundbreaking Office of Alternative Medicine, which will investigate and evaluate treatments that were previously dismissed out of hand. A landmark study published in the January 1993 *New England Journal of Medicine* confirmed that up to one-third of Americans use alternative treatments. And Bill Moyers brought us a PBS series called "Healing and the Mind." Some insurance companies are beginning to cover these alternatives. The time has come for us to educate ourselves about all our available options—and that includes alternative medicine, which offers a gentler approach to healing that complements conventional care.

CHAPTER 1

Rethinking the Nature of Menopause and Aging

Is menopause devil or angel? Or is it both? It depends on whom you talk to.

For some women, such as Sonja, menopause is smooth sailing—a barely noticeable ripple in their lives: "Except for a few hot flashes, I hardly feel a thing. It's no big deal." Others feel they are being tossed on a stormy sea, buffeted by sudden hot flashes, exhaustion, sleepless nights, Jekyll-and-Hyde mood swings, and a nonexistent sex life. Anne Marie speaks for this group when she says, "Menopause is the worst thing that ever happened to me." Still others view the transition as an adventure, a period of welcome change. Patty finds that "menopause for me feels like a positive change—every hot flash takes me closer to the more powerful and wiser woman I am becoming."

The same holds true for the aging process and the years beyond menopause. Menopause marks the point at which many women first say, "Hey, I'm getting older!" But what this fact *means* varies from individual to individual. Some women are not concerned at all that the bulk of their lives is in the past. Others become upset and keenly feel the beginning of a slide down an inevitable slope into physical and emotional decay. Still others seem to enjoy life all the more—they're not getting older, they're getting better, wiser, more accomplished. Wrinkles are not something to be despised, covered up, or at best tolerated—they're to be celebrated. As Eleanor, a former Peace Corps worker, says, "Hey, I've been through a lot to get my face to look this way!"

The Turning Point

For better or worse, most women intuitively recognize menopause as a significant turning point in their lives. It marks the beginning of a whole new phase with potentially far-reaching changes. Although "the change" is a normal transition and to be expected, our society tends to both ignore and exaggerate its importance. Because we are so youth-oriented, we downplay the positive aspects and play up the negatives. Instead of viewing menopause as a chance to let go of monthly bleeding, our culture views it as an end of reproduction and sexual desirability. Instead of portraying menopause as a new start, it is presented as the end of a vital phase in our lives. We confuse being *reproductive* with being *productive,* and *giving life* with being *full of life.*

The fact is: Menopause is going to happen anyway, so why not consider the transition to be a positive one? You experience many such turning points including puberty, your first sexual relationship, marriage, leaving home, becoming a parent, watching your children grow independent, beginning and ending relationships, changing jobs—and now, menopause.

During such times of transition, you are presented with an opportunity to change or reinforce the way you view the world, your relationship to it and to other people, and your physical and emotional health. Rather than the end of youth, menopause can be your opportunity to heal past illnesses and regenerate yourself physically, emotionally, and spiritually. Menopause and the years beyond are frequently the best years of a woman's life.

Together with a trusted physician, you can decide how you will handle menopause and aging. Will you use hormone replacement therapy? Will you begin to take better care of yourself? Now's the time to make changes in your life—and perhaps your attitude—that build a strong foundation for better health and well-being. These simple changes may not only stave off premature, unnatural aging, but improve your health in general and give you more vitality than you did in the first half of your existence. While aging begins and the seeds for serious degenerative conditions are sown before menopause occurs, midlife is not too late to make a difference.

The Positive Side of Menopause and Aging

Menopause is not a medical condition or disease. It's not something to be dreaded, but rather can be a time of physical, spiritual, and emotional growth and freedom. If you're skeptical, think about all the positive physical changes brought about by menopause:

No more menstrual cramps; no more bleeding and tampons or pads; no more extra laundry or embarrassing leaks; no more discomfort during ovulation; no more PMS with its swollen tender breasts, abdominal bloating, and mood swings. "My periods were always so heavy and I had terrible cramps," recalls Pauline, a forty-six-year-old approaching menopause. "When I think about all the medication I took every month, the time I lost—I can't wait to be rid of all that." Plus: No more fears of pregnancy, no more messing with birth control devices. And if you have endometriosis, migraine headaches, fibroid tumors, or fibrocystic breasts, these tend to disappear or lessen dramatically after menopause (unless you supplement with too much estrogen).

Some women experience a diminished sexuality and find they enjoy their newfound freedom from the distractions of sexual interest and activity. Others, such as Melissa, notice the opposite. She was thrilled to find menopause increased her sex drive and sees this as a benefit. "Menopause changed my life," she says. "I feel so free now—of pregnancy, periods, and kids—and I'm enjoying sex more than I ever did."

Studies have shown that, as we age, our body image stabilizes. Rather than the nitpicking, hypercritical "I hate my hips" attitude, we become more accepting of our appearance as we mature. Rita Freedman, Ph.D., a body-image consultant, says that contrary to popular wisdom, women over forty-five have the highest ratings of feeling sexually attractive. She believes that as a woman becomes older, she realizes she is more than the sum of her physical attraction; she is also a wife, mother, worker. Once you stop defining yourself in relation to what men want, or how younger women look, you can get a better sense of your own value and self-worth. You are not defined solely by your looks, and character takes precedence.

Many women choose this time to get in touch with their inner selves and rediscover long-cherished hopes and dreams—or create totally new ones. You can reclaim your life, if you've had children and they're grown and gone. You can make your time your own—and decide to spend it doing what you *want* to do, rather than what you *have* to do. Perhaps you'll quit that boring job, end a meaningless marriage, stop being a slave to your kids, move to an exciting city, or wear flowing purple clothes. With maybe thirty years left to go, you have time to go back to school, start a second (or first, or third) career, enjoy another intimate relationship, travel to far-off lands you've always wanted to see.

And what about the wisdom and equanimity that comes with maturity? You've earned a worldliness and sophistication that would be unnatural and disturbing in a twenty-year-old. You've learned how ephemeral youthful beauty is, and can let your inner beauty shine through, a beauty based on inner strength, wisdom, and experience.

The potential for positive change goes beyond the personal. Our society is at a turning point as well, because of the increase in the proportion of the aging population. According to the U.S. Census Bureau, 15 million American women will turn fifty (the age when most women experience menopause) by the year 2000. They will join the 35 million women who are already over age fifty, bringing the total to 50 million. The average lifespan of today's woman is about seventy-eight years—and that means she will live about thirty years, or nearly one-third of her life, beyond menopause.

Yes, But . . . Problems and Concerns with Menopause and Aging

We do not mean to say that there aren't menopause symptoms that may cause discomfort or embarrassment, and that in some women these can be quite severe. Not every woman is able to face getting older, sagging skin, and approaching mortality with calm and good cheer. But as you'll see, American women (and women in most other Western countries) suffer more from menopause-related problems than do women in many other parts of the world. And they are at higher risk for serious age-related conditions such as osteoporosis, cardiovascular disease, breast cancer, and diabetes. These conditions and diseases are not a natural part of the aging process. They are mainly "Western diseases" caused by our "Western lifestyles" and our attitude toward aging—and this means they can largely be prevented.

What Happens During Menopause and Aging?

Before you decide to make the life changes that put a positive spin on menopause and aging, it helps to have some understanding of how they occur. This basic knowledge will also help you understand how they affect you and enable you to talk intelligently with your physician about menopause and age-related problems and their treatment.

Menstruation and Menopause

Your *endocrine system* (see ''The Major Endocrine Glands'') consists of glands that secrete chemical messengers called *hormones.* Hormones travel through your body via blood and lymph to all the body fluids in and around the cells of all your tissues. Almost all our cells have receptors on their surfaces; hormones fit into these receptors like a key fits inside a lock, which in turn turns on a particular function of the cell. Hormones from four endocrine glands in particular—the *adrenals, hypothalamus, pituitary,* and *ovaries*—hold sway over your reproductive organs. The endocrine glands not only communicate with your organs, but also communicate and influence each other.

The hypothalamus is the master gland. The size of a walnut, it is located in your brain and is responsible for triggering your thyroid, adrenal, and ovarian hormone activity. This in turn regulates your menstrual period. It secretes *gonadotropin-releasing hormone (GnRH)* to stimulate your pituitary, a pea-sized gland also located in your brain. The pituitary then secretes *follicle-stimulating hormone (FSH)* and *luteinizing hormone (LH).* During the first half of your cycle, FSH stimulates *follicles* to grow and begin secreting *estrogen.* The follicles are the bubbles, or flexible egg shells, which surround the egg itself in fluid. Estrogen is a very powerful important hormone that does many things, including thickening the lining of your uterus *(endometrium),* in preparation for possible implantation of a fertilized egg.

As the egg follicles grow, they continue to secrete estrogen. About halfway through your cycle, the estrogen reaches its peak, signaling the hypothalamus to tell the pituitary to stop producing FSH and produce a surge of LH. The LH causes one egg to *ovulate,* or be released from your ovary. The egg floats out in your pelvis and, if all goes as planned, is picked up by one of your *fallopian tubes,* beginning its journey to your uterus for possible fertilization. Some women

The Major Endocrine Glands

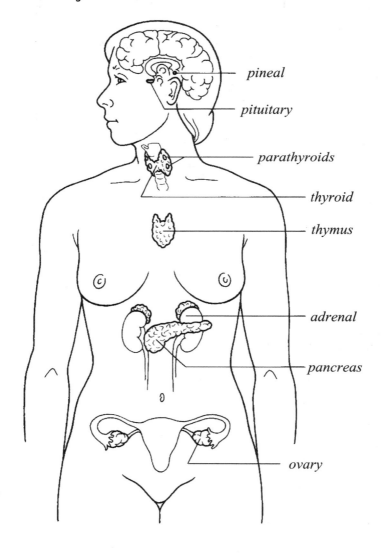

pineal

pituitary

parathyroids

thyroid

thymus

adrenal

pancreas

ovary

are aware of ovulation because they feel a brief midcycle pelvic cramp.

During the second half of your cycle, the empty sac-like structure on the ovary left behind by the egg forms a temporary gland called the *corpus luteum* (''yellow body'' because of its color). This secretes some estrogen and another major female hormone called *progesterone*. The progesterone stimulates a thicker buildup of your endometrium as further preparation for a possible fertilized egg and pregnancy. If the egg is fertilized, estrogen and progesterone continue to be secreted by the corpus luteum until the placenta takes over to continue endometrial buildup and nourish the developing embryo.

If the egg is not fertilized, the corpus luteum shrivels up and stops secreting estrogen and progesterone. The sudden drop in hormonal support in turn allows the endometrium to wither. As endometrial cells die, the body sheds them along with blood that had nourished them, a process called *menstruation*. The low levels of estrogen and progesterone signal the production of FSH and the cycle begins again. Unless a woman becomes pregnant, this process is repeated every month, for an average of thirty years or so.

Until menopause, that is. Then the process begins to change, essentially because you run out of eggs. As is the case with every woman, you started out with two million eggs in your ovaries when you were born. This number diminished to less than half a million by the time you reached puberty. All through adulthood your egg supply continues to dwindle until by age fifty, you have only a few eggs left, and they may or may not respond to FSH and LH. After menopause, there are no eggs and you will no longer be able to become pregnant.

As your egg supply diminishes, the production of estrogen and progesterone becomes erratic and the dips cause the hypothalamus to signal the pituitary to produce more and more FSH and LH in an attempt to stimulate your few sluggish egg follicles. This sometimes works, and sometimes doesn't, resulting in irregular periods. Your doctor may use high blood levels of LH and/or FSH to determine how close you are to menopause. Eventually even the extra effort can't stimulate eggs to produce enough estrogen, mature, and ovulate. Without the corpus luteum, there's too little estrogen and progesterone, and too little endometrium to slough off. Periods become lighter and farther apart, and eventually stop completely—our reproductive clock has run out.

The Stages of Menopause

Strictly speaking, menopause is your final menstrual period—an event you can determine only in retrospect. Although most people use the term *menopause* to identify the years surrounding this event, what we commonly refer to as menopause actually has several phases.

Premenopause occurs before menopause and is the time during which brain hormones FSH and LH begin to increase and ovarian hormones estrogen and progesterone begin to decrease. Menstrual periods may begin to become irregular. Most women become premenopausal after age forty.

Perimenopause is the term used to identify the approximately two years before and after your final period, and is the time when most of the physical signs of menopause occur, such as hot flashes and irregular periods. In some women, perimenopause lasts longer.

Menopause is your final menstrual flow; this can only be identified with certainty one year after the fact. The average age of menopause in the United States is around fifty.

Postmenopause, or the *climacteric,* refers to the years after your last menstrual period. Your body continues to undergo hormone-related changes, but these tend to be more gradual and subtle.

Although it's impossible to predict when you will experience menopause, there are some guidelines. You'll probably undergo menopause around the age your mother did, unless you've smoked quite a bit, which hastens menopause. Hysterectomy can hasten menopause too, and so can giving birth to twins; women with low income and education also tend to have an earlier menopause, but we're not sure why. Being overweight, on the other hand, helps delay it. In the United States, the timing for natural menopause (as opposed to menopause brought on by surgery or medical treatment) breaks down like this:

Percentage of women who reach menopause . . .	by age . . .
10	38
30	44
50	49
99.9	55

Is Menopause Nature's Mistake?

The prevalent medical view holds that nature didn't mean for us to live long after our reproductive days are over. Throughout much of history, women died before menopause because of disease, childbirth, infections, and a slew of other medical problems that Western medical care can now cure or prevent. As recently as 1900, American and European women lived to an average of only forty-five.

Others say menopause and the climacteric are nature's way of being smart. Perhaps menopause evolved in humans because by giving us a period of life when we could no longer reproduce, it freed us to help raise late-born children and grandchildren without the dangers or distractions of additional pregnancies or more of our own young ones. It allowed us to accumulate more wisdom and gave us time to transmit cultural knowledge to the next generation.

Healthy menopausal women often have plenty of hormones for everything *but* childbearing. Nature continues to provide us with estrogen, only at lower levels. After our ovaries no longer produce significant amounts of estrogen, the adrenal glands, when healthy, take over. They produce hormones, such as androstenedione, which are converted into estrogen by fat cells and in other parts of your body such as muscle, liver, kidney, brain. The estrogen produced by extra fat cells may explain why many women who weigh more are reported to have an easier time adjusting to menopause. As we'll see in Chapter 6, it may also help explain why obesity is related to breast cancer.

Menopause and Aging—What Can You Expect?

A glance at the A-to-Z listings in Chapter 5 may cause you to faint, but you can relax: no woman experiences all the possible symptoms, and most women experience only a few of the signs of menopause. Still, there's a lot of confusion about midlife symptoms—what's due to hormonal shifts and estrogen withdrawal, and what's due to aging? It's an important distinction because hormonal changes are only one aspect of aging. Tinkering with our hormones would logically affect hormone-related symptoms, but not solve all our problems. To help clarify the picture, here's a closer look at what estrogen does.

Estrogen is the term used to refer to a group of sex steroids; both men and women produce estrogen, but women generally produce more. Of the three types of estrogen, *estradiol* is the most powerful; it is produced primarily by egg follicles in your ovaries. In addition to its role in the reproductive/menstrual cycle, estradiol affects many other parts of your body. It stimulates the development of your breasts, and keeps your uterus, vagina, urinary tract, and surrounding pelvic muscles and tissues toned and firm. Estrogen also influences your central nervous system, bones, hair, and skin.

During menopause, fluctuating hormones lead to a group of fairly predictable symptoms in many women, but the frequency and intensity vary considerably. The most common and most noticeable are:

Changes in menstrual periods. These are experienced by every woman—but they typically begin with more frequent shorter and lighter periods which change to an irregular flow perhaps followed by heavy periods. Usually periods arrive less and less frequently and gradually diminish, but some women just stop abruptly. (*See* "Heavy Periods," page 185, and "Irregular Periods," page 205.)

Hot flashes or flushes. The most notorious symptom, hot flashes or flushes are experienced by about 75–80 percent of American women; these may happen frequently and leave you drenched, or you may experience only a few mild episodes and that's it. (*See* "Hot Flashes," page 190.)

Vaginal changes. These include thinning of the vaginal walls and vulva and lack of lubrication which may make intercourse uncomfortable, or cause discomfort even if you're not having vaginal sex. The pH balance in your vagina changes, increasing your risk of vaginal infections. (*See* Chapter 7 and "Vaginitis," page 236.)

Bladder problems. This often occurs because the urinary tract tissues grow weak and thin, and the surrounding muscles lose bulk and strength. You may have trouble controlling your urine and develop more frequent bladder infections. (*See* "Incontinence," page 195, and "Urinary Tract and Bladder Infections," page 228.)

Sleep disturbances. These may be due to hot flashes that occur at night, or to low estrogen affecting the stage of sleep during which dreams occur. This stage, also called REM sleep (rapid eye movement), is believed to be the most restful stage of the sleep cycle. (*See* "Insomnia," page 198, and "Night Sweats," page 222.)

Fatigue. This is the number one problem that women at the MEND Clinic complain about. It may have a myriad of contributing causes, and wreak havoc with your personal and professional life. (*See* "Fatigue and Low Energy," page 167.)

Emotional and mental changes. There's very little scientific information or agreement about why some women, such as Ellen, notice
they get "real nasty at times—snapping at my friends, in a bad
mood—I feel exhausted, muddle-brained. I just don't feel like me."
Some changes may be due to hormonal effects on your nervous system. And certainly physical problems such as hot flashes that disturb
sleep (night sweats) can leave many women grumpy. But new evidence suggests we've been too quick to blame menopause for midlife
mental and emotional changes. Recent studies show that depression,
for example, is not rampant among menopausal women, and stress
factors such as adult children returning to the home, or caring for
aging parents, or career changes are more likely to be at the root of
depression. (*See* "Confusion, Forgetfulness, and Poor Concentration," page 139; "Moodiness, Mood Swings, and Irritability," page
219; and "Depression," page 145.)

Loss of sex drive. Lowered hormones may be directly or indirectly
related. Lowered libido may be due in part to vaginal atrophy—discomfort during intercourse is definitely not an aphrodisiac. Fatigue and
emotional difficulties experienced at midlife may also play a part. (*See*
"Loss of Sexual Desire," page 208; "Painful Intercourse," page 223;
and Chapter 7: "Enjoying Sex During Menopause and Beyond.")

Increased risk of serious disease. While these and other symptoms
of menopause may affect your quality of life now, heart disease, osteoporosis, breast cancer, and diabetes all increase after menopause.
Many of these diseases have subtle or no symptoms until they are
quite advanced. However we often find early signs and can decrease
our risks, as you'll see in Chapter 6.

Aging

Many of the symptoms blamed on menopause are probably due to
aging, rather than loss of estrogen or progesterone per se. However, as
mentioned earlier, since lowered hormones is part of the aging process, it's often difficult to separate one mechanism from the other.
Nevertheless, it's likely that such changes such as weight gain and
"middle-age spread," wrinkles, loss of skin tone, creaky joints, and a
decrease in energy are signs of wear and tear and a natural slowing
down of the body's systems, independent of hormonal shifts. However, they are not independent of lifestyle, attitude, and environmental
factors.

Although science has been studying aging for decades, we're still not sure what aging actually is, let alone what causes it. One theory is that to a certain extent aging is genetically preprogrammed: our cells are destined to give out according to a fixed timetable—witness our dwindling supply of eggs.

One influence on aging seems to be cellular damage by toxic oxygen molecules called *free radicals*. The free radical molecules are missing an electron, and they try to replace their missing electrons by robbing electrons from molecules in healthy cells. Then the robbed molecule tries to rob another electron, and so on, creating a damaging free radical chain reaction in our bodies. The damage cripples our cells in several ways. It injures the cell membrane and the genetic material contained in DNA (deoxyribonucleic acid). As a result, cells die, malfunction, and replicate themselves imperfectly. Eventually, entire organs and organ systems work less well than they used to.

This accumulation of tissue damage may explain at least some of the signs of aging such as sags and wrinkles, age spots, failing eyesight, weak muscles and poor stamina, and poor memory. Excessive free radical damage has been linked with abnormal, accelerated aging and many degenerative diseases and conditions such as cancer, heart disease, immune dysfunction, arthritis, lack of energy and stamina, failing memory and concentration, and even diabetes and osteoporosis.

Free radicals are created in our bodies by environmental pollution, radiation, stress, poor nutrition, and our own metabolism. We need some free radicals for normal metabolism and our bodies have mechanisms for controlling them so they don't get out of hand (like keeping a beach fire within a fire ring) with *antioxidants*. Antioxidants are enzymes the body produces or nutrients such as vitamins C and E and beta-carotene; their molecules are capable of losing electrons and "quenching" free radicals without starting a chain reaction. But this system can be overwhelmed by excessive free radicals, which end up injuring our cells. If you'd like a fuller explanation of free radicals and antioxidants, refer to *The Natural Health Guide to Antioxidants* (listed in Appendix D, "Bibliography and Recommended Reading").

What's Normal?

In the United States, we tend to make a big deal out of the symptoms of menopause, and there's a whole industry devoted to "antiaging.'' We often mistake menopausal symptoms and signs of aging that are ''expected,'' ''average,'' or ''common'' with what's ''normal.'' But the doom and gloom surrounding menopause appears to be exaggerated. In the first place, there is little evidence that most women are plagued by the dozens of symptoms that have been associated with the change of life. In the second place, there is a huge variation in the number and severity of the symptoms that do occur. It seems that women in the United States and some other industrialized Western countries suffer much more from menopause and aging than women in many other parts of the world—as well as a higher incidence of heart disease, breast cancer, osteoporosis, and diabetes.

Risk Factors for Difficult Menopause

A 1993 survey of 2,000 readers conducted by *Prevention* magazine and Columbia University found that the older you are at menopause, the less likely you'll be bothered by symptoms:

Age at menopause	Percentage of women who have problems
40–44	33
45–49	21
50–54	18
55 or older*	6

Another factor is your hormonal history. It's more likely you'll have a problem menopause if you've had:

• irregular periods.
• premenstrual syndrome.
• difficult pregnancy, labor, or delivery.
• medical treatment that affects hormones, such as chemotherapy, the ''antiestrogen'' cancer drug tamoxifen, or a hysterectomy, which plunges you into ''instant'' menopause, often with dramatic symptoms.

---

* Menopause that occurs at fifty-five or older is considered to be late or delayed.

Menopause Attitudes Around the World

There are many cultures where women look forward to menopause, and where reaching menopause means an elevation in status. For example, in South Africa, older Indian women are free to enter Hindu temples and participate in rituals once menstruation has ceased. In Thailand, there is an expensive celebration at menopause, indicating a new status and respect. A study of Sikh women living in Canada found that the women perceive menopause as a positive event in their lives, and another study conducted in Israel astonished the researchers when they found that women across five cultures (Muslim Arabs, immigrant Jews born in Africa, Persia, Turkey, and Central Europe) unanimously welcomed menopause.

By way of contrast, a survey of 505 middle-class women aged thirty-five to fifty across the United States conveyed a disturbing picture: There was no sense of achievement or elevated status associated with menopause, and the focus was on menopause as a disease. However, older American women tend to have a more positive or neutral attitude toward menopause than younger women and men. Interestingly, many black women in the United States are reported to have a positive attitude toward menopause and some have referred to menopausal distress as a white middle-class thing.

Menopause and Aging: A Worldwide View

When we look at statistics on menopause symptoms and age-related conditions in the United States and compare them with the experiences of women in other countries, we see some rather startling differences.

Menopause

Across the world, we see vast differences in the types of menopausal symptoms women experience, as well as in the severity. Figures vary as to the prevalence of hot flashes, the most common symptom associated with menopause: Other studies found they occurred in only 24% of the women polled, while in other studies, up to 93% of the women experienced them. In a U.S. study of 126 women,

64% had hot flashes for 1 to 5 years; 26% had them for 6 to 10 years; and 10% for more than 11 years.

In many countries, women experience healthy, positive menopause without taking additional estrogen. For example: Women of the Colombian tropical forest report symptom-free menopause. Asian women as a whole see menopause as less of an event. Hot flashes are rarely reported among menopausal women in Japan—in fact there is no word for "hot flash" in either the Japanese or the Navaho language. As we show on page 16, symptom-free menopause is more common than you might expect. Even in the United States, we notice a great variety in menopause experience. According to a reader survey published in 1993 by *Prevention* magazine, American women who reported fewer symptoms exercised frequently, ate a low-fat vegetarian diet that included soybean foods (high in plant estrogens—*see* Chapter 4), and felt less stressed out.

Heart Disease

When we compare the prevalence of heart disease in women, we also see that in some countries, women tend to have healthy hearts and in other countries they do not. In many parts of the world older women (and men) suffer much less heart disease than Americans do. In the United States, 63% of all women aged sixty-five and over die of diseases of the circulatory system. Contrast that with Thailand's rate of only 7%. Even in the United States the high incidence of coronary heart disease is a relatively new phenomenon, being barely known at the turn of the century. Today it is the major killer in America among both women and men. Altogether, twenty-three countries have a lower death rate from heart disease than do we. (*See* Chapter 6.)

Osteoporosis

Looking at anthropological data from around the world, we see that osteoporosis occurs in some areas much more than in others. While the United States has one of the highest osteoporosis rates in the world—over 300 hip fractures per 100,000 women per year—there are other areas where this disorder is relatively rare, even among older people. As you'll see in Chapter 6, the inhabitants of Singapore, Hong Kong, and the Bantu of South Africa have extremely low rates of osteoporotic fracture—from a low of 14 per 100,000 women to a high of 87.

Menopause Symptoms Around the World

Menopause is a physical, biological event in our lives, but it is also a cultural and social event. All these factors affect how we experience menopause. It's no coincidence that, in countries where menopause is not a negative event, the people have a healthier cultural attitude as well as a healthier lifestyle.

- Asian women generally, and Japanese and Indonesian women particularly, report far fewer hot flashes than their Western counterparts. In Taiwan, only one out of five women experiences hot flashes during menopause. In China, only 5% of women report menopause symptoms.
- In India, anthropologists report that among 483 women of one caste, there was none of the depression, dizziness, incapacitation, or any other symptom commonly associated with menopause in our culture.
- Mayan women in Mexico report no menopausal symptoms except irregular menstrual periods.
- Arabs and North African women suffer few or no menopausal problems.
- Greek and Mayan women both report better sex with menopause.
- In Botswana, Africa, women reported that the most frequent menopause symptom was increased sex drive (in 64% of the women). The least frequent was painful intercourse (4%).
- In Australia, women have quite positive feelings about menopause; 70% felt good-natured and only 4% felt depressed.
- In Holland, 80% of women get hot flashes, which can continue for 10 years in 35% of the women.
- A summary of studies in the United States and Great Britain found that 16% of women were totally symptom-free; 74% experienced some discomfort; and 10% complain of severe symptoms.

On the other hand, Norway has the highest rate (421 per 100,000); Sweden, Finland, and New Zealand whites have rates approaching or exceeding ours. Statistical studies indicate that this is not merely due to the longer life expectancy in Western countries. In fact, British researchers recently analyzed the bone density of 87 females buried between 1792 and 1852. When they compared the density of 300 present-day women, they found that women living 200 and 300 years ago had stronger bones than contemporary women. Some progress!

Breast Cancer
With breast cancer we see the same pattern—Western countries generally have the highest death rate. For example, England and Wales have the dubious distinction of having the highest rate (about 29 deaths per 100,000 women per year), followed closely by Denmark (28), the Netherlands (27), and Canada (24). The United States has the sixteenth highest rate among 46 countries (22 deaths per 100,000). In Japan and Taiwan, the breast cancer incidence rate is about six times lower than in the United States for women aged 50—and for postmenopausal women it is *twenty times* lower. There's good evidence that this is not genetic—second- and third-generation descendants of Chinese and Japanese people living in Western countries and eating a Western diet have breast cancer rates similar to the white women living there.

Diabetes
Again, diabetes is not a universal phenomenon. According to one study, in industrialized countries, 3–10% of the people have diabetes, but an average of only 1% get it in traditional societies. However, as they become exposed and acculturated to the Western way of eating, diabetes flourishes.

The Underlying Causes of Menopause Problems and Aging Disorders
If naturally occurring lower estrogen levels were solely to blame for menopausal difficulties of age-related disorders, why is it that women in certain other parts of the world don't experience them to the degree that many American women seem to? Why do some studies show that sex hormones are similar in postmenopausal women both with and without osteoporosis, and with and without hot flashes? And why

would studies done at the Mayo Clinic and in Canada and Japan show that osteoporosis can begin way before menopause? Clearly, estrogen is not the only factor and estrogen replacement therapy is not the only answer. Even so, many physicians rely on estrogen replacement as the primary solution to menopause and age-related conditions such as osteoporosis.

Take Care of Your Adrenal Glands

To understand why estrogen from your ovaries isn't solely to blame, you need to learn a bit about hormones in general, and the endocrine system that produces them. Our bodies produce many other hormones besides estrogen, and our ovaries aren't the only source of estrogen. Hormones are chemicals that deliver messages to start or stop a multitude of biochemical reactions. Released directly into the bloodstream, hormones travel all over the body and are taken up by the cells that have *receptors* for that particular hormone. The hormone slips into its receptor site on the cell membrane, much as a key slips into a lock, and delivers its message.

All of your endocrine glands—the pituitary, thyroid, parathyroid, pineal, adrenals, ovaries, liver, and pancreas—are related to menopause and late-life health. Of the dozens of hormones we produce, nine of them are major sex hormones: three *estrogens* (estradiol, estrone, and estriol), several *androgens* (including testosterone), and *progesterone.* Under normal, healthy conditions, our bodies are able to maintain a continuous and adequate supply of the various hormones, which work together in delicate balance. Too much of one, too little of another, and the whole system is thrown off, in sometimes subtle— and sometimes dramatic—ways.

Although there's so much emphasis on ovarian estrogen, in actuality *your postmenopausal health depends heavily upon the health of your adrenal glands.* The amount of estrogen produced by your ovaries may drop by as much as 75 percent at menopause. The focus then shifts to your adrenals, which become the source for the vast majority of your postmenopausal estrogen. That's why it's important for you to make sure you have healthy adrenals during the years surrounding menopause—if you have sufficient adrenal hormones, your estrogen levels remain adequate and your menopause will be symptom-free.

Unfortunately, today's stressful, high-octane lifestyles overstimulate our adrenals. Your revved-up glands produce too much glucocorticoid hormones, and this can wreak havoc with your bones. Eventually, after years of overactivity, it appears that adrenals can become exhausted, leading to adrenal insufficiency. Or adrenal insufficiency may be due to therapy with cortisone or other drugs, or to poor nutrition (under stress, your adrenals gobble up vitamin C), contributing to menopause difficulties and health problems.

Several studies show that bone loss accelerates in Western women during menopause, but this may be linked to poor adrenal functioning. When the ovaries go into retirement, the adrenals should be able to take over, but are often not healthy enough to do this. If you trust that a woman's estrogen production is gauged to her body's needs, then the universal decrease in estrogen production after a woman's reproductive years would be a benefit, and not a detriment—to the species, and perhaps the woman. Seen from a wider perspective, less estrogen is needed because we no longer need its primary function—to allow and regulate reproduction. Interestingly, prolonged exposure to high levels of estrogen produced by the body has been linked with higher breast cancer risk, so lowering estrogen as we age is actually protective. The estrogen produced by healthy adrenals is adequate for estrogen receptors in the bone and elsewhere, but does not overstimulate the sex organs such as the uterus (and perhaps the breasts).

The MEND Clinic Program: A Healthy Approach to Menopause and Aging

Lifestyle, social, and cultural factors—in addition to genetic factors—are responsible for the hormonal imbalance behind menopausal problems and for the current epidemic of chronic and deadly degenerative disease among women of the United States and many other modernized countries. While many women may have the resilience to withstand abuses in their youth, by age forty our past begins to catch up with us, making a natural transition such as menopause difficult. The MEND Clinic program recommends life changes that bring us closer to some aspects of the lifestyles of women who live in low-risk countries and allow us to harness and enhance our body's natural ability to maximize health rather than expecting a single powerful magic bullet to counteract all the detrimental effects of an unhealthy lifestyle.

Our comprehensive, holistic program provides you with specific measures you can take to prevent and treat most menopausal complaints and reduce the risk of serious diseases associated with aging. There are three overlapping approaches to the program. You may stick with just the first approach or move on to the second or third. How far up the ladder you go depends upon the intensity and tenacity of your menopausal symptoms, and your individual level of concern about and risk for serious disease. Before beginning the program, turn to Chapter 6 and do the self-assessments to determine your level of risk for serious age-related diseases.

Approach 1: The Balanced Life Plan

Following this program, as outlined in Chapter 2, includes basic lifestyle guidelines and is the most important component because it acts as a foundation. We encourage every woman to embrace these basics which set the stage for health by providing the life-supporting raw materials and environment, and let nature do the rest. The nutritional changes, exercise guidelines, and other lifestyle factors all help you reestablish balance and experience normal menopausal well-being and overall health while reducing your risk of serious disease. Unless you are at high risk for serious disease, this is the safest step you can take.

These lifestyle changes may be all you need if you are experiencing mild menopausal changes and are at normal risk for age-related diseases. For example, a patient of Dr. Maas's simply stopped drinking coffee and Cokes and started taking half-hour walks every day. Her headaches disappeared and she slept better; she had more energy and felt less achy. By cutting out sweets and prioritizing an active social life and cultivating friendships with a healthier groups of people, she stopped her blood pressure medication.

Approach 2: Natural Therapies

These therapies, as described in Chapter 3, include nutritional supplements, herbs, massage, and relaxation techniques. Continue with the lifestyle changes in Approach 1, but add one or more of these therapies if the Balanced Life Plan doesn't solve your menopausal problems or if you are at higher-than-average risk for serious age-related diseases. You can administer these therapies yourself or work with a professional natural health care practitioner to address specific symptoms or reduce risk of disease. These therapies are generally safe when used as directed, but there may be some undesirable side effects. Dr. Brown had a patient who was doing better after she made lifestyle changes, but still had some residual problems. All she needed to do was add alfalfa and vitamin E supplements, and all her symptoms cleared up. One of Dr. Maas's patients was able to clear up her mood swings and fatigue after beginning a complete multivitamin supplement program.

Approach 3: Hormone Replacement

Taking hormones, either prescription or nonprescription, synthetic or natural, is your third option (*see* Chapter 4). Although you risk experiencing side effects, the risks may be worth the benefits if natural therapies don't help enough or if you are at very high risk for age-related diseases. However, even naturally derived hormones are not well tested. Therefore, we advise that you work with a physician familiar with nonprescription hormone products and to report any problems, and follow your progress with appropriate diagnostic tests.

We believe that if the first two approaches don't alleviate your symptoms, you shouldn't continue to suffer or remain at high risk for serious medical problems if hormone replacement therapy (HRT) can help. HRT may be a good alternative, and may be needed only temporarily to help you get through a certain time. The important thing is to take charge of your life, and to keep your body and mind healthy through the midlife years and beyond. Beginning with the next chapter, you can do exactly that.

CHAPTER 2

The Balanced Life Plan

Chapter 1 has shown you that menopausal difficulties, the premature aging that we see in our culture, and our major killer diseases are not inevitable. This chapter will show you how our health-building program will help:

- relieve, prevent, and minimize most menopause-related symptoms.
- lower your risk of heart disease, osteoporosis, diabetes, and cancer—and even minimize or reverse some of these once they have begun.
- improve your all-around health and make you fitter, stronger, more energetic, and less likely to show signs of premature aging.
- if you are premenopausal, prepare yourself physically, mentally, and emotionally so you can enjoy a more normal transition to your later years.

Our Balanced Life Plan is tailored to the needs of women as individuals and emphasizes the why and how of restoring hormonal balance and how to adjust other factors that influence menopausal problems and serious age-related diseases. Our program is designed to encourage your body to optimally produce, use, and break down hormones—and at the same time optimize your health in general. It consists of five components, most of which are straightforward changes you can accomplish on your own. They are the following:

1. Maximize nourishing foods.
2. Minimize antinutrients.
3. Be physically active.
4. Relax and manage stress.
5. Establish a partnership with your doctor(s).

In addition, there are a few other lifestyle habits that we discuss. All are important, and all work together synergistically to enhance each other's effects. But don't panic: You don't need to change everything at once. Incorporate parts of our program into your life gradually.

Even if you only cut down on "antinutrients" such as sugar and caffeine, you may be amazed at how much better you feel and how quickly this happens. Such was the case with Mary, who was particularly sensitive to sugar and coffee. A forty-eight-year-old teacher, she came to Dr. Brown complaining of hot flashes, fatigue, and other problems that were interfering with her ability to work. When she looked at her diet, she realized how much coffee she was drinking to jump-start her during the day and how much sugar she was eating to give her an energy boost. She stopped both these habits and her symptoms vanished. In fact, she started feeling so good that she began slipping off the program—a cup of coffee here, a cookie there—and her symptoms slowly returned . . . until she started eating smart again.

When and How to Start?
It's never too late! The time to start is *now*—whatever your age. It's also true that the earlier begun in life, the greater the impact on health in later years. Scientists have found fatty deposits in the arteries of children, setting them up for heart disease as adults. Children and adolescents who have built optimally healthy bones will have stronger bones through menopause and old age. That's why we encourage you to raise your daughters and granddaughters to consider their future health, and hope you'll help the next generation build health early.

To begin, familiarize yourself with the program by reading this chapter all the way through. Then, identify the areas in which you most need to change and prioritize them. Find at least one and prefer-ably two priorities in each of the five areas. For example, your highest priority may be to quit smoking, or reduce your meat intake to 4 ounces a day or less, or to walk three times a week. Be realistic—what are you ready to do *now*? What are you likely to follow through with? Begin with the things most likely to set you up for success. That sets up an atmosphere of satisfaction and confidence and higher level of health that will motivate you to take the next step.

You'll notice that we spend most of our time discussing food and nutrition. All problems can't be blamed on diet, but nourishing the body is the cornerstone of any health-building program. Eating good food is not only one of life's greatest pleasures, but also one of the easiest ways to create our own good health every day. Yet many American women have a love-hate relationship with food. We use food as a drug, to lift us physically and psychologically. We consume junk food to keep us going and think as long as a woman is thin, walking, and talking, she's okay. Somehow her amazing body sur-vives—but is she thriving?

As you grow older, it is especially important to pay attention to what you eat. Certain foods and nutrients affect menopause symp-toms, affect your risk of serious disease, and influence the aging pro-cess. Cells aged by antinutrients such as sugar and caffeine become less efficient at repair and regeneration. So, you need to be particu-larly careful to eat food that supplies cells with the nutrients they need to function as well as possible and avoid antinutrients. At the same time, metabolism slows down at midlife, so you require fewer calories to maintain your weight. This means you need to emphasize foods that are high in essential nutrients but lower in calories than during the earlier part of your life.

The Standard American Diet (SAD)

The way most Americans eat certainly is "sad"—numerous surveys show that, despite our wealth as a nation, our intake of certain nutrients is appallingly inadequate, while our intake of others is way too high. Simply put, the average diet in this country is too low in nourishing vitamins, minerals, and fiber; and too high in fat, protein, and refined starches and sugars.

Women are at higher risk of undernourishment because they con-sume less food than men, and because they tend to go on extreme diets in order to lose weight. This is a culture that believes you can't be too thin or too rich—yet women, the chief family cooks, are habituated to serving rich, fatty foods in caring for their family. This is the daily dilemma women face, and we want to assure you that you can feel so much better once you start changing your eating patterns.

1. Maximize Nourishing Foods

A nourishing diet is high in vitamins, minerals, complex carbohydrates, fiber, and other essential nutrients which we can't make ourselves, such as essential fatty acids which the typical American diet sorely lacks. *Vitamin and minerals* are called "micronutrients" because, compared with other nutrients, we require relatively small amounts. Vitamins and minerals are substances that help activate chemicals reactions that are vital to life, from digesting food to forming bone to laughing at silly jokes.

One group of vitamins in particular—the antioxidants beta-carotene (a precursor of vitamin A), vitamin C, and vitamin E—has created quite a stir because it appears they might help prevent aging and degenerative diseases at the cellular level. Antioxidants protect cells and tissue from the cumulative damage caused by free radical oxidation. Oxidation is the chemical process we see in action when cut fruit turns brown or fat turns rancid. (*See* Chapter 1 for information about free radicals, and Chapter 3 for more information about antioxidant supplements.)

So, vitamins and minerals are essential—but how much are you getting and is that enough? Let's begin by looking at the RDAs (recommended dietary allowances). The RDAs, established by the National Academy of Sciences, defines the levels of the essential vitamins and minerals adequate to prevent deficiency diseases. The problem is, they do not necessarily guarantee optimum health, only that we won't die of a deficiency such as scurvy or beriberi. Even so, according to a recent U.S. Department of Agriculture survey, which studied the three-day food intake of 21,500 people, *not one single person* consumed 100 percent of the RDA for the ten nutrients included in the survey.

It's ironic that we have the wealth to eat well, but we don't, and our health suffers for it. For example, low calcium intakes are linked with an increased risk of osteoporosis. Many studies associate low intakes of vitamins such as vitamin C, E, and beta-carotene with cancer, heart disease, and age-related conditions such as cataracts and arthritis. The handy "Nutrient Table of Vitamins and Minerals," in Chapter 3, pages 61–64, lists the major vitamins and minerals we need to be healthy, along with the best food sources, the RDA, and the optimal amount for supplementation.

We've seen many women who have subclinical deficiencies and just "don't feel right." Vegans (women who eat vegetable foods only) who don't take supplements can be low in such nutrients as vitamin B-12, which is hard to obtain from vegetable foods. These women complain that they are depressed and fall into an energy slump in the afternoon, but show no clinical signs of any disease or deficiency, other than low blood levels of this vitamin. Other classic signs of subclinical deficiencies are leg cramps (calcium deficiency), or bleeding gums (a sign of vitamin C deficiency), or cravings for sweets (chromium deficiency). Nutrient deficiencies are shockingly common and do not show up in the typical laboratory profiles ordered by physicians.

Starches and fiber are carbohydrates—macronutrients needed to fuel the body and create energy. Such complex carbohydrates are found in whole grains, beans, nuts, fruits, and vegetables. The body digests these complex molecular structures slowly, making these foods more filling than simple sugars, which are digested quickly and cause a rapid rise and fall of blood sugar levels. In addition, such starchy foods are generally relatively high in vitamins and minerals. They also contain more fiber than simple sugars and refined carbohydrates such as white bread; fiber aids the digestion, prevents constipation and hemorrhoids, and helps prevent colon cancer and possibly breast cancer. Fiber also lowers cholesterol and blood sugar and thus may also protect you from heart disease and diabetes.

Most of the food you eat should be complex carbohydrates—aim for about 60 percent of your total calories. Drink plenty of additional fluids to help the fiber move smoothly through your digestive tract.

While, on the one hand, we eat too much fat in general in this country, on the other hand, *essential fatty acids* are rather sparse in the typical American diet. Called essential because they are essential for health and because our bodies cannot manufacture them, these substances have many remarkable qualities. Essential fatty acids are used in forming and balancing a group of hormone-like substances called prostaglandins, which regulate inflammation. Essential fatty acids are found in every cell of our bodies and bring fluidity to the cell membranes, which regulate every system of the body. Adequate essential fatty acids are needed to maintain the cardiovascular, reproductive, immune, and central nervous systems. Deficiencies have been linked with many diseases including heart disease, cancer, arthritis, allergies, and several immunological disorders.

There are two known essential fatty acids: linolenic acid (also called the omega-3 fatty acids) and linoleic acid (omega-6). Omega-3 fatty acids are found in varying amounts in seeds, nuts, and beans and the oils made from them, including flax seed, hemp, canola, soy, and walnut; in dark green leafy vegetables; and in fatty fish such as herring, salmon, cod, and tuna. Omega-6 acids are found in seeds, nuts, and beans and the oils made from them, including flax seed, safflower, sunflower, hemp, soybean, walnut, pumpkin, and sesame; evening primrose oil, and borage and black currant oil, are also rich in omega-6 fatty acids and are available primarily as supplements.

2. Minimize Antinutrients

Antinutrients is a term we use to describe a substance that works against good nutrition, in some cases by depleting the body of health-building nutrients. Some antinutrients such as protein and saturated fat are health-building nutrients, but are harmful when eaten in excessive amounts. Others such as caffeine, alcohol, and tobacco are harmful in themselves. They are addictive substances that we use in excess to make us feel good temporarily. It's a challenge to kick the antinutrient habit, but it's well worth it because of the payback you'll get in better health and long-term well-being.

Americans eat not only too much protein and fats, but also unhealthy types of these foods. Adequate *protein* is essential to health because it is needed to repair and replace cells and is the building block for much of our structure including our bones, as well as for biochemicals such as enzymes and brain chemicals. The vast majority of Americans consume far too much protein. The RDA average for women is 44–50 g (grams) per day. The actual average intake is nearly 100 g. This is about twice the RDA and nearly four times that recommended by the World Health Organization.

Eating too much protein contributes to a host of health problems including heart disease, colon cancer, and constipation. Excessive protein—particularly animal protein—contributes to osteoporosis because it actually washes calcium out of the body and depletes bones of this vital mineral. Excess protein is especially dangerous if combined with a low calcium intake, a common scenario in the United States. Most of the protein we consume comes from animal products such as beef, chicken, turkey, pork, fish, eggs, milk, and cheese. Because protein is so concentrated in animal products, cutting your intake of these foods is by far the best way to bring your protein down to a healthier level. Replacing some animal proteins with vegetable proteins is wise, too, because vegetable sources can contain more vitamins, minerals, carbohydrates, and fiber; cause less calcium to be lost in the urine; and come "packaged" without the saturated fat found in animal products.

Vegetarians generally consume a relatively low protein diet and many have greater bone density than meat eaters. Countries with lower protein consumption generally have lower rates of osteoporosis than Western countries where animal protein is abundant. You'd be wise to keep your protein down to about 15 percent of your total calories—think of it more as a condiment than as the star attraction of a meal.

Fat is needed by your body to carry the fat-soluble vitamins A, D, E, and K through the system, and to absorb minerals. Fats are also a part of our cell membranes and are needed to produce hormones.

As a nation, we consume far too much fat—the equivalent of 6–8 tablespoons daily yet we consume too few essential fatty acids. All we really need is the equivalent of about 1 tablespoon of high-quality fats per day and this can be obtained from a whole foods diet with the addition of small amounts of high-quality cooking oils and salad dressings made with appropriate oils and fresh nuts. There are three main types of fats, and the Standard American Diet tends to favor the least healthy types:

• *Saturated fat* tends to raise cholesterol and is implicated in cardiovascular disease. Recent studies link breast and ovarian cancer to a diet high in saturated fats. Animal products are the main source of saturated fats, but some vegetable oils such as palm and coconut oil also contain saturated fat. You can tell when something is saturated fat because it remains solid at room temperature. Hydrogenated vegetable oils have been chemically changed into saturated fats by adding hydrogen atoms; they are used in margarine and processed foods such as pastries and baked goods to increase shelf life.

• *Polyunsaturated fats* appear to lower cholesterol in the blood and may be less promoting of heart disease than are saturated fats; however, both saturated and unsaturated fats are implicated in many types of cancer including colon, breast, and uterus. Part of the mechanism may be due to this type of fat's vulnerability to oxidation by free radicals, so do not heat polyunsaturated fats because this forms free radicals. Vegetable oils such as corn, sunflower, and sesame are high in polyunsaturated fats.

• *Monounsaturated fats* seem to be beneficial in that they actually lower LDL (the bad cholesterol), while raising HDL cholesterol (the good kind). The oleic acid in olive oil appears to protect fats from oxidative damage from free radicals. In addition to olive oil, peanut oil contains monounsaturated fats, as do avocados and cashews.

The Standard American Diet gets 40 percent of its calories from fat—much of it saturated fat. Cutting down on fat would not only help you lose weight, but help reduce your risk of cardiovascular disease, osteoporosis, many cancers, diabetes, stroke, and high blood pressure. Most women should limit their fat intake to 40 g or less per day. If you want to lose weight, limit yourself to 30 g or less. Those at higher than normal risk for fat-related diseases should aim even lower to 20 g per day.

The simplest way to cut down on fat is to emphasize whole, fresh, unprocessed foods such as vegetables, fruit, and whole grains. You'll get an added bonus of more vitamins, minerals, starch, and fiber; many studies suggest that it's the combination of low fat and high micronutrients that lowers risk of serious disease the most. Avoid adding unhealthy fat to foods—such as margarine and mayonnaise—and cook foods using a minimum of fat. When you cook with fats, use more stable types such as butter and olive oil, and for uncooked dressings use cold-pressed polyunsaturated oil such as canola. Low-fat products abound, but read the labels of prepared foods carefully to check the type of fat and actual fat grams per serving. To find out more about fat and how to eat less of it, read any of Covert Baily's books, such as *Fit or Fat?*

Sugar is a highly refined carbohydrate, and Americans eat an average of 120–150 pounds of sugar and other sweeteners every year. Our collective sweet tooth is a health problem, for many reasons. Sugar contains no nutrients other than calories; if your body doesn't spend them as energy, they turn into fat. In addition, as your body uses sugar to create energy or as the excess is converted to be stored as fat, it depletes its own stores of nutrients, including B vitamins and the minerals chromium, zinc, and copper. High sugar intake also increases the excretion of nutrients such as calcium, magnesium, and chromium; sugar also limits our ability to absorb calcium. Sugar often causes women to retain water, adding to menopausal symptoms such as bloating and cramping, and also increases hot flashes in some women. Studies show that our high sugar intake contributes to and worsens a wide range of degenerative diseases including diabetes, arthritis, tooth decay, heart disease, and osteoporosis. Dr. Maas has known several women with arthritis whose pain decreased so much that they no longer needed pain medication or surgery. All they did was avoid certain foods, particularly sugar.

To cut down on sugar, emphasize fresh fruit instead of baked goods and candy and use natural sweeteners such as stevia. It's best not to try to appease or tease a sweet tooth, but if you have an overwhelming craving, try carrots—though high in sugar, they are also rich in antioxidants. We find that the trick to quitting the sugar habit is to consider it to be "too sweet" or "unhealthy" rather than a treat that you are denying yourself. Be aware of any feelings of deprivation which may arise, and consciously set about providing other means of satisfaction—affection, verbal communication, exercise, giving yourself a massage, or eating a healthier snack. Once you've gotten into the habit of using these other ideas, sweets will really begin to taste too sweet to eat. And you'll feel so much better physically (and so much worse when you "cheat") because you've cleaned out your system.

You probably know that sweets and treats such as cookies, candies, pastries, and soft drinks are high in sugar: For example, a piece of chocolate cake contains 15 teaspoons of sugar. But you may be surprised to learn that many other common foods that we consider to be "healthy" or that don't really taste sweet are also high in sugar. For example, 12 ounces of colas and sodas contain 7–9 teaspoons of sugar; but apple cider contains almost as much—6 teaspoons. Here's another surprise: One ounce of fudge contains 4.5 teaspoons of sugar—but the equivalent amount of jam contains 4–6 teaspoons!

Salt, or sodium chloride, is a mineral needed to maintain water balance in our cells. However, modern Americans consume far more than the 2,000 mg needed each day: from twelve to thirty-six times more than we need! Most of the sodium sneaks into our diet from processed foods, rather than the salt shaker. A serving of canned soup may contain 1,500 mg of sodium.

Too much sodium contributes to high blood pressure in many people. Because it encourages your body to retain too much water, it may aggravate premenstrual symptoms such as bloating, headaches, breast tenderness, and irritability. Excess sodium causes calcium to be excreted in the urine, contributing to osteoporosis; sodium may also contribute to hot flashes.

Presumably because salt was scarce during most of human existence on earth, we evolved a sodium-conserving mechanism. Today salt is no longer so precious, but we still conserve sodium in our bodies—and as our kidneys age and slow down, we conserve even more. To cut down on sodium, eat fewer processed foods and read labels carefully. Reduce the salt you use in cooking and seasoning; gradually substitute herbs, spices, fresh or powdered garlic, and lemon juice.

Caffeine is clearly America's favorite drug. It's found in coffee, black and green tea, cola drinks, chocolate, and many prescription and nonprescription medications. We like it because it perks us up and helps us think more clearly and quickly. The down side is that in some people, caffeine causes "coffee nerves," anxiety, heart palpitations, sleep disturbances, gastrointestinal problems, urinary tract inflammation, and breast tenderness. More bad news: Since caffeine causes tiny blood vessels in your skin to constrict, it can raise your blood pressure and your body temperature and worsen hot flashes. Because it acts as a diuretic, it pushes your kidneys into overdrive and depletes your body of many nutrients including vitamin C, the B complex, calcium, magnesium, and zinc. As little as 300 mg of caffeine (the amount in two mugs of coffee) can cause a considerable loss of calcium, thus contributing to osteoporosis.

Coffee and other caffeine-containing beverages are deeply imbedded in our culture. Over 80 percent of the adults in the United States consume caffeine regularly—an average of 43 gallons of coffee and tea per person each year. The average American drinks more soft drinks than water, many of which contain caffeine. A recent study at

Johns Hopkins University suggests that some people become chemically dependent on caffeine, similar to other psychoactive substances. Because of these factors, it can be very difficult to kick the caffeine habit. Unless you have stomach pains, heart palpitations, or other urgent problems which mandate quitting abruptly, set a quit date you know you can comfortably keep. The most successful technique involves tapering off gradually to limit withdrawal symptoms such as headache and lethargy. Each day, cut down by one-fourth the amount of coffee, cola, or tea you've been drinking. For example, if you drink three cups a day, take five days to quit. Switch to water-processed decaffeinated coffee as an interim, or substitute decaf for part of your regular coffee and taper off that way. Keep alternative beverages handy—such as Caffix, Inka, or Pero (cereal-based instant beverages) or herbal teas—to sip instead. Although they don't have the sinful bite of real coffee, they do have their own unique flavors that can be quite delicious and much better than your typical fast-food coffees.

Caffeine is sneaky—as the following list shows, you'll find it in varying amounts in many common beverages and medications.

Coffee, 5 oz:	automatic drip	110–150 mg
	percolated	64–124
	decaffeinated	2–6
Black tea, 5 oz:	brewed, one minute	9–33
	brewed, five minutes	20–50
	iced, in can, 12 oz	22–36
Soft drinks, 12 oz:	colas	36–48
	ginger ale	0
	Dr Pepper	38
	Mountain Dew	54
	7-Up	0
Chocolate	baking (1 oz)	35
	milk chocolate (1 oz)	6
	chocolate milk	6–10
Nonprescription drugs	Exedrin	65
	Anacin	35
	Midol	32
	NoDoz	100

Alcohol has a relaxing effect, acts as a "social lubricant," and enhances our enjoyment of food. Used in moderation, it appears to raise the level of "good" cholesterol in the blood (HDL). Studies done with men indicate that moderate drinkers live longer than teetotalers. But it also has many negative effects, especially if consumed in excess. Alcohol depletes many B vitamins and minerals from the body and contributes to osteoporosis. It interferes with the way our bodies utilize vitamins and metabolize carbohydrates. It can wreak havoc with our efforts to eat a healthier diet, since it weakens our resolve to stay away from junk food, increases our appetite, or may cause us to forget to eat at all! Excess alcohol damages the liver, reducing its ability to metabolize anything, including hormones; it can be toxic to your heart and nervous system. A recent study, published in 1995 in the *Journal of the National Cancer Institute,* found that postmenopausal women who take more than two drinks a day produce higher levels of estrogens believed to have a role in breast cancer development; alcohol has been linked with an increased risk of breast cancer and other cancers. Alcohol has been shown to trigger hot flashes, accelerate aging of the skin, worsen premenstrual syndrome, and cause depression and sleep disturbances.

If you use alcohol at all, limit yourself to 4 ounces of wine, 10 ounces of beer, or 1 ounce of hard liquor once or twice a week. Substitute light or nonalcoholic beverages such as wine coolers, "near beer," iced tea drinks, and spritzers made with wine or fruit juice. If you drink frequently and especially if you get drunk to numb your problems, we strongly recommend that you get a "reality check" from your doctor or an alcoholic support group. This could be the single most important step you can take for your health.

Cigarette smoking is associated with a host of health problems. Smoking kills 300,000 Americans annually, and cuts 10–15 years off life expectancy. Unlike an occasional glass of wine or beer, even light smoking is bad for you—each cigarette shortens life by five minutes. Smokers are ten times more likely to develop lung cancer than nonsmokers; two times more likely to develop heart disease. Cigarette smoke is also related to emphysema, chronic bronchitis, gum disease, and cancer of the mouth, throat, and bowel. It places an extra burden on the liver, which must detoxify the constituents of smoke such as cadmium, lead, and nicotine. Smoking depletes the body of several nutrients such as vitamin C and interferes with calcium absorption.

These are of concern to everyone, but cigarette smoking also has some effects of particular concern to the midlife woman. It is linked with earlier onset of menopause, possibly because smoking decreases estrogen production of the ovaries. Smoking is sufficiently antiestrogenic that it cancels out the benefits of estrogen therapy. It also appears to cancel out the cardiovascular benefits of exercise. It constricts your blood vessels and intensifies and lengthens the duration of hot flashes, and it's a factor in excessive menstrual bleeding and cervical cancer. Smoking increases your risk of osteoporosis and bone fractures and slows the healing process once a fracture has occurred.

Smoking makes you look and feel older than your years. A recent study out of the Oregon Health Sciences University found that smoking made women age sixty-five and up feel older—they were less able to walk, climb stairs, or even get up out of a chair—and this may increase their risk for injuries from falls. Puffing cigarettes has a detrimental effect on your skin and worsens wrinkles, especially around the mouth.

Roughly one-third of all adult Americans smoke; although smoking has decreased overall, it has been steadily rising among young women, setting them up for problems in midlife and beyond. Nicotine is one of the most addictive drugs there is—it can both relax you when you're anxious and rev you up when you're tired. It depresses the appetite and increases metabolism and is a popular weight control crutch. Like caffeine, cigarettes become thoroughly ingrained in a person's social life and personal identity, adding to the difficulty of quitting. In addition to changing your self-image, giving up cigarettes can be a huge and happy event, or a nerve-racking trial. Many women have strong, deeply hidden emotional issues which supported their coping this way to begin with. We can't overstate how much adequate psychological support can help in these instances.

Nine out of ten former smokers say they quit without any professional help, often going "cold turkey." Most ex-smokers have tried several times before finally succeeding, so don't give up if at first you fail. Consider the nicotine patch—it's not a cure-all but has been a helpful adjunct for people who can't seem to quit on their own. Group programs can help; contact your local hospital, American Cancer Society, American Lung Association, or a commercial program such as Smokenders. Replacing cigarettes with other healthful habits such as taking a 5-minute walk or deep-breathing yoga break sounds simplistic, but many people find they do work. Be aware that "secondhand smoke" is also dangerous to your health. The evidence is not as well established as for firsthand smoke, and the tobacco industry supports public relations campaigns to downplay these effects. However, *Consumer Reports* evaluated the evidence as of January 1995, and concluded that there is a consistent case that secondhand smoke causes lung cancer and is strongly linked with many other ills including asthma and bronchitis in children, and probably heart disease in adults. The annual death toll from secondhand cigarette smoking is about 43,000—on a par with motor-vehicle accidents or breast cancer.

Better Eating Guidelines

We've already suggested some ways to make food changes, but how do these tips translate into a daily eating pattern? Why can't you just take supplements? As controversial as this subject is, there is consensus that we should satisfy most of our nutritional needs through food. Science is still discovering new compounds in foods, so how can they put in a pill something that hasn't been discovered yet?

So, in revamping your eating patterns, use the following four basic principles as your guide: (1) Emphasize whole, fresh foods; (2) limit fatty foods; (3) limit animal products; and (4) consider taking nutritional supplements if you suspect that food isn't supplying you with the nutrients you need, owing to inadequate intake, improper absorption, and metabolic problems such as high stress (*see* Chapter 3). These work hand in hand to ensure you're eating foods high in health-building nutrients and low in health-robbing antinutrients.

To help you create healthy eating habits, refer to our Daily Eating Pattern Guidelines (shown on pages 36–37). This easy-to-read chart shows you the type of daily eating pattern we recommend. It gives you a general idea of the food groups and the amount of each to aim for each day. Be aware that even if you follow these guidelines faithfully, it's still very very difficult to meet the RDAs through just food alone. Half of all women consume less than 1,500 calories a day, a level where it is next to impossible to create meals which provide the RDA of the main nutrients necessary for optimum health.

Daily Eating Pattern Guidelines

Whole grains
> At least 2 cups, plus 1–2 slices of whole grain bread, if desired: brown rice, oats, corn, millet, barley, buckwheat, amaranth, quinoa, wheat, triticale, rye.

Low-Starch Vegetables
> 3–4 cups of low-starch vegetables such as broccoli, carrots, spinach, lettuce, onions, celery, string beans, artichoke, summer squash, endive, cabbage, cucumbers, asparagus, chard, peppers, parsley, sprouts, tomatoes (include 1 cup of high-calcium leafy greens such as collards, kale, dandelion and turnip greens, or bok choy).

Starchy Vegetables
> 1–2 servings ($\frac{1}{2}$ cup each) of potatoes, yams, sweet potatoes, parsnips, winter squash, turnips.

Beans
> 1 or more $\frac{1}{2}$-cup servings: split peas, lentils, kidney beans, navy beans, chickpeas, aduki beans, black beans, white beans, mung or soy beans, tofu.

Meat, Fish, Poultry
> Limit to one 4–5-ounce serving per day, or less; fish is preferable; fresh lean meats such as turkey or chicken in moderation.

Dairy
> 0–3 servings; one serving is 1 cup of low-fat or fat-free milk, yogurt; $\frac{1}{2}$ cup cottage cheese; 1 ounce cheese.

Fresh fruit
> $\frac{1}{2}$–2 cups per day

Essential fats
> 2–3 teaspoons of unrefined from whole beans, nuts, seeds or oils such as flax seed, canola, safflower, or sesame; from fish. Refrigerate all oils.

Other Oils
> Olive oil is not high in essential oils but is stable and an overall acceptable oil. Butter is good for sauteing; it is saturated and, unlike polyunsaturated oil, is not damaged by heat.

Nuts and seeds
> $\frac{1}{8}$–$\frac{1}{4}$ cup of fresh, unsalted nuts and seeds or nut butter if de-

sired. Home roasted sunflower, sesame, or pumpkin seeds are a delicious snack or garnish.

Water

At least eight 8-ounce glasses; purified or spring water is preferred.

How to Eat Better: Saying Good-bye to Old Habits

Food is a highly charged emotional issue. It seems it's always time to eat: to help comfort us during times of stress, and to help us celebrate happy events. At the same time women are inundated with contradictory messages: women's magazines often provide both a weight loss diet and a section of luscious dessert recipes!

So it's not surprising that women have a bizarre relationship with food and so many struggle their entire lives to reach or maintain a desirable weight. Most heavy women use food almost like a drug to provide emotional comfort.

"Dieting" is not the answer—only a few women lose weight permanently by going on "diets." A change in attitude comes first, and then habits have a chance to change naturally toward nourishing, health-building foods and away from health-robbing ones. Many women have found the following suggestions helpful:

- To find out why you're eating too much, or too much health-robbing food, keep a food diary for at least 2 weeks. Write down what you eat, where you ate, and why.
- "Catch" the thought that occurs before your decision to eat. Ask yourself, "Am I hungry?" If not, learn to sit with any discomfort or unpleasant emotions or urges without acting on them. Our culture is intolerant of discomfort—where did we learn that life should be without the "chewier" feelings?
- Eat because you're hungry, not because you're bored, or anxious, or the clock says it's mealtime. Stop eating just before you feel completely full—it takes about 15 minutes for your brain to realize your stomach is satisfied.
- Eat all your food mindfully—not while watching TV, reading, or working. Appreciating the sensual aspects of eating delicious food helps you become satisfied with less quantity. Whenever you think, "I can't believe I ate the whole thing," it's probably because your mind was somewhere else.

- Some women need a lot of structure in their food plan. If you are very compulsive—certain feelings or foods trigger overeating—you may need to eliminate certain foods completely. Sweet, fatty, salty, or yeasty foods trigger binges in some women and should be avoided even in small doses until they normalize their relationship with foods. (This may take months or years.) Also, some women need to eat by the clock, especially if they are hypoglycemic or tend to skip meals, or graze while on automatic pilot.
- Evaluate the role that other people play in your eating habits. Avoid people who eat badly and reinforce your unhealthy eating behavior. Tell your family you will be eating a healthier diet and won't be cooking or buying unhealthy foods for them, either. (Their health will improve too.)
- Consider joining a support group such as Overeaters Anonymous for emotional support; or read one of the better healthy eating books such as *Why Weight? A Guide to Breaking Free from Compulsive Eating,* by Geneen Roth (Dutton, 1989); or *It's Not Your Fault You're Fat Diet* by Marshal Mandell (Harper & Row, 1983).
- Exercise to reverse the tendency of lean body mass (muscle) to be replaced by fat—something that seems to occur with aging and lower metabolism. (Later in this chapter we explain the why's and how-to's of getting more physical exercise.) Exercise decreases nervous appetite and increases self-esteem.

Menopause and Food Allergies or Sensitivities

At the MEND Clinic, we find that adverse reactions to food are extremely common and can cause a surprising variety of symptoms, some of which appear to be related to menopause. Such reactions may be *food allergies*—an inappropriate response by the immune system is involved. A food particle leaks from the gut into the bloodstream without being fully digested and the immune system sees this harmless food particle as a potential invader. White blood cells, blood vessels, and even distant organs such as the adrenal glands respond amid a torrent of biochemicals including histamines, which produce allergic symptoms.

Or a reaction may be due to *food intolerances or sensitivities*—the immune system is not directly involved. The body may respond directly to specific compounds in a food, such as when a person flushes after eating sulfates. Or foods may have an indirect effect or excite an already existing propensity, such as sugar triggering a yeast overgrowth, or coffee triggering hot flashes. Or there may be an enzyme deficiency as in lactose intolerance or a lack of pancreatic enzymes, leading to gas and bloating, or a blood sugar reaction leading to weakness, hunger, and the like.

It is likely that 60–80 percent of our population suffers from one or more food allergies or sensitivities. Typically recognized symptoms are headache, sinus congestion, runny nose, cramping, diarrhea, and skin eruptions. Less well-known reactions include edema, sore throat, heart palpitations, anxiety, fatigue, mood swings, joint pain, irritable bowel syndrome, and migraine.

Eggs, corn, chocolate, dairy, wheat, soy, citrus, peanuts, food additives, and preservatives are the top ten offenders. Dairy is a single culprit 80 percent of the time. If you suspect you might have a food allergy or sensitivity, be sure to have your symptoms checked by a physician to make sure you don't have an underlying medical problem. Then, on your own or working with your doctor, become a nutrition detective by using the simple elimination and challenge procedure described in Appendix B.

3. Be Physically Active

Our bodies are meant to move, although you'd hardly know it judging by our sedentary lifestyles. Attention all couch potatoes, desk potatoes, and car potatoes: It's time to get moving. "Use it or lose it" was never truer than at middle age. The benefits of regular exercise are almost endless, and along with eating well, being physically active is your ticket to a more vibrant, healthier life through menopause and way beyond. It is the number one key factor in preventing osteoporosis. If lowered risk of serious disease, lessened menopause symptoms, and improved energy levels, moods, and self-esteem sound good to you—you'd better get up and go.

What Exercise Does for You

- Oxygenates your entire body, boosting circulation and giving you energy.
- Helps you handle stress better, and gives you a psychological lift and general sense of well-being.
- Helps you live longer and healthier, since exercise is linked with

reduction in heart disease, cancer, diabetes, and osteoporosis. One theory is that exercise lays the foundation for optimism and that helps us live longer!

• Improves sleep.

• Helps normalize hormones; reduces menstrual cramps, premenstrual syndrome, and hot flashes; helps adrenals convert androgens to estrone, the major source of estrogen after menopause.

• Helps normalize your weight by burning calories, speeding up your metabolism, and controlling appetite.

• Improves your nutrition because it allows you to consume more wholesome food without gaining weight, as well as enhancing digestion and absorption. It balances your appetite over time, and as you feel better, you'll crave healthier food.

• Replaces flabby fat with firm, conditioned muscles, which look better and burn more calories.

• Helps you look healthier and younger because you'll be stronger and more flexible and able to move with greater ease, energy, and confidence. Exercise boosts circulation, imparting better skin tone, fewer blemishes, and a healthy glow.

• Helps you stay ''clear'' and get more done for the amount of time you put in—the time you spend exercising is never time lost.

Getting Started

Perhaps you've been physically active all your life—don't stop now! As long as you feel well and able, continue what you're doing, letting your body signal you whether it's time to change the intensity or duration of your activity. But if you're an absolute beginner, you'll be glad to hear that you don't have to exhaust yourself or spend all your spare time (and spare change) at the gym to reap the benefits of an active lifestyle.

Walking is the easiest, simplest, and best way to kick off a more active life; it's also a terrific mainstay no matter what else you do. Let your body be your guide and begin slowly, gradually increasing the distance and/or the intensity with which you cover the same distance. A good goal is brisk walking for two or three miles every other day; every day is preferable. A recent study from Tufts University found that women who walk at least a mile a day delay onset of bone loss by up to seven years.

To keep yourself interested and motivated, try to choose a pleasant, interesting route—a tree-lined street, a riverwalk, or a commercial street with a variety of interesting shops, buildings, and people. Feel free to slow to a stroll, or stop to chat or shop, as long as you cover the distance.

Should you decide to go beyond walking, choose from the astounding variety of clubs, classes, books, and workout tapes available. Dr. Maas has produced movement videotapes (see Resources). Whatever you choose, make sure you enjoy it, or can learn to enjoy it. It's often tough to find the time to exercise, and it's tougher still to stick with something that you consider a bore or a chore. Today you have many options to choose from, so there's really no excuse.

Aim for a variety of activities because that will condition all the parts of your body while keeping boredom at bay. It will also reduce the chance of injury from overusing one part of your body. A complete program exercises your heart, lungs, and major muscles; these are called *aerobic* exercises because they increase the flow of circulation, bringing fresh oxygen to the working muscles. Examples of aerobic exercise include brisk walking, jogging, running, aerobic dancing, skating, swimming, jumping rope, stair climbing, bicycling, rowing, ball sports, and skiing.

Your program should also include activities that *condition and strengthen* many different muscle groups. Many aerobic activities do this, but if not, you may fill in any gaps with weight lifting, push-ups and sit-ups, and/or exercise machines. A recent study done at Tufts University found that 45 minutes of high-intensity strength training exercises twice a week (on a pneumatic resistance machine) may help you avoid bone fractures. The women in the study, aged fifty to seventy, not only *increased* bone mass which may make bones stronger, but also increased muscle mass, improved strength and balance, and were more motivated to participate in spontaneous physical activity. In contrast, most conventional hormone replacement and nutritional approaches have been able only to maintain or slow the loss of bone.

Finally, be sure to include stretching activities that keep your joints limber and muscles long and lithe and may help release pain and tension: yoga, stretches, dance, and martial arts all fill the bill and often help condition your heart and muscles as well. (*See also* Chapter

3, page 96, for the benefits of gentler forms of activity such as yoga.) Conditioning and limbering exercises are good ways to begin and end your aerobic sessions. Be sure to incorporate 5-minute warm-ups and cool-downs in your program to ease your body into and out of a workout and lessen the chance of injury and tightness.

In addition to—or as a substitute for—a formal exercise program, look for ways to informally add more activity to your life. New recommendations by the U.S. Centers for Disease Control and the American College of Sports Medicine have broadened the traditional view of exercising for fitness. Although they agree that every adult should be physically active for 30 minutes or more every day, they also emphasize that the accumulation of short bouts of moderate-intensity physical activity could add up to the 30 minutes. The panel of experts concluded: "An active lifestyle does not require a regimented, vigorous exercise program. Instead, small changes that increase daily physical activity will enable individuals to reduce their risk of chronic heart disease and may contribute to enhanced quality of life."

So, take a walk during a lunchtime break; if you can, walk or bike at least part of the way to your workplace or when doing errands; take the stairs instead of the elevator (think of it as a free StairMaster!). Gardening, riding a stationary bike while watching TV, raking leaves, dancing, and playing actively with children all count, if performed at an intensity corresponding to brisk walking. This is good news indeed for women who don't get a thrill out of a workout, or don't mind missing that aerobic rush of intense activity, or simply get discouraged by formal exercise.

It's also important for anyone with a sedentary job to take frequent stretch and activity breaks. This not only reduces mental stress and strain, but helps counteract the stiffness and shortening of muscles and ligaments that we begin to feel as we get older.

Sticking with It

Once you become active, chances are you'll feel so much better that you won't need much convincing to keep it up. As one convert observes, "Hey, I knew it was going to be hard to start exercising—but nobody told me it's also hard to stop!" Still, even the most gung-ho Olympic wanna-be occasionally falls off the wagon and could use a few supportive hints:

• Unless you're the solo type, or use your runs or swims as a mental respite or "think time," find a partner—or several—to join you. There's nothing like the right walking pal to motivate you, keep you from slipping off your routine, and provide an added fun social dimension.

• Formally set aside a specific time in your schedule for exercise, write it in your datebook (think of it as making an appointment with your body), and stick to it. We recommend that you do aerobic exercise at least three times a week for a minimum of thirty minutes each time.

• Instead of watching TV or reading a trashy novel (or eating that chocolate cake), join a community garden, help restore a natural habitat or park, play volleyball, go bowling, shoot some baskets, take a hike, fly a kite. Who knows? In addition to conditioning your body, you might make a new friend or two.

After a month or so, take stock: How do you feel? How do you look? Are you more relaxed, energetic, limber? Are you stronger, do you have more endurance, are you sleeping better? Another gauge is your resting pulse rate. Take your pulse rate during inactivity (*see* box, pages 44–45) before beginning your program. Then periodically check your resting rate—it should drop down as an indication of your improved fitness. When fifty-four-year-old Phyllis began her aerobics class, she could barely make it through and her resting pulse was 97; six months later, she was keeping up in class and her pulse had dropped to 78; a year later, it had dropped to around 60.

Note: Before you begin a new exercise program, please check with your doctor and get a complete physical exam and discuss your intended plan. Some exercises may be inadvisable or need to be modified if you have an established condition such as severe osteoporosis or arthritis. To be safe, stop any exercise if you experience persistent pain anywhere or soreness in your joints. Always be comfortable— learn to tell the difference between a stretch and a strain.

Aerobics: Get Fit, Burn Fat, Take Pulse

In order to get the most out of aerobic exercise and avoid strain and injury, do it regularly (at least three times a week), for a specific duration (20–30 minutes or more) without stopping. You also should reach a certain intensity, which is indicated by your heart rate during exercise.

To see whether you are within the recommended heart rate for your age *(training heart rate),* take a moment during your exercise session to determine your pulse rate. You may need to slow your exercise pace as you take your pulse, but try not to come to a complete halt for too long. Place the tips of the first three fingers of your hand on your carotid artery, located about 1 inch below your ear, or at the inside of your wrist, 1 inch above the crease. Don't use your thumb because it has its own prominent pulse. Press lightly until you feel the throb; count the beats for six seconds, then add a zero to find the rate per minute.

Using the chart below, compare your heart rate to the recommended rate for your age range. If you exercise at the low end (60% of your maximum heart rate), you're burning mostly fat calories, but slowly. If you're at the high end (80%), you're burning calories more quickly, but they will be both fat calories and calories stored as glycogen (a sugar) in the muscles. Both rates of intensity confer cardiovascular benefits, but if you're at the low end, you need to exercise for longer periods to enjoy them. For example, jogging at 80% intensity for 20 minutes is on a par with brisk walking at 60% intensity for 40 minutes. If you are beginning an exercise program, however, start at 60% and work your way up.

Training Rate Ranges

Age	*60% (low)*	*70% (medium)*	*80% (high)*
20	120	140	160
30	114	133	152
40	108	126	146
50	102	119	140
60	96	112	128
70	90	105	120

> Or use the following formula: Take 220, subtract your age, then multiply by 60%, 70%, or 80% to get your low-, medium-, or high-intensity training rate.

4. Relax and Manage Stress

Did you know that the world is turning around on its axis faster and faster and every day is measurably shorter than the last? Of course, we're talking about a fraction of a second, but for most women, every day does *seem* shorter than the last. We have so much more to do, and less and less "free time." Our lives are bursting with endless details and obligations and deadlines and sometimes conflicting priorities. What is a woman to do when there's too much to do? Relax!

We've been hearing for some time about stress—but what is it and how does it affect us? When we perceive something to be stressful, an internal alarm goes off, triggering a cascade of physiological changes that was originally described by Hans Selye in the 1940s as the "fight or flight" response. Adrenaline floods into the bloodstream, the heart beats faster, digestion screeches to a halt, muscles tense up, blood pressure skyrockets, the brain and senses become hyperalert. This response is designed to enable to us fight for our lives or to get us away from the danger as fast as possible. It worked well for our ancestors because their stressors were mainly of the saber-toothed tiger variety. Stresses were immediate and short-lived, and once the dangerous situation was over, the body had time to return to normal.

Today life is not so simple or clear-cut. Instead of saber-toothed tigers, we're constantly barraged by little day-to-day hassles—job insecurity or frustration, exasperating children, or traffic jams—that are difficult to fight or escape from. Nor is the stress response so simple and clear-cut. We now know that the way a person responds to stressful situations depends in part on the way a person has learned to cope. The more stress we perceive, and the less able we are to cope with it, the less we are able to recover from it, and the less we are able to deal with new stressors. Prolonged stress wreaks all sorts of havoc: it can contribute to fatigue, diabetes, hypertension, ulcers, loss of libido, and reduced resistance to disease. Emotional upset can throw our periods off-kilter—nature's ancient way to reduce pregnancy during difficult times such as famine, exhaustion, or extreme physical exertion. When we are stressed out, our brain doesn't stimulate the ovaries, ovulation may not occur, and our ovarian hormones may become imbalanced. As a result, periods become irregular in some women; in others, they become lighter or heavier or stop completely. By affecting hormones, stress can also make menopause more difficult and accelerate aging. In turn, going through menopause and getting older can make life seem more stressful, creating a health-sapping feedback loop. Recently, stress has also been shown to contribute to osteoporosis.

Stress affects your ability to work, to think clearly, and to have satisfying social relationships. In animal experiments, stress has accelerated aging and death, hastened the spread of cancer, and promoted heart attacks. No wonder women who are already overstressed find it difficult to cope with aging and the transition of menopause!

You can't control all the stress-causing factors in your life, but by following these suggestions, you can control some of them, as well as minimize their affect on you physiologically. If you find stress is still a problem, consider trying some of the natural mind-body therapies discussed in the next chapter.

Take Stock, Take Action

One thing you can do is to evaluate your life stressors and change what you can. If your job is bringing you down, what can you do to fix it? Talk to your boss? Get more training and education so you can change jobs? What about your social relationships? Is something bothering you or are you unsatisfied? If you are taking care of an elderly parent, can you enlist someone to share the burden? Like so many women, you may be conditioned to ignore or conceal your feelings. Although maintaining the status quo may seem the safest thing to do, consider that now might be the time to be brave, take the plunge, and bring troubles into the open.

Negative Stress or Positive Stress?

Another approach you may find helpful is to try to change the way you react to things you normally find stressful. Although everyone would probably prefer not to have their car totaled, some women become greatly upset when this happens, while others remain calm and treat it as if it were the merest of ripples in their lives. Such variations in stress response occur because the broadest definition of a stressful event is any type of change or unexpected event. Your reaction to changes may be positive, negative, or neutral. People with "hardy" personalities are able to weather changes with equanimity, and even zest. What some people would consider major tragedies they perceive as minor inconveniences or perhaps challenges to be met with energy and enthusiasm. While resistance to stress depends a good deal upon your childhood experiences, you can develop more optimism and hardiness at any point in life.

How you perceive any event in your life influences your reaction to it and determines mood and, eventually, health. What does a particular stressful event mean to you? Do you see the glass as being half empty or half full? We all tell ourselves "stories" to explain why something is happening. What story did you make up about why something went in a way you didn't want it to? Pessimists expect bad things to happen and tend to dwell on them when they do. A pessimistic interpretation of losing a job might be: "This will ruin my whole life; no one hires a woman my age. I'll never pay all my bills and I'll die in a gutter because nobody loves me anyway." Pessimists perceive stress as something that is unpredictable and out of their control. Optimists expect good things to happen; they seek them out and remember them. They interpret "bad" events differently, thinking, "This too shall pass, and it will probably set me free to find a job I like better." Try to find the lesson inherent in any situation, no matter how painful. Instead of the negative thought, look for a positive affirmative thought to help you avoid a recurrence. For example, instead of concluding, "Never trust anyone," you could think, "I can tell when someone is trying to take advantage of me, and I can easily and tactfully find ways to protect my interests, which are always valid."

There are several techniques to begin shifting from a tendency to react to stress negatively, to a more neutral or positive response. Try the suggestions given on page 48, adapted from the book *Healthy Pleasures,* by David Sobel and Robert Ornstein. With time, you'll evoke a healthier response, without suppressing your feelings and risking an explosive reaction later on. When something stressful happens to you:

- Avoid thinking in all-or-none terms. Be on the lookout for words like *all* or *completely:* You are not totally stupid, and everyone else is not totally brilliant.
- Don't assume every situation is the same. They are not—and you always have the option of reacting differently.
- Don't confuse a rare occurrence with a high probability. You will probably not get fired for being late one more time; but you probably will be reprimanded.
- Don't assume the worst possible outcome. If you lose that client, it may not be the catastrophe you imagine it to be.
- Look for your strengths. In any situation, you probably show elements of both weakness and strength.
- Avoid blaming yourself for something that is beyond your control. Although we should accept personal responsibility when it's appropriate, blaming yourself for a party ruined by rain is not one of those times.
- Don't expect perfection in yourself and in others. Expecting perfection is a setup for failure and disappointment. Everyone should do their best and strive to improve, but we learn more from our mistakes than from our successes.
- Imagine how you could have handled the situation differently. Think about how these alternative reactions would make you feel, and how you can use them to do better next time.
- Ask yourself: What difference will this make in a week, a year, or ten years? Some things just aren't that important when you take the long view.

Cultivate Closeness

You might be surprised to learn that a lack of close, supportive social relationships can be as damaging to health as cigarette smoking, a diet of junk food, or a sedentary lifestyle. That's why having close, intimate friends and significant others can be the most rewarding thing you can do for your health. Humans are social animals and need to feel connected with others, and feel warmly toward them. Studies suggest that isolation from other people and feelings of hostility damage the heart and that people who feel apart from their fellow humans are more likely to die of heart disease. When established relationships are disrupted, owing for example, to divorce or the death of a loved one, physical health also suffers.

If loneliness kills, then togetherness heals. Couples who live together are better off healthwise than people living alone without much social support. A happy marriage is particularly conducive to better health and longevity—but more so for men than for women. This may be because women tend to give more support than they get. Fortunately for them, women seem to be more adept at forming and maintaining close social ties with other women and relatives outside their marriage, and this confers great health benefits.

Even loving an animal is good for your health: People with pets report fewer minor health problems. Animals may help prevent heart disease—studies show that blood pressure drops sharply when people pet a cat or dog and pet owners have markedly lower the cholesterol and triglyceride levels. What's more, people with pets who have already had a heart attack live longer than those who don't.

Work Some, Play Some

Take a good look at your life: Do you balance periods of challenging work with "down" times of rest and relaxation, of great and little pleasures? If not, you're not taking good care of yourself. Having a purpose in life such as a satisfying job tends to make people happier and healthier. But lest you feel guilty about taking a Caribbean vacation: One study showed that taking a vacation reduced fatigue (surprise), digestive problems, insomnia, and loss of libido by 50 percent.

As Sobel and Ornstein write, "Doing 'nothing' and just hanging out is a vital part of self-renewal." In their book they provide the scientific evidence for incorporating many other healthy pleasures into our lives. Laughing, eating delicious food, sex, music, and connecting with nature make us feel good and bestow relaxation and thus health and longevity. Advocates of common sense and moderation, they point out that people with stressful jobs need an outlet for their frustrations, not more frustration. Being forced to adhere to a strict diet, for example, actually worsened the health profile of hassled male executives, who saw this as one less thing they could control.

Even experimental rats show less stress when they can gnaw on a piece of wood or are given something to eat or drink or a wheel to play on. So forgive yourself your binges. Although such habits such as overeating under stress may seem unhealthy, they may be the best you can do to deal with stress at any time, considering the information you have and your past experience. You can always try to do better next time.

Helping others, for love or money, is also linked with more robust health. Situations where there are clear boundaries to your responsibilities and where you give for the sake of giving, out of respect for yourself and for others, are the most rewarding. Make getting enough sleep a high priority, even if this requires a daily nap; sleep appears to be needed to maintain a healthy immune system and a fully functioning body and brain.

5. *Establish a Partnership with Your Doctor(s) and Other Health Providers*

Much of menopausal care is self-care: you can learn about your options, take care of yourself, know what you need for your own comfort and to decrease your risk of disease in the future, and be able to convey your concerns to your physicians and any other health providers you may have.

A doctor can be your best source of information, helping you to interpret information, making treatment decisions, and diagnosing serious disease. He or she can also administer lab tests to better determine your risk factors for serious disease and monitor the effectiveness of and potential side effects of hormonal or other medical treatment.

To develop the kind of relationship you want, see how the physician responds to your questions. Does he or she give and receive feedback if a treatment isn't working, or there are side effects or new problems that need attention? Does he or she feel comfortable giving you a referral to another doctor if necessary for a second opinion or if you've had a change of heart and want to switch to someone else? If the two of you see things differently about natural therapies, for example, don't give up right away. Educate yourself. The more you understand how natural therapies work, and the more valid support you can present for your views, the more gracefully and convincingly you can discuss your options.

Know what you can and cannot expect of your doctor. Doctors are rightly leery of kooks and quacks, and sometimes need to repair the damage done by those health practitioners who have not shared the rigors of medical school and postgraduate training. However, excluding vast realms of treatment options because they ''weren't taught at

Cornell''—which one specialist gave Dr. Maas as his reason for not "believing in" alternative medicine—is simply shortsighted. Fortunately, more and more doctors are perking up their ears and learning from—and with—their educated patients. Bear in mind that if you want your doctor to read the literature you give him or her, it should be as "scientific" as possible. By that we mean it should be from a reputable source; the larger the number of patients in the study, the better; and there should be no strong bias against the establishment or conventional medical treatment.

It's important for both you and your doctor to be able to calmly discuss the pros and cons before you make a treatment decision. However, if your longtime doctor is not helping you through a difficult menopause, or you still don't feel comfortable with him or her despite your efforts, or you're not getting as much advice as you'd like about reducing risk factors or specific treatments such as hormone therapy or natural alternatives, you should ask for a referral to another physician and explain why. Today, there are specialists in treating menopause and aging women, menopause clinics, and endocrine specialists who have the particular knowledge you need. (You may still want him or her to be your primary physician to coordinate your care.)

Unfortunately, under the current health insurance system you may not have much choice. If you belong to an HMO, you may find yourself in an impersonal clinic setting, and have access only to doctors who are under such pressure to see so many patients that he or she can only spare each patient ten minutes' worth of attention. The reality is, you may have to pay more out of your own pocket to get the kind of care you want, especially if you want someone who is knowledgeable about natural therapies. (*See* Appendix C, "Resources," for names of holistic, osteopathic, and naturopathic physicians' associations.)

Support groups provide a forum for you to share your experiences, questions, and knowledge. There are also newsletters that keep you up-to-date about the latest development in menopause treatment. (*See* Appendix C, "Resources.")

Medical Tests and Physical Exam

We recommend that you see your physician once a year, more often if you're on medication or hormone therapy and/or you are having problems. If you are at average risk for serious disease, the visit should include a yearly physical exam with a breast exam and pelvic exam even if you've had a hysterectomy and a blood pressure test to detect hypertension. The American College of Obstetrics and Gynecology recommends that most women get a Pap smear every year. Other health providers recommend Pap tests every two to three years after a run of annual tests with normal results. Other tests vary, depending on your medical history, family history, and other risk factors. You may be given a urine test and blood tests for anemia, diabetes, liver and kidney problems and other abnormalities such as high cholesterol.

If you are age fifty or older, you should have a mammogram 2 years in a row; if they are negative, then every 2 or 3 years, depending on your risk factors and the physical exam. You should have colorectal screening to detect bowel or rectal cancer. A chest X-ray is advisable only if you are at high risk for or have symptoms of lung cancer or heart disease.

You may want to have a baseline bone density scan done of your spine and hip; they cost around $250 for hip and spine measurements and around $125 for just one site. Ideally, you should have one if you are concerned about your bone health or you are about to begin a treatment program because you are at high risk for osteoporosis (*see* Chapter 6). Follow-up measurements to gauge the success of your efforts are usually done annually. If possible, follow-ups should be done on the same type of equipment because test results can vary from place to place and are impossible to compare. You should be aware that this test uses ionizing radiation, as does mammography. As of this writing, the DEXA scanner is considered to be the state-of-the art bone scan device because it is highly accurate and uses the lowest levels of radiation. Understandably, exposure to unnecessary radiation from any diagnostic or monitoring test is a concern for many women. As a safeguard, make sure that the facility meets the guidelines for the standard established by your state. And be sure to ask your doctor if the procedure is necessary; if you are at high risk for a serious disease, the risk from radiation pales in comparison with the risk of a disease being missed early.

When it comes to osteoporosis prevention, the new urinary tests measuring bone breakdown rate are radiation free and likely to be very useful. These simple urine tests can distinguish those who are losing a normal amount of bone from those who are ''fast losers.''

Fast losers need to take corrective steps to slow bone loss and the success of these corrective measures is easily evaluated by follow-up urine tests. For more information about where to get these tests, *see* Resources section.

CHAPTER 3

Using Natural Therapies

No one knows for sure, but chances are there are many more women using natural therapies to manage symptoms of menopause and slow the aging process than are using prescription hormones. From nutritional supplements to massage, these therapies work, often at least as well as hormones. So, if you would like to go beyond the Balanced Life Plan outlined in the previous chapter, this chapter is for you. We introduce you to the most popular and effective natural therapies that are commonly available in the United States: nutritional supplements, herbal therapy, homeopathy, accupressure and traditional Chinese medicine, aromatherapy, the touching therapies (massage, osteopathy, and chiropractic), and mind/body therapies. We first give you background information about how each therapy works, and then explain how to buy the remedies, how to prepare them, and how to use them. Once you have become acquainted with this basic information, you'll be ready to turn to the A-to-Z chapter for information about which therapies to use for specific symptoms or complaints.

Some of the following therapies, such as herbal therapy or homeopathy, are ''medicinal'' in that they introduce nonfood substances into the body. Some, such as massage and chiropractic, work their magic by hands-on manipulation of body tissue. Still others, such as relaxation and meditation, unleash the power of the mind to influence the body. However, they are all natural since they help to normalize your body's functions. Some natural remedies are slower and subtler than Western medicine, so give them time to work. Natural approaches complement, but do not take the place of, a health-building lifestyle and appropriate medical care. All therapies will work best when you also follow our Balanced Life Plan in Chapter 2.

A Word to the Wise

There are dozens of natural therapies from a host of different cultures which have helped women around the world manage menopausal and other symptoms. Many of the natural remedies are based on centuries of use and observation, and we're learning more about these therapies as more studies are being done. These therapies are generally quite safe. But remember: Just because a remedy is considered to be "natural" doesn't mean it is *guaranteed* to be safe. Some are quite powerful and some have serious side effects if taken inappropriately or in toxic amounts. There have been some adverse effects reported with the use of herbs. For example, ginseng may cause abnormal uterine bleeding and, along with other herbal remedies, it has not been approved by the Food and Drug Administration. We don't know all the compounds that herbs contain, nor do we know specific risks and benefits.

If you are under a doctor's care for a specific illness or are taking medication, make sure you discuss these approaches with your health care provider before beginning any new therapy. You will also need professional medical care for physical exams, laboratory tests, mammograms, and understanding the full spectrum of medical options. Women with a history of hormone-related conditions, cancer (especially breast cancer), or other serious medical conditions should also consult a professional for guidance.

Self-care or Professional Guidance?

Since they are generally safe for most women when used as recommended, and the results will guide you, natural therapies lend themselves to self-care. Books, classes, and an increasing number of knowledgeable professionals can also advise you about dosages, interactions, and expected results. We recommend seeing a professional particularly if you have moderate to severe symptoms, or have given self-care a try but haven't gotten satisfactory results. Endocrine imbalances are especially complicated and have strong physiological and emotional effects which sometimes require a more experienced hand at managing.

Unfortunately, there is no nationally recognized standard degree, licensing procedure, or certification for practitioners of many of these approaches, so finding a reputable practitioner can be a challenge. However, there is an increasing number of certifying programs and boards for some such as homeopathy, acupuncture, and herbal therapy. Ask your physician or other trusted health care professional for a referral; or ask a friend or relative who has gotten good results. Alternatively, you can refer to Appendix C, ''Resources,'' and contact the appropriate professional associations for lists of qualified individuals in your geographical area.

With all the options in alternative medicine, how do you know which is right for you? Some women find that one particular approach just feels natural to them, and it does work beautifully. For example, you may prefer to take just nutritional supplements to relieve your hot flashes—if your osteoporosis and heart disease risk is low, that's all you may need. Other women may need to experiment and find the right approach or the combination of approaches through trial and error. Often you need a combination to cover several symptoms or mechanisms of action simultaneously, or to take advantage of their synergistic effects.

For example, a client of Dr. Brown's named Ellen was bothered by as many as fifteen hot flashes a day. She began with changing her diet; she then added herbs and she told Dr. Brown that her hot flashes decreased by about 75 percent. But she still was bothered by night sweats—up to three or four—so she added a homeopathic remedy and in three weeks she slept through the night and had no more daytime hot flashes either.

Some women are able to stop taking prescription estrogen—or avoid taking it in the first place—when they add glandular extracts to strengthen their adrenal glands. Although Dr. Maas supports women who find and follow what feels good to them, she is generally reluctant to recommend glandulars because these preparations vary in quality and content and because although she has seen that some people are helped by these agents, others get worse.

Nutritional Supplements for Added Protection

You walk into a health food store, and feel overwhelmed by the walls of supplements. Or you have a friend who swears by a certain multivitamin-and-mineral supplement. New articles are always coming out touting this vitamin or that. Should you take supplements? Which ones? Are just calcium and vitamin C enough? What nutritional supplements can help minimize menopausal symptoms or slow aging? How much should you take? Are supplements dangerous? Here are the answers you need to take supplements safely and to get the most out of them.

Who Needs Supplements?

The experts agree: The food you eat is your *primary* source for these nutrients. Some respected groups, such as the American Heart Association, and many nutrition experts believe food can and should be our *only* source. Supplements aren't necessary if we just eat a "balanced diet"—a few say that supplements are dangerous. At the same time, evidence is building that even in America it is very difficult to eat what is, in the most conservative eyes, a "balanced diet" adequate in all the essential vitamins, minerals, and fatty acids. We feel that supplements are critical in some cases, rarely undesirable for others (for whatever reasons), but it is *always* up to the woman to decide for herself. We recommend that you educate yourself and then consider trying supplements to see if they help you.

We certainly won't pretend that vitamins (or certain foods, either) will solve all your menopause problems or help you live forever. Adelle Davis, one of the early advocates of supplementation, died of cancer. On the other hand, both Dr. Maas and Dr. Brown have hundreds of patients for whom nutritional supplementation has solved their menopausal and other problems. And more and more researchers and nutritionists are taking supplements themselves. Since this is still a hotly debated subject, we present you with the information we feel has firm scientific support and then let you decide for yourself.

It takes planning to eat a balanced diet. A large survey showed that less than 10 percent of the population eats the recommended five servings of fruits and vegetables. We convince ourselves that our lives are too busy and unpredictable, and that good food isn't always available. In addition, a diet that satisfies the RDAs (recommended daily allowances) of vitamins and minerals is based on 2,000 calories—too high for most women to maintain their weight, even if they are active.

Which orange? Foods vary tremendously in their nutrient content. The vitamin C content of your orange juice may not be as high as the food charts say. Nutrient content varies depending on the growing conditions, how the crop was fertilized, and when it was harvested. Shipping, storing, preparing all reduce the nutrient content of foods. For example, in the fall, a freshly harvested potato has 30 mg of vitamin C, but this drops down to 8 mg by spring and to 0 in summer. English studies found that some Brussels sprouts have 64 times the chromium of others, and some wheat had thirty-six times more than other types of wheat. Organic foods have higher levels of nutrients and fewer pesticides, some of which can influence estrogen in the body.

Individual requirements. We all are born with our individual biological blueprints which includes nutrient requirements and predisposition to diseases. In addition, we are under an unprecedented amount of physical stress from our polluted environment, and psychological stress from our complicated, hectic lives. Such stresses are known to deplete the body of nutrients, and we have evidence that supplemental nutrients help protect us against damage from such stresses. Furthermore, diseases and disorders—and many medical treatments themselves, even antacids, fiber supplements, and birth control pills—affect nutrient absorption and requirements, as does aging.

The RDAs are not enough. The RDAs were set up to prevent deficiency diseases such as pellagra, beriberi, and scurvy. Although the RDAs were a significant step in improving nutrition in this country, many respected authorities no longer believe the RDAs are really adequate for every person. For example, two prestigious publications, *The Journal of the American Medical Association* and *The University of California at Berkeley Wellness Letter,* recently recommended that Americans should take at least some nutritional supplements. *The Wellness Letter* stated, ". . . even if you do eat a very healthy diet . . . it's unlikely you will get the high levels . . . many authorities think you need."

It's possible that the RDAs may be adequate for some people. But we believe that some RDAs—vitamin C, the B vitamins—are ridiculously low. Others may be adequate—calcium, vitamin D, vitamin K, and possibly zinc—for the average healthy person who does not have any long-standing deficiencies. However, the RDAs were designed to prevent deficiency diseases and fall far short of creating and maintaining optimum health; nor are they adequate if you have health problems and are trying to recover your health. So many of our patients feel better when taking supplements greater than RDA levels that it's clear that amounts above the RDA are needed by some people.

How Supplements Can Help

To have optimal health and to correct an illness or long-standing deficiency, you may need higher amounts of vitamins and minerals than even the best diet can supply. Scientific evidence is growing that certain supplements can give us added protection and stronger health. Most of the positive studies using supplements (rather than food) involve the antioxidant nutrients which, as explained in Chapter 2, protect our cells from free radical damage. Studies suggest that doses in excess of the RDA for the antioxidant nutrients vitamins E, C, and A and beta-carotene, and the minerals zinc and selenium are particularly useful to reduce the risk of many diseases and conditions, including premature aging and death, cardiovascular disease, many types of cancer, diabetes, cataracts and other degenerative eye problems, arthritis, and possibly osteoporosis. There's even some evidence that supplements can reverse these diseases or help slow the progression once they are established. In one large study, 50 mg supplements of beta-carotene taken every other day cut the incidence of heart attacks, strokes, and deaths related to heart disease in half. Another study showed that vitamin C supplements enhanced immunity in elderly adults, as did 800 IU of vitamin E. Still other studies show that calcium, magnesium, zinc, and vitamin D supplements help stave off osteoporosis. In some studies, nutritional supplements actually helped reverse osteoporosis—while prescription estrogen only halts the progression. And 400–800 IU of vitamin E has been shown to reduce hot flashes; because vitamin E is found only in vegetable oils, this amount is impossible to get from a healthy low-fat diet, and is difficult to get even in a high fat diet.

How to Begin

The "Nutrient Table of Vitamins and Minerals" (pages 61–64) gives a range of safe recommended dosages for the best-known nutrients. We show you both the RDA, and the optimum intake. The optimum intake amounts are based on the most current research studies published in professional journals, our own experiences in our clinical practices, and the experiences of other well-respected clinicians. We do not believe that more is always better where nutrition is concerned. The range of optimum amounts we recommend may seem high to those who follow the RDAs, but these dosages are beneficial for many women and they are safe. If you have any questions or concerns, we advise you to work with a knowledgeable nutritionist or physician knowledgeable in nutritional sciences.

Before deciding on your level of supplementation, ask yourself the following questions:

1. Am I at high risk for serious diseases (*see* Chapter 6 for self-assessments)?
2. Do I follow a healthy diet? Do I generally follow the recommendations in Chapter 2?
3. Is my lifestyle a healthy one? Do I avoid cigarette smoke, alcohol, and coffee? Do I take time to relax? Do I live in a polluted area or am I exposed to toxic chemicals at work or at home?
4. Have I followed the Balanced Life Plan for six weeks and do I still have symptoms?
5. How severe are my symptoms? Can I wait for the Balanced Life Plan to have an effect or do I need relief sooner?

The more severe your symptoms and the higher your risk for serious disease, the more important it is to involve the help of a practitioner knowledgeable in using supplements to meet your particular needs. Overdoing zinc, iron, copper, and several other nutrients can be damaging. Since vitamins and minerals typically work together, we recommend that you look for a multiple vitamin-mineral formula as your foundation. You may want to take a multivitamin with just the RDAs; other women find they don't get relief until they increase their dosage to meet the optimum intake range. These nutrients mostly affect changes that are slow or impossible to detect, but are hugely important in preventing deadly diseases such as cardiovascular disease and osteoporosis.

For specific problems or concerns. If you are at very high risk for disease, or if you have specific symptoms that are bothering you, check with your doctor or a knowledgeable nutritional counselor. You may want to take higher amounts of certain nutrients than suggested as optimum intake. Turn to Chapter 5 for an A-to-Z listing of specific symptoms for details on taking higher therapeutic amounts of these nutritional supplements where appropriate. Then just take a separate supplement of the additional amount needed in addition to your basic formula.

Nutrient Table of Vitamins and Minerals

Nutrient	RDA, 1989*	Optimum Intake†	Good Food Sources
Boron	No RDA	3–4 mg	Soy meal, raisins, prunes, dates, apples, peaches, peanuts, almonds, hazelnuts, alfalfa, parsley
Calcium	800–1,200 mg	1,000–1,500 mg	Seaweeds; leafy greens, especially bok choy, dandelion and turnip greens, and kale; dairy foods; salmon and sardines, especially with bones; scallops; oysters; shrimp; sesame seeds; soybean nuts; almonds
Chromium	50–200 mcg	200 mcg	Brewer's yeast, meat, cheese, whole grains, beer, prunes, plums, pears, apples, rhubarb
Copper	2–3 mg	2–3 mg	Selected meats such as liver and lamb, nuts, dried beans
Fatty Acids Omega-6	none	9–30 grams	Oils as evening primrose, safflower, sunflower, grape seed oil, corn, flax oil, pumpkin seed oil, soy, walnut, wheat germ

Nutrient	RDA, 1989*	Optimum Intake†	Good Food Sources
Omega-3	none	6 grams	Cold water fish such as salmon, cod, mackerel, tuna, and oils such as flax, pumpkin, soy, walnut
Folic Acid	180–200 mcg	400–800 mcg	Brewer's yeast, bran, chicken giblets, beef liver, green leafy vegetables especially turnip greens, asparagus, avocados, collards and lettuce, fortified cereals and breads, black-eyed peas, lima beans
Iodine	150 mcg	150–300 mcg	Iodized salt, seafoods, saltwater fish, kelp and seaweeds
Iron	10–15 mg	10–18 mg	Seaweed, spirulina, amaranth, tuna, chicken and beef liver, oysters, clams, dried peaches and pears, raisins, beet greens, asparagus, parsley, whole grain or enriched breads and cereals
Magnesium	280–350 mg	500–800 mg	Seafood, fish, split peas, lentils, wild rice, kelp, spinach
Manganese	2.5–5 mg	15 mg	Avocado, whole grains especially wheat germ, whole oats, brown rice, seaweed
Niacin	15–19 mg	25–300 mg	Avocado, many vegetables, beans, peanuts, fish, poultry, liver, kidney, brown rice, fortified cereals
Pantothenic Acid	4–7 mg	100–200 mg	Meat and eggs, yogurt, dried beans, brussels sprouts, sweet potatoes

Nutrient	RDA, 1989*	Optimum Intake†	Good Food Sources
Phosphorus	800–1,200 mg	800–1,200 mg	Dairy products, meats, nuts and seeds, grains, vegetables
Potassium	1,875–5,625 mg	4,000–5,625 mg	Kelp; seaweed; fish; scallops; whole grains; dairy foods; vegetables especially avocado, Swiss chard, bamboo shoots, and baked potatoes; melon; legumes especially pinto, lima, soy beans
Pyridoxine	1.6–2 mg	25–50 mg	Beans, turnips, avocados, kale, apples, bananas, dehydrated prunes, raisins, watermelon, poultry, turkey giblets, mackerel, red snapper, trout
Riboflavin	1.3–1.7 mg	25–50 mg	Wild rice, unrefined whole grains, organ meats, seaweed, spirulina, nori, dark green, leafy vegetables
Selenium	50–200 mcg	100–200 mcg	Seafood, meats, eggs
Thiamin	1–1.5 mg	25–100 mg	Unrefined whole grains, beef kidney, pork, brewer's yeast, seaweed, spirulina, dried sunflower seeds
Vitamin A	800–1,000 IU	8,000 IU	Green and yellow vegetables, especially sweet potatoes, carrots, and spinach; liver and giblets, especially beef; fish liver oil; fruits, especially mango, papaya, cantaloupe, and apricot
Vitamin B-12	2 mcg	25–300 mcg	Meats, especially beef liver, heart and tongue, seafood, especially herring and mackerel, some cheeses, blue-green algae

Nutrient	RDA, 1989*	Optimum Intake†	Good Food Sources
Vitamin C	60 mg	1,000–3,000 mg	Vegetables, especially green; fruits, especially berries and citrus
Vitamin D	5–10 IU	400 IU	Fish liver oils, seafood, organ meats, eggs, vitamin D–fortified dairy products
Vitamin E	8–10 mg	400 IU	Cold-pressed vegetable oils; whole grains; hazelnuts; sunflower seeds; dark green leafy vegetables, especially kale and collards; legumes, especially kidney beans
Vitamin K	70–140 mcg	150–500 mcg	Green leafy vegetables, especially kale, turnip greens, spinach, broccoli, lettuce, cabbage
Zinc	12–15 mg	22 mg	Oysters, seafood, organ meats and flesh foods, whole grains, bran, wheat germ, fortified cereals, beans

If you have any major health problems or a special health need, consult your physician about proper nutrient dosage.

* RDA values are for nonpregnant, nonlactating adults. For nutrients without RDAs, the designated "safe and adequate" levels were used.
† Partially adapted from Werbach, Nutritional Influences on Illness, Third Line Press, 1989; Lieberman and Bruning, The Real Vitamin and Mineral Book: Going Beyond the RDAs, Avery, 1990; and Udo, Fats and Oils, Alive Books, 1991. Treatment level doses should be used under guidance of your health care professional.
Copyright by Susan E. Brown, The Nutrition Detective, 1995. Reprinted by permission.

How to Buy and Take Nutritional Supplements

There are several nutritional formulas especially designed for women going through menopause; some also include herbs that help relieve symptoms as well. When buying and using supplements, keep in mind the following:

- Try to divide the dosage throughout the day to increase effectiveness. For example, if you are taking 1,500 mg of vitamin C, take 500 mg three times a day.
- Take most supplements with meals; this also increases absorption and prevents indigestion or "tasting" the vitamins later.
- Give them time to work—three or four weeks are usually enough to judge if supplements are working; or if you are still menstruating, at least two cycles. It may take 3 to 6 months to halt and reverse symptoms of degeneration such as arthritis—and remember, many serious diseases such as cardiovascular disease and osteoporosis are "silent" so there are no tell-tale symptoms to monitor.
- Some experts believe that you should buy only "natural" vitamins because synthetic ones are less effective. Others feel you are paying extra money for nothing. Keep in mind that the accepted definition of a "natural" nutrient is one that has a chemical structure the same as that found in nature. We can synthesize such chemicals easily, yet they are labeled "natural" because it is believed the body can't tell the difference. However, some products are more biocompatible than others—that is, they are more easily absorbed and therefore better used by the body. For example, there is evidence that this is true of the naturally occurring form of vitamin E. Another possible exception is if you are buying supplements that are *really* natural—that is, concentrations of foods that are naturally high in certain nutrients. However, in most cases, high potencies are difficult to get in natural form. We simply advise you to avoid buying your supplements in pharmacies or typical grocery stores, and favor health food stores. They have a greater variety and you are more likely to get products that contain nutrients in their most potent form.
- Store supplements in a cool, dark, dry place—not the refrigerator, which is damp. Supplements have a limited shelf life, so toss them after the expiration date.

Other Nutritional Supplements
Garlic. As we said in Chapter 2, including garlic in your diet may have many beneficial effects. Garlic has been shown to protect the heart and nervous system, enhance the immune system, prevent and treat infection, and help lower the risk of cancer. Garlic also comes in

supplement form, which many people find more convenient because supplements are often odorless. Generally, 200 mg per day is the recommended level of supplementation.

Essential fatty acids. (These were also discussed in Chapter 2.) If you choose to add supplements to your intake of EFAs from food, we recommend a starting dose of 250 mg per day of EPA from fish oil, and 45 mg of GLA from evening primrose oil, borage oil, or black currant oil. A tablespoon of flax seed oil is an excellent source of all EFAs.

Gamma-oryzanol. A component of rice bran oil, this substance has been shown to be effective in a broad range of symptoms and disorders. These include menopausal symptoms including hot flashes, chills, heart palpitations, dizziness, insomnia, fatigue, and digestive problems such as nausea, diarrhea, and constipation. Symptoms take from 1 to 8 weeks to clear up. It has also been found to lower serum cholesterol. Treatment doses range from 20 to 300 mg per day. Because it is not reported to affect hormone levels, gamma-oryzanol appears to be a safe alternative for women who for medical reasons, such as breast cancer, do not want to take estrogen.

Glandular supplements. The use of animal glands as natural remedies began in ancient times. Animal organs were used in ancient Egypt, India, and China. According to the Greek poet Homer, Achilles ate the bone marrow of lions in order to increase his strength. Many indigenous peoples recognize the healing power of organs such as the liver, heart, kidneys, gizzard, giblets, sweetbreads, and tongue as a concentrated source of nutrients. Indeed, we now know that they contain generous amounts of iron, vitamin A, B vitamins, protein, phosphorous, potassium, zinc, and copper.

Glandular supplements used today are prepared from animal glands—usually from cows or pigs—and come packaged in a variety of ways. The glandulars most commonly used for menopausal concerns are those made from ovaries, pituitary, and adrenal glands. Glandulars are sometimes mixed with supportive vitamins, minerals, herbs, and other plant substances. Some practitioners report that extracts of ovarian tissue seem to help with menopausal symptoms perhaps by nourishing the ovary and enhancing its function. Drs. Brown and Maas have found that adrenal glandulars are particularly helpful during menopause (sometimes combined with Siberian ginseng), especially for women who are under stress or who have a tendency to low blood sugar.

Glandular products contain active hormone or hydrolyzed hormones which can be rebuilt by our bodies to make our own hormones. Glandulars are powerful and sometimes unpredictable. At the MEND Clinic, we have seen several people get anxiety reactions from adrenal extract. So we feel they should be used judiciously, and obtained from reputable organic suppliers.

Precautions

As a general rule, it's best not to take a supplement of just one nutrient. Nutrients typically work synergistically and frequently depend on one another to work best. For example, you need adequate amounts of calcium and magnesium plus other minerals and vitamin D to slow osteoporosis. In addition, taking large doses of one nutrient can create an imbalance in your body. If you take only vitamin B-12 for example, it competes with other B vitamins to be absorbed in your intestine, and an excess of B-12 could create a deficiency in the others. The B's usually work together.

Remember, nutritional supplements are just that—*supplements* to a healthful, balanced diet and active lifestyle, not *substitutes*. Taking supplements is not a license to slather margarine over everything, lie around eating junk food, or smoke cigarettes.

If you have a diagnosed disease or illness, are taking medication, or are otherwise under the care of a physician, consult a medical professional before taking supplements. Some supplements may interact with medication or cause problems. The dosages we recommend have been found to be safe in the vast majority of people; however, be alert for any possible side effects or unusual sensitivities.

Herbal Therapy

As you'll see in Chapter 5, "A-to-Z of Natural Remedies for Common Conditions of Menopause and Aging," many herbs can be useful at this time of your life. You may feel naturally attracted to or curious about herbs. In many traditional cultures, it is the women who know the medicinal uses of the plants in their region. As nurses and mothers, they learn from their elders and pass to the next generation the useful knowledge our present mainstream culture is now reclaiming.

Herbal lore isn't generally part of our culture, so before using any herb to treat a specific complaint, you need to learn the basics about herbal therapy. Although "herbs" technically refers to the above-ground parts of plants, we use the term to include all plant parts as well as mushroom remedies which might be more accurately referred to as "botanical substances."

Herbs have been called part of "nature's pharmacy." Although their action can be similar to modern drugs, herbal remedies are generally gentler and safer. Many of the drugs used in conventional medicine are derived from herbs—for example, digitalis is made from foxglove, and aspirin was originally made from the white willow. Some drugs are *synthetic*—they are synthesized from separate elements. Other drugs are *semisynthetic*—the original ingredients may come from plants, for example, but they are in some way altered so they can be patented. Such patented drugs undergo rigorous testing before they can be approved by the Food and Drug Administration, a process that costs millions of dollars. The pharmaceutical manufacturer must prove a drug is safe and effective according to established scientific criteria. The benefit of such costly, arduous testing is the hope of finding a "magic bullet" to fill a specific medical niche: a drug that targets a specific problem, fixes it, and then leaves the body without wreaking too much havoc.

Many people don't realize that although much of our knowledge of herbs comes from folk medicine, herbs have also been studied scientifically, and in many cases, we know the mechanisms of action. Some herbal agents were tested long ago and these fascinating studies exist in old medical texts. And more and more herbs are being tested by manufacturers and naturopathic doctors, especially in other countries.

A pilot study conducted in 1993 by naturopathic doctor Tori Hudson looked at the effects of several herbs on perimenopausal women. The herbs were *Glycyrrhiza glabra* root, *Arctium lappa* root, *Dioscoria villosa, Angelica sinensis,* and *Leonurus cardiaca.* The main symptoms were hot flashes, insomnia, mood changes, and vaginal dryness. After three months on the treatment, all the women in the test group reported a reduction in the severity of their menopausal symptoms, versus only 6% of the women receiving a placebo. And 71% of the test group reported fewer symptoms, versus 17% of the placebo group. In addition, cholesterol levels were decreased significantly in the test group. Dr. Hudson concluded that "selected botanicals appear to have a positive effect on some menopausal symptoms'' and that more research is needed on herbs, particularly regarding their effects on cholesterol ''due to the publicized effects of estrogen replacement therapy on cardiovascular health.''

How Do Herbs Work?

Herbs usually have dual or multiple positive effects. Therefore, herbs are usually prescribed differently than conventional medicines—rather than treat one isolated symptom, herbs are generally used more holistically to balance the whole person. There also seems to be something beyond what we can scientifically measure at this point in time, and which imbues healing power to herbs and many other natural remedies. We hope that someday we will be better able to understand this and be able to explain it to our patients and readers. In the meantime, some herbalists explain this power as the life force— the energy or vibration—of the plant itself, which increases and redirects the energy of the person taking the herb.

Also in contrast to conventional medicine, rather than isolating the ''active agent,'' herbalism uses the whole plant or whole parts of the plant such as leaves, flowers, or roots. Frequently, plants contain constituents which work together synergistically. Sometimes using the whole plant helps decrease the side effects that may occur when using isolated components.

Herbs function in several different ways, and some function in more than one way, to alleviate menopausal difficulties. Many of the herbs used for menopausal problems contain plant *hormones* (phytosterols). They are not exactly like human hormones, but rather natural forms of hormones that either function as weaker versions of human hormones, or that can be converted into hormones by your body. For example, black cohosh has been used in clinical practice for over thirty-five years, especially in Germany. It has been clearly documented that a component of black cohosh binds to estrogen receptors on our cells and acts like a weak estrogen. A randomized double-blind study proved that 4 mg of black cohosh per day was superior to that of the usual daily dose of prescription conjugated estrogens (0.625 mg) such as Premarin in relieving menopausal symptoms.

Herbs are frequently nourishing and can be considered to be food. For example, alfalfa is high in *minerals* (calcium, magnesium) and vitamins (A, B complex, C, D, E, and K) that support normal function. Some herbs and plants are known for their *antioxidant* properties. *Ginseng* is nearly in a class by itself, and is one of the most frequently recommended herbs for women during the menopause years. It is an all-round tonic and rejuvenator; known as an *adaptogen,* ginseng helps your body to adapt and normalize its functioning. Certain herbs are helpful in *strengthening the liver.* These are useful if you are taking hormones or any medication which is metabolized by the liver. In fact, many of the herbs that were thought to affect the body because of their plant estrogens actually appear to affect the body's own estrogen primarily by helping the liver metabolize it. These are just some of the many herbs and the ways that they work; you'll find many others listed for use in treating specific symptoms in the A-to-Z chapter.

How to Buy and Use Herbs

You can buy herbs and herbal formulas at health food stores, food co-ops, herb stores, and farmers' markets, as well as from health practitioners and mail-order companies. When buying loose dried plants, look for a bright color and a strong flavor and aroma. Avoid any that look or smell moldy, or rancid or are gray in color. These are then used to prepare teas, decoctions, infusions, tinctures, extracts, and pills and capsules. Freeze-dried or tincture forms from reputable companies are usually much more effective, and tincture forms have a very long shelf life. Other forms, even stored in a dark, dry place, should be replaced after one year (mark the expiration date on the container).

Herbal teas are brewed for a short time and are an easy and pleasant way to take herbs. To make tea, pour boiling water over the loose herbs, which may be in a tea basket or a teabag. Generally, about 1–2 teaspoons of herb per cup of water is recommended; or you may use 1 ounce of herb per pint of water. Let steep for 5–10 minutes and remove the herbs from the water before drinking (longer steeping results in a bitter brew). Teas are the least concentrated form and are useful mostly for mild symptoms and as substitutes for coffee or sodas. For medicinal purposes, you may make a stronger cup of tea by tripling or quadrupling the usual amount of herbs (three tea bags) and steeping for a full ten minutes; this is more equivalent to the more potent decoctions or infusions described next.

Begin cautiously and drink only half a cup the first time. If you experience no adverse reaction, you can gradually increase the amount you drink. Generally, a dose is 1 cup.

Decoctions are made by boiling the herb. Break up the hard, woody parts of plants—stems, roots, and bark—into small pieces so there is a greater surface area for the healing chemicals to be more readily released into the water. Add 1 ounce of the herb to 4 cups of water; boil for about 10 minutes until the water is reduced down to 3 cups. Next add the rest of the plant—leaves and flowers—and cover and steep for another 10 minutes. Strain the mixture and store in your refrigerator for up to 3 or 4 days. Generally, the dose is 1–3 cups per day. (Note: If you are using a combination of herbs to prepare a decoction, use 1 ounce of the total combined herbs, not 1 ounce of each single herb.)

Infusions are made by pouring boiling water over the dried flowers or leaves of the herb. Be sure to break them up or crush them first in a clean cloth. Use 1 ounce of herb and 3 cups of boiling water. Cover and let steep for 20–30 minutes. Strain and refrigerate for up to 3 or 4 days. The usual dose is 1 to 2 cups per day. (Note: If you are using a combination of herbs to prepare an infusion, use 1 ounce of the total combined herbs, not 1 ounce of each single herb.)

Tinctures are concentrated preparations of herbs which have been preserved in alcohol. Most people get their tinctures from an herbalist or herb company. It's possible to make your own tincture by combining 5 ounces of 100 proof vodka or Everclear ethyl alcohol and 1 ounce of the herb in a small sterile airtight glass bottle. Over the course of 2–6 weeks, the qualities of the herb are released into the alcohol. Alcohol-based tinctures last almost indefinitely if stored in a cool, dark place; some are made with cider vinegar or glycerine, which remains potent for about a year. You take tinctures by the drop—about 10–30 drops three times a day—or by the teaspoon— about 1 teaspoon per day. Taking the tincture as drops straight from the bottle dropper under your tongue will get them into your system the fastest, but the alcohol makes it unpleasant to take herbs this way. Most women prefer to add the tincture to a small amount of boiled water to make a beverage—the hot water will evaporate the alcohol.

Extracts are also highly concentrated preparations of herbs, but unlike tinctures, they are prepared with water. Commercially prepared extracts last several weeks under refrigeration because they have glycerine or alcohol added as preservatives.

Capsules, tablets, and powders contain dried herbs and are convenient for busy people. Some herbalists dislike capsules and pills because they feel the active constituents are not as readily available to your body in this form. There's no guarantee that your digestive system will release the healing agents to the same degree as the heat, water, and alcohol used in preparing the above forms. Doses vary widely—generally 2 capsules or tablets 2 or 3 times a day. Follow the directions on the bottle unless advised otherwise by an experienced doctor or herbalist.

Most herbs are best taken along with meals. Take one dose of the specified herbal preparation 2 or 3 times a day for chronic conditions and one dose every 2 or 3 hours for acute conditions. For chronic conditions, you usually need to take the herb faithfully for at least 2 or 3 weeks to obtain the desired effect, but this depends on the problem and the herb. If you don't notice any improvement, try another herb. Although there may be several possible herbs for you to choose from, try to find the one that most closely relates to all your complaints. If that doesn't work, then move on to the next.

Dosage: Unless directed otherwise—either by the labeling on an herbal product, your practitioner, or by this book under the listings for specific complaints—follow the generally recommended dosages suggested above.

Combination Formulas

Herbs may be used singly, but are often used in combination to produce a more effective result. You may purchase herbs singly and combine them yourself. The following herbal combination is recommended by herbalist Jason Elias for general menopausal symptoms:

1 part:	dandelion
2 parts:	vitex agnus-castus
1 part:	motherwort
1 part:	St. Johnswort

Make a decoction (*see* page 71) by boiling the dandelion root in 1½ pints of water for 10 minutes, and reduce it to 1 pint. Add the other herbs, cover, and steep for another 10 minutes. Strain. Use 1 ounce of the total combined herbs, and drink 1–2 cups a day of this combination for intermittent three-month periods, taking off at least two weeks in between.

Or you may prefer to buy a commercially prepared formula, in which herbs effective for menopausal symptoms are already combined. We have found the following commercially prepared formulas to be most effective and reliable for balancing hormones (*see* Appendix C, "Resources," for suppliers of these products):

- From Vitality Works Herbals: Fem Complex (dong quai, chaste tree, false unicorn, black cohosh, cramp bark, licorice, red raspberry, sarsaparilla, wild yam, ginger; Energy (American ginseng, Siberian ginseng, Chinese ginseng, ginkgo, gotu kola, fo-ti, licorice, and cayenne).
- From NF Formulas: Spectra Gyn-PMS (dong quai, wild yam, damiana, squaw vine, black cohosh, vitamin B-6, ovarian concentrate, and pituitary concentrate); Spectra 305-E and Spectra 305-P (wild yam, dong quai, damiana, squaw vine, black cohosh, vitamin B-6, and either pomegranate seed, which contains plant estrogen [in 305-E], or chaste tree, which contains progesterone [in 305-P]).
- From Phyto Pharmica: Remifemin, which contains a standardized amount of the most potent component of the herb *Cimicfuga racemosa;* and FemTone, which contains plant extracts of dong quai, chaste berry, licorice root, vitamin C and bioflavonoids.

Because menopause is a transition that takes years to complete, you may need to take herbs for a long time. Therefore, we usually recommend that menopausal women consult a professional trained in herbal medicine, such as a holistic medical doctor (M.D. or D.O.), acupuncturist, or naturopath, for ongoing monitoring and evaluation.

Herbs from the East

A 5,000-year-old system of medicine from India called Ayurveda also incorporates herbalism. Ayurveda, which means something like "the science of life" or "the science of living to a ripe old age," evolved from Hindu philosophy and religion. It is one of the oldest healing arts in the world. Much of Ayurveda focuses on balancing your body type with specific foods and living practices. They also use herbs, and Ayurvedic herbal formulas in tablet form are available from health professionals and through the mail (*see* Appendix C, "Resources"). One company makes four Ayurvedic formulas created specifically for women, including two for women at midlife that help nourish and balance the hormones. Others are formulated to act as antioxidants, to aid digestion, to relieve insomnia and nervousness, and to improve mental clarity.

Traditional Chinese medicine (discussed later in this chapter) also relies on herbs to help restore balance to women who are having menopausal and other difficulties. Chinese medicines have been used for thousands of years; they are inexpensive and remarkably effective. These usually are formulas that the practitioner specifically combines for each individual patient; the loose herbs and other natural substances are boiled to make a strong tea. There are also patent remedies that are available without a prescription in health food stores and in Chinese pharmacies. These are often imported: the quality varies and the contents may be unreliable; you may be getting active hormones (such as steroids) and other strong medicines in these inexpensive nonprescription products. They are safest and most effective when taken under the advice of a professional trained in traditional Chinese medicine.

Precautions

There have been reports of mislabeling of herbs, and quality and potency can vary depending on harvesting, handling, and storage. Therefore, be sure to buy herbs only from the most reputable sources you can find. Because they are made according to certain standards, many practitioners recommend tinctures, extracts and freeze-dried products as the safest and most effective forms of herbal remedies. The suppliers listed in Appendix C, "Resources," are recommended.

- Remember to use caution when self-prescribing herbs. In some people certain herbs may cause undesirable reactions. Begin with the lowest recommended dosage and increase gradually as needed. The most common symptoms of herb intolerance are nausea, vomiting, diarrhea, or allergic reactions; however, these are rare and extremely variable depending on both the herb and the individual. If you notice any questionable reaction, discontinue the herb(s) at once. If your reaction is severe, call your local Poison Control Center and go to the emergency room of the nearest hospital. *If you are under the care of a physician or have a particular medical condition, you should consult with your doctor before taking any herbal therapy.*

- Read the manufacturer's recommendations carefully, and make sure there is detailed information on appropriate dosages.
- If you are over sixty-five, stick to the lowest dosage recommended.
- Some herbs should be avoided or used under the guidance of a professional if you have a chronic illness or diagnosed medical problem; for example, women with hypoglycemia (low blood sugar) should know that goldenseal lowers blood sugar. And since many of the herbs used for menopausal discomforts contain estrogenic substances, you should not use them if your medical history indicates they may harm you. For example, some of those containing plant hormones can stimulate uterine bleeding or worsen endometriosis or fibroids. Some may also stimulate breast and uterine tissue, which is a concern for women who have a history of estrogen-sensitive cancers, or a high risk for them. The most commonly used herbs in this category are alfalfa flowers and leaves, red clover flowers and leaves, black cohosh root, hops flowers, licorice root, sage leaves, sweet briar hips or leaf buds, pomegranate seeds; chaste tree/vitex berries, sarsaparilla root, wild yam root, and yarrow flowers and leaves.
- Some of these have unclear mechanisms of action and some are both estrogenic and progesteronic. Although usually safe, it is best to combine herbs with prescription or over-the-counter medication only with professional guidance; some herbs may contain similar substances and could result in an overdose. If you have any questions or doubts, contact a knowledgeable herb specialist for advice.

Homeopathy

Homeopathy is often confused with herbal therapy, but it is founded on completely different principles. Homeopathic remedies use substances from plants, and also from the animal and mineral world. It is a 200-year-old system of medicine that is based on the principle that "like cures like." This principle grew out of the time-honored observation that substances that cause harmful symptoms in healthy people can, in much diluted doses, cure similar symptoms in sick people.

In the late 1700s a German physician named Samuel Hahnemann studied many substances in this manner and formalized this healing system, which he called homeopathy (from the Greek words *homeo* meaning "similar" and *pathos* meaning "disease").

Hahnemann also invented the process of potentization that is used to make homeopathic remedies safer and more effective. During this process, the original active substance is diluted, usually in a solution of distilled water or grain alcohol. The substance is diluted again and again—sometimes up to thousands of times. Most scientists are skeptical that something so diluted can have an effect. In many remedies not even a single molecule of the original substance remains! Still, homeopathy has been used for over 200 years and is growing in popularity in the United States. It is the fastest-growing medicine in the world. Several recent studies provide evidence that homeopathy is effective in treating a wide range of health problems. Homeopathy works very well in young children and animals as well as in skeptical adults—you don't have to believe in it for it to work, and you have little to lose since homeopathic remedies are very low in cost, and adverse effects are extremely unlikely in common potencies.

Homeopathy offers help and healing without the side effects of drugs or prescription hormones. Homeopathy can be curative—after treatment your symptoms may be gone for good. Many other forms of medicines, including herbs, are merely palliative—they just relieve the immediate symptoms temporarily and you need to repeat the medicine each time they return.

Judyth Reichenberg-Ullman, a naturopathic physician practicing in Seattle, Washington, says, "I have found homeopathy to be effective at least eighty percent of the time in relieving menopausal symptoms." Correctly prescribed individual therapies work best, but a 1989 survey of a German homeopathic product shows that even a combination remedy, which is not tailored to the individual, can help the majority of women. The product, called Mulimen (developed by a German company named Fides and manufactured in the United States by BHI), was rated by doctors to be "very good" for relieving menopausal symptoms in nearly 60 percent of the women taking part in the survey. Women experienced improvement in hot flashes, depressive moods, and nervousness/irritability. The product is also successful in relieving premenstrual symptoms.

How Homeopathy Works

Even homeopaths don't all agree on how homeopathy works. The prevalent theory is that when the remedy is prepared or potentized, the shaking "imprints" a memory of the remedy's energy pattern on the molecules of water or alcohol. This retains the active substance's pure essence while preventing any harmful effects which the active molecules themselves may cause. For example, arsenic is normally a poison, but is harmless when it is diluted homeopathically. Homeopathy, therefore, somehow communicates its healing message on an energy level rather than a material level.

According to homeopathy, symptoms are not the enemy, and they are not the disorder itself. Rather, they are signs that your body is trying to deal with an underlying disorder or imbalance and therefore should not be suppressed. According to the principle of like curing like, taking a remedy that matches the symptoms of your illness stimulates and strengthens your body's innate healing power. Eventually your body no longer needs the symptoms and they fade away naturally. Dr. Maas was initially skeptical of homeopathy until she saw many examples of its effectiveness. Since then, she chooses homeopathy as her most potent avenue of treatment in many cases.

Choosing a Homeopathic Remedy

Homeopathy recognizes that your symptoms are not just physical—they can also exist on an emotional and mental plane, and that all three planes are interrelated. Homeopathic remedies are therefore prescribed according to your unique overall *pattern* of symptoms and general individual characteristics. There's no one universal remedy for hot flashes, for example, because women differ from one another and so do their hot flashes. You may have hot flashes that affect your whole body and night sweats accompanied by depression and loss of energy. Another woman may have hot flashes primarily affecting the top half of her body combined with irritability and nervousness. They would require different homeopathic remedies to be treated most effectively.

Homeopathic remedies come in several forms: in small tablets or pellets that contain a tiny amount of sugar, liquids that contain tiny amounts of alcohol; and gels and liquid tinctures to apply locally, for example, to soothe joint and muscle aches and pains or lubricate a dry vagina. They also come in different potencies; for self-care, lower potencies in the range of 6C to 12C* are usually recommended. Professional homeopaths usually prescribe higher potencies of 30C and more to treat deep-seated underlying conditions, long-term or strong symptoms, or severe emergencies. You can buy single or combination remedies. Single remedies are more personalized and more potent than combination remedies, but are trickier to prescribe correctly.

Single Remedies. There are about 200 to 300 commonly used single remedies, each with their own symptom pattern. To be most effective, you need to choose a remedy carefully to get the best match. As explained earlier, one remedy might help your friend's hot flashes but have absolutely no effect on yours.

The A-to-Z listings in Chapter 5 include brief descriptions of symptom patterns for the most commonly used remedies for each complaint. Please bear in mind that these are only approximations of the full symptom patterns, and if one remedy isn't effective, try another. If none of our suggestions work, don't give up on homeopathy. Prescribing the right single remedy is a challenge—there are entire guidebooks books written for the general audience (*see* Appendix D) and we encourage you to study one or more if you'd like to get the most out of this healing system. And remember, if you are taking medication or are otherwise under the care of a physician for a specific disease or illness, you should consult with your medical professional before taking any homeopathic remedy.

Combination Remedies. An alternative is to try one of the combination remedies available, which are more user-friendly. You'll find combination products for menopause in general as well as for specific conditions such as insomnia or nervousness or fatigue. Combination products contain two or more of the single remedies that are most often used to treat that symptom or condition. Therefore, this "shotgun" approach increases the chance that a product will contain the remedy you need, but at a low potency. Because it is difficult to assess all the new companies who are introducing homeopathic remedies, we recommend you choose products made by established companies with a good track record—these include Boericke and Tafel, Boiron, Stan-

---

* The number preceding "C" indicates how many hundred times a remedy has been diluted. The most dilute remedies are the most potent—the exact opposite of what one might expect.

dard Homeopathic, and Medicine from Nature, which is new but founded by Dana Ullman, a well-respected homeopath and educator. We also like the two combination products made by BHI called Feminine and Mulimen and the Menopausal Relief Formula from Natra-Bio; and those from Heel Pharmaceuticals called Hormeel, Klimaktheel, Nervoheel, and Ovarium Compositum.

As is the case with single remedies, if you don't get relief from a particular combination, don't give up on homeopathy. You may need to try another brand or two until you find the proper "fit." And if you still fail to see benefits, don't give up on homeopathy altogether—the combinations may not contain the particular remedy you require. You may need to consult a homeopathic physician for help in finding the right remedy.

How to Take Homeopathic Remedies

Follow the dosage directions on the product label—generally 2–3 pills or 5–10 drops equal one dose. After taking a homeopathic remedy, you may notice some changes right away, or it may take time for symptoms to gradually improve.

Homeopathy comes with its own set of rules to follow. Some—such as caveats against touching the remedy, or drinking coffee—may seem illogical to the average person. And admittedly, there are differences of opinion in the profession as to how strictly you need to adhere to the rules. However, the consensus is that to be safe and give homeopathy the best chance of working, it's best to follow these guidelines:

1. The frequency of the dosage depends on the intensity of the symptoms: severe symptoms that come on suddenly such as hot flashes may require one dose every 5 minutes; a slowly developing headache may need the remedy every 3–4 hours. As the symptoms improve or disappear, increase the interval between doses or stop the medication. Start again if the same symptoms return. However, if there has been no response after six doses, stop the remedy and switch to another. You increase the potency by taking the same small dose more frequently—taking more pellets or drops per dose won't increase the potency.

2. Avoid touching the remedy with your hands, especially if you are giving the remedy to another person. Rather, tip the required number of pellets into the container cap and then into your

mouth; if tablets are blister-packed, pop them directly into your mouth. Touching the remedy could contaminate or inactivate it.

3. Avoid eating or drinking anything but chlorine-free water for 15 minutes to a half hour before and after taking the remedy. And allow the remedy to dissolve slowly under your tongue so it is absorbed directly through your mucosa. Some combination tablets instruct you to chew them instead.

4. Store homeopathic remedies in the original container, away from heat, sunlight, and strong-smelling substances that might contaminate them; the list includes perfumes, camphor and eucalyptus (found in many cosmetics and other items that inhabit the medicine chest such as Tiger Balm, Vick's products, and lip balms), and moth balls; some also advise against drinking strong herbal teas or ingesting mint-containing products including toothpaste.

5. Avoid drinking coffee around the time of treatment—preferably at least within 24 hours. Coffee may counteract the remedy's effect by acting as an antidote, or by otherwise slowing the healing process.

Seeing a Professional Homeopath

Most homeopathy in the United States is self-administered; according to the National Center for Homeopathy, there are only about 2,500 homeopaths in this country and about 1,000 of them are conventional doctors who have ''converted.'' Licensing and certification standards vary from state to state; your best bet is to find a health practitioner— medical doctor, nurse practitioner, etc.—who is licensed to practice in your state and ask where the practitioner studied homeopathy and how long he or she has been practicing it. It takes diligence, experience, and good intuition to succeed regularly as a homeopath.

Your first visit may last over an hour and the homeopath will ask a barrage of questions, some of which may seem unusual compared with the symptom-and-causality-related questions of a typical medical interview. The homeopath not only will ask questions about your physical symptoms, but will want to know details about your emotional and mental symptoms as well as idiosyncracies such as food and weather preferences, quality of sleep, your moods, and dreams.

You may need only a single dose of the right remedy to restore balance and normalize menopause. Or you may respond more slowly—over several months or more—and require a series of remedies, or vary the potency, dosage, or frequency of the remedy to complete the healing process.

Acupressure and Traditional Chinese Medicine (TCM)

Traditional Chinese medicine (TCM) consists primarily of acupuncture, acupressure and massage, and herbal therapy (see the earlier discussion on herbal remedies in this chapter). Still mysterious to most Westerners, this system of medicine has been used in the Eastern part of the world for over five thousand years.

TCM is based on the notion that an energy force called Chi or Qi (and pronounced "chee") flows through your body. You also have two life forces called Yin and Yang, and your Chi moves constantly between them. When your Yin and Yang are balanced, you are healthy. When they are out of balance, your Chi energy is disturbed, which leads to ill health.

The flow of Chi may be disturbed in a number of ways, primarily poor nutrition, lack of exercise, pollution, insufficient rest and sleep, inability to manage stress, pressure, and negative emotions. If your Chi is insufficient or weak, it may lead to fatigue, depression, or bloating. If your Chi is imbalanced (too much in part of the body, not enough in another), this can lead to any number of problems including hypertension, headache, painful menstruation and difficult menopause.

TCM is concerned with restoring the balance of Yin and Yang and the flow of Chi. Acupuncturists often successfully treat a wide variety of conditions, including menopause-related symptoms, painful menstruation, premenstrual syndrome, headaches, high blood pressure, depression, stress, and insomnia. The World Health Organization reported that acupuncture is able to successfully treat over forty diseases. It is widely used in China and other Far Eastern countries as anesthesia during surgery and childbirth. In the West, it is used very successfully in clinics to help people give up smoking, alcohol, and drugs.

In the right hands, TCM can be an effective alternative to conventional medical treatment. Anne Marie, a grade school teacher, had been troubled by a heavy, painful menstrual flow ever since age twelve when her periods began. In her late forties, her periods became irregular, prolonging her premenstrual syndrome symptoms. She had had breast cancer, so hormone replacement therapy was out, and all her doctor could offer was a strong diuretic. "Feeling bloated, crampy, and cranky for two weeks premenstrually was one thing," she says, "but being premenstrual for three months was too much!" A nurse practitioner with a similar problem had gotten good results from acupuncture and recommended that Anne Marie give traditional Chinese medicine a try. A few days after her first acupuncture treatment, Anne Marie's period started to flow, bringing instant relief from her prolonged PMS. Weekly acupuncture treatments were required until her health was fully restored. She occasionally needed to take Chinese herbs as well, which she says tasted like "a prune juice-and-beer cocktail." She now has acupuncture once a month to maintain her newfound equilibrium.

How Traditional Chinese Medicine Works

Practitioners of traditional Chinese medicine explain that its effectiveness derives from the balancing of energy flow ("Chi"), which may be too weak, too strong, or blocked. The Chi flows through your body in a series of pathways called *meridians.* Each meridian runs the entire length of your body and passes through a major organ, which gives the meridian its name. (These meridian organs do not always correspond to the physical organs of conventional anatomy.)

Your energy flow is accessible at certain key points on your body, and can be manipulated by inserting small sterile needles at the points (acupuncture) or by pressing on them (acupressure). Acupuncture points can be anywhere on the meridian and are rarely located on the part of your body that needs treatment—that's why a hormone imbalance may be corrected by placing needles in your foot!

Your Chi may also be influenced by certain herbs and other natural substances such as various types of eggs, insect parts, minerals, hormones, and organ parts.

The Chinese medicine system is highly developed and is difficult for most Westerners to understand. What are we to make of a Chinese herbal formula that says it addresses menopausal imbalances of Liver Blood, Kidney Yin and Yang, Heart Blood, and Spleen Deficiency with Floating Yang in the Upper Body and Fluid Dryness in the Lower, plus complications of Liver Qi Stagnation? One theory that some conventional physicians do accept is that stimulating the acupuncture points releases brain chemicals called endorphins, which are our own natural painkillers. However, there is far more to Chinese medicine and it deserves more respect than this common explanation. Acupuncture requires professional care. However, you may want to try acupressure on yourself, or ask a friend to help you, provided you follow the directions and precautions provided below.

Seeing a professional trained in traditional Chinese medicine. If you see an acupuncturist or traditional Chinese doctor, your visit may or may not include the kind of physical exam you are accustomed to. Rather, the diagnosis may be based more on his or her closely observing your skin and tongue, listening to your breathing and quality of voice, and taking several pulses which relate to organs and functions of your body. He or she may also interview you at length about your physical and emotional symptoms and how they relate to events in your life such as stresses and time of day. All these tools offer clues to the state of your Chi. However, some of the best Chinese doctors can't speak or understand English. Although they may insert needles without much preliminary discussion, in Dr. Maas's experience, the therapy still works! She also has observed that American acupuncturists are usually gentler, but their acupuncture can be equally effective.

Acupuncturists insert sterile, hair-thin needles on specific points of your meridians. Acupuncture may or may not be comfortable, depending on the point and its need for treatment and/or its proximity to a superficial nerve. You may feel pressure, numbness, a slight pinch, or a tingling "zingy" sensation when the needle reaches the Chi. Sometimes it is outright painful—but only momentarily—if the needle grazes a nerve or sore point. Sessions last a half hour to an hour. They are usually relaxing and often people doze off and awake refreshed.

You will usually need to make several visits, since this form of therapy acts gradually for most chronic problems and is adjusted according to the progress you are making. Several sessions are usually required to achieve noticeable, lasting results. Some women find they need to have acupuncture or other treatment on an ongoing basis, usually once a month, to keep their health in balance, and their symptoms under control. (*Note:* To avoid blood-borne diseases, make sure your acupuncturist uses presterilized disposable needles in sealed packages or sterilizes the needles in an autoclave [sterilizing machine]).

Acupressure. This involves applying pressure to the acupuncture points using primarily the fingers and hands, rather than inserting needles. There are sixteen different methods of manipulating the points, including pushing, twisting, patting, rolling, pressing, and rubbing. You may have acupressure done professionally, or you may safely try a simplified form of it on yourself or another person. Specific acupressure points are shown in the A-to-Z listings of individual complaints. When points occur on both sides of the body, press both points, simultaneously if possible.

When applying acupressure, use the tip of your index or middle finger or thumb to apply the basic technique of pressure and rotation. Press to a point that is beyond pleasure but short of pain. Press for as long as indicated, while rotating your finger two or three cycles per second. Try to relax as you work and exhale slowly as you release the pressure. (*Note:* Do not do acupressure before or after eating a heavy meal, while bathing in hot water, or within four hours after taking any drug or medication including alcohol.)

Aromatherapy

Aromatherapy takes advantage of our sense of smell to help heal us on physical, emotional, mental, and spiritual levels. The Egyptians and other ancient peoples used fragrant oils, herbs, flowers, and other natural substances to treat and comfort one another. Today, modern aromatherapy is helping women with insomnia, anxiety, panic attacks, back pain, migraines, food cravings, lack of sexual desire, fatigue, and other discomforts of menopause. Aromatherapy is often used simultaneously with massage therapy, chiropractic, or acupuncture.

How Does Aromatherapy Work?

Aromatherapy uses essential oils, which some regard as plant *pheromones* (hormones or other substances released by a living thing that gets a response from another). They are more than perfumes—they affect the most ancient part of our brain in the limbic system. This is where our basic life processes—breathing, heart rate, temperature, and blood sugar levels—are regulated. It is also the seat of emotions related to survival such as sexual desire and the "fight or flight" response. This is why smells can so powerfully affect your moods and well-being, and have subtle physiological effects as well.

How to Buy and Use Essential Oils

While there are professionals who offer aromatherapy, including massage therapists who use scented oils during a massage, anyone can experiment with essential oils. They are sold in tiny bottles in health food stores, aroma shops, and food co-ops as well as through the mail. Some companies make combinations blended to relieve specific symptoms, such as headache.

You need only a drop or two at a time, depending on the concentration of the oil—sometimes they are ''cut'' with a carrier oil. Well-sealed, fragrant oils have a long shelf life. Make sure you buy only pure and natural oils (not synthetic) made specifically for healing purposes.

There are many ways you can use essential oils, singly or in combination:

- You can dilute them with a less aromatic carrier oil such as jojoba, almond, or avocado. Use about 4–10 drops of scent per ounce of carrier oil and rub the dilution on your skin.
- You can put them in your bath water, or in a foot bath. Use 6–8 drops of oil per bathtub of water. Add the oil while the water is running into the tub, and soak for about twenty minutes. Be careful, since the oil is slippery.
- You can add an essential oil to a steam vaporizer, and let the heat diffuse the aroma throughout the room.
- Simplest of all is to sniff them right from the bottle, or from a cotton ball.
- You can make a compress, which is often used to relieve pain and swelling. To make a compress, fill a basin with water as hot as you can stand to touch. Add 4–5 drops of essential oil. Dip a folded towel or cloth into the basin so the cloth picks up the oil. Squeeze out the excess water and apply the compress to the painful area. This is especially good for backaches. Make cold compresses the same way, using water as cold as you can stand (add ice cubes if need be); cold compresses are useful for sciatica and headaches.

As you experiment with aromatherapy, remember that smells effect people differently and this is influenced by any associations you may have with a particular scent. Dr. Maas uses a combination of rose oil to open the heart, sandlewood to center the spirit, tangerine to enliven the mind, and ylang-ylang to calm and clarify. *Note:* Some people are allergic to certain essential oils. Take a sniff and test each one on a small spot on the back of your hand before purchasing or using on more delicate skin surfaces. Some oils may cause adverse effects in women with certain conditions such as epilepsy or high blood pressure, so check with a knowledgeable professional if you have any of these problems. Essential oils are sometimes used internally, but since some can be harmful, we advise that you avoid internal use unless you are under a knowledgeable professional's care.

The Touching Therapies

Touching is one of the oldest and simplest natural therapies; in our minds, it is also frequently the most effective of all. We are all healers in the making. Dr. Maas often teaches her patients a hands-on technique to use on their family members and themselves. There's increasing evidence that we respond to human touch throughout our lives. Many human and animal studies have demonstrated our basic need for touch for mental, physical, and emotional growth. Touch therapies, from Swedish massage to Chi Gong in China to therapeutic touch, have helped relieve symptoms of pain and stress as well as measurable benefits in blood pressure, heart rate, and muscle tension. In one experiment, animals that were touched early in life grew old more gracefully, lost fewer brain cells, and retained more of their memory in later years. Experiments at McGill University suggest that touch produces less long-term brain damage from stress hormones.

Another experiment involved a group of patients with chronic muscle tension, body aches, and pain who failed to find relief with conventional drugs. They were treated with ten sessions of massage. Most reported a marked reduction in their symptoms, and researchers found massage slowed their heart rate, lowered their muscle tension, and decreased their stress response.

Massage

Massage works on the soft tissues of the body—muscles and ligaments—to soothe taut, tired muscles, stimulate sluggish circulation, and enhance the function of the nervous system. It helps minimize headaches, ease insomnia, and lower blood pressure. Depending on the technique used, massage can make you feel more alert and energetic or calmer and more relaxed. It can help you recover from injury and illness and leave you with an overall sense of well-being. Many recipients of massage say the sheer pleasure they feel after a good massage is itself therapeutic.

There are many types of massage, and each practitioner has his or her own style. Swedish massage is the form most commonly used in Western countries. It consists of rhythmic stroking, lifting, rolling, pressing, and kneading movements. The movements may be light and soothing or deep and firm. Swedish massage is usually performed on a nude subject and uses massage oils so the practitioner's hands glide smoothly. Shiatsu massage was developed in Japan and combines massage with acupressure (*see* "Acupressure and Traditional Chinese Medicine," page 81). It can be done through your clothing and does not require oils. There are many other forms of body work, including Polarity Massage, Jin Shin, Trager, Therapeutic Touch, Rolfing, and more.

To get the most from a massage, let yourself settle into the working surface. Breathe deeply and slowly, inhaling and exhaling in sync with the massage strokes. Try to surrender completely and let your limbs and head be moved and lifted passively, rather than trying to "help" the giver. Let her or him know what feels good—and what feels uncomfortable, but avoid talking unnecessarily. Take the opportunity to concentrate on your body's experience rather than submit to the urge to chat. If memories or feelings arise, this may be a safe place to talk about your personal issues. Many a massage is conducted in the midst of sighs, groans, moans, revelations, tears, yawns, and snores.

To find a good professional massage practitioner, ask for a reference from a health professional, friend, or relative. Sometimes massage schools will provide massages by their students for free or at reduced rates. It's usually risky to respond to advertisements for massage services, but if you have no other resource, be sure to ask for references and to see the practitioner's certificate or license. Because of the intimate nature of this form of therapy, it is very difficult to relax if you have any doubts about the practitioner's credentials or motives.

Another possibility is to trade massage with a friend or intimate.

There are many good massage books and videos available to get you started. As one woman said, "Massage is one of the nicest things you can do for a person." Another remarked, "I would have strangled my cat if it weren't for my monthly massages." There are also a variety of at-home massage aids such as back rollers, foot rollers, and rubber balls sold through catalogs and at health food stores. If the wooden rolling-pin-type devices used along the spine are too hard for comfort, Dr. Maas recommends rolling your back over an inflatable or Styrofoam boat bumper or tennis balls.

Spinal Manipulation

Osteopathy comes from the Greek words *osteo* (meaning "bone") and *pathy* (meaning "disease"). This system of healing was founded by Dr. Andrew Taylor Still in the 1870s. Osteopaths (D.O.s) are fully trained medical doctors and are licensed in all fifty states. The difference between D.O.s and M.D.s is that D.O.s have additional training in the structure and correct biomechanism of the musculoskeletal structure—bones, joints, ligaments, tendons, muscles, and connective tissue. They study how these structures relate to organ system functions and how to affect health through manipulation of the physical body. The majority of osteopaths practice primary family medicine, although there are many who specialize in other fields. Osteopaths who practice manipulation focus on the function of the body and use many different techniques to improve the flow of blood and lymph, improve nerve balance and muscle tone, increase the range and fluidity of motion, and unblock subtle body energy pulsations.

Osteopaths work on the premise that all our parts are interrelated, and they treat the whole body as a unit. Since they are trained in conventional medicine and diagnosis, they can diagnose and treat all aspects of health, including those related to menopause and aging. Research has shown that musculoskeletal abnormalities can affect the lungs, heart, stomach, intestines, bladder, and uterus. Osteopathic manipulation can help treat many conditions including headache, menstrual pains, heart disease, and digestive problems.

Chiropractic, like osteopathy, is a form of manipulative therapy. Developed in the late 1800s by David Palmer, the term derives from the Greek words *chiro* (meaning "hand") and *practic* (meaning "action"). As is the case with osteopathy, chiropractic involves manipulating the musculoskeletal system structures of the body to restore freedom and balance; some chiropractors provide nutritional guidance as well. However, they are not trained as conventional physicians. Licensing requirements and the services they are permitted to provide vary from state to state.

Mind-Body Therapies

These therapies are all based on the well-accepted observation that the thoughts in your mind have an enormous effect on your body. There's even a tongue-twisting name for a new field of scientific investigation of the mind-body connection: psychoneuroimmunology, or PNI. PNI studies the interaction between the mind, nervous system, immune system, and endocrine system and acknowledges the unity of our complex interacting parts.

Early mind-body studies showed that people were more likely to become ill after suffering severe emotional trauma; recent studies have been able to actually measure the dip in immune defenses. In one study, the immune cells of students dropped significantly during exam week, presumably because of the extra stress. In another, rats were taught to shut down their own immune systems by conditioning alone. And perhaps most startling of all, a Stanford University Medical Center psychiatrist who set out to disprove the mind-body link provided strong evidence that it does exist. In the study, women with advanced breast cancer attended support groups in which they shared feelings and information and learned simple relaxation techniques. When compared with women who did not attend the groups, the supported women were less depressed, felt less pain, had a more positive out-look—and lived twice as long. Two of the women were still alive and disease-free 10 years later, but none of the unsupported women survived. Many scientists suspect that the mind-body connection is involved in the documented spontaneous remissions from cancer and many other diseases that are miraculous and appear otherwise inexplicable.

How Do Mind-Body Therapies Work?

We don't know yet exactly how the mind and body influence each other, but the chemistry of emotions is part of the picture. According to Deepak Chopra, attitude is the single most important influence on longevity. He writes in his book *Ageless Body, Timeless Mind* that for every thought and emotion, there is a corresponding physical molecule. For example, when you feel fear, it is accompanied by molecules of the hormone adrenaline, causing the stress response described in Chapter 2. We feed ourselves food three times a day—and look how much that affects our well-being. We "feed" ourselves thoughts all day long, so it's no surprise that this also affects us physically, sometimes obviously and sometimes with a great deal of subtlety. Has the idea of food ever made your mouth water? Does the very thought of Sean Connery make your heart beat faster? These are but two simple examples of the mind-body at work.

Mental messages affect all systems and organs including your endocrine system, immune system, circulatory system, and digestive system. Twenty-four hours a day, complex chemical "conversations" are taking place between your nervous system and many parts of your body. Another possible explanation for mind-body effects derives from the new physics, which tells us that mind and matter are different forms of energy. Recent thinking sees thought and body as two manifestations of the self at any given time. If you are interested in exploring this incredible phenomenon further, you may wish to read *Ageless Body, Timeless Mind,* in which Deepak Chopra discusses how some people may be able to transform conscious energy (thoughts) into matter. Deep relaxation exercises have profound effects on your mental, emotional, and physical health. Dr. Maas knows meditation to be her single most powerful discipline in healing of herself and of others. She has found no disorder—physical, mental, emotional—that is not eased by meditation. Even as a nutritionist, Dr. Brown regularly teaches meditation to maximize clients' health potential. Spiritual awakening, regardless of religious persuasion, grows from an open, relaxed sensibility. The relaxation tools that follow are simple and anyone, no matter how stressed out, can learn them. They are designed to be at least pleasant, and are often extremely enjoyable. They may even be blissful, especially if you are unconstrained by time and let your mind settle into focus, and if you give yourself time to practice.

There are many books and tapes devoted to all kinds of relaxation and meditation techniques (*see* Appendix C), and excellent teachers in nonsectarian disciplines such as Mindfulness, Transcendental Meditation, and Chi Gong. It is common in the Far East for a student of meditation to study many forms and systems. We encourage you to experiment—although the study of a meditation system does not necessarily involve adoption of a religion, there is quite a bit of ritual, faith, and aesthetic variation among the forms. You can get a good feeling as to whether a particular form is right for you by glancing at the literature, talking to the people involved, or visiting a meeting or ceremony.

Relaxation Therapies

It is never too late to decrease your stress and the deleterious effects we described in Chapter 2. The skills you develop now can reverse hormone imbalances and improve menopausal symptoms, as well as positively affect your immune system, your cardiovascular system, and other body processes to make you less susceptible to degenerative diseases.

We all can have the skills and make the time to relax as a normal part of our daily lives. Yes: you corporate wizards and high-rollers— part of the maturing process is to learn to balance work, play, and self-care. Do your hobbies, exercise, and sleep routines counteract your stress? Women frequently tell Dr. Maas that they are so caught up in their responsibilities they just don't know *how* to let go. Many of the other natural therapies mentioned in this chapter help you cope with stress. However, the natural therapies that follow are designed particularly to help you easily and effectively reduce your stress and bring you the benefits of increased peace of mind and greater ability to concentrate, relate to others, and balance emotions. These therapies can open you up to further personal growth as well as decrease the symptoms of menopause.

Deep Breathing

This simple technique helps reduce anxiety, depression, nervous-ness, muscle tension, and fatigue. In one study it helped women re-duce their hot flashes by 50 percent. It may be included as a component of total body muscle relaxation, meditation, and yoga. Loose-fitting, comfortable clothes and dark, quiet surroundings help, but are not required. You can try this anywhere, any time you need to "take five."

1. To begin, sit or lie down in a comfortable position. Rest one hand over your abdomen and one on your upper chest. Take a few slow breaths and notice where your breath goes—does your chest rise and fall but not your abdomen? Or does your abdomen move alone? Which rises or falls first?
2. Next, breathe in slowly through your nose, attempting to fill your abdomen first, by lowering your diaphragm. This may take several tries for some women—imagine your abdomen is a balloon.
3. Once your abdomen is filled, keep inhaling and fill your chest, allowing it to rise.
4. Exhale slowly through your mouth, first emptying your chest and then your abdomen.
5. Repeat the inhalation and exhalation, trying to slow the breath even more. This should feel like a wave of air, rhythmically entering and leaving your body.

Only breathing in should require any effort—allow the air to flow out on its own as you let the weight of your chest and abdomen relax down.

Total Body Muscle Relaxation

This is another basic technique that builds on the above breathing exercise. It is based on alternately tensing and relaxing your muscles. It effectively slows your breathing and heart rate, leaving you rested and refreshed. Give yourself a half hour to begin, and as you become adept, you may reduce the time to twenty or fifteen minutes. Begin in a warm, quiet room; disconnect the telephone if possible.

1. Lying down, close your eyes and take a few deep breaths. Begin the deep breathing exercise described above and try to maintain it throughout the relaxation.
2. Focus your attention on your right foot and point your toes very hard. Hold for one slow breath and then let it go completely limp. Work up your right leg by flexing and relaxing your foot, tensing and relaxing your calf, and then tensing your thigh by pulling up your kneecap and then letting it go, enjoying the contrast between the two sensations. Then do your left foot and leg.
3. Now squeeze and relax your buttocks, waist, back, chest, right hand and arm, left hand and arm, shoulders, neck, and scalp.

Include your face, opening your mouth and eyes wide, then scrunching them tight before completely relaxing those muscles.
4. Finally, stretch your arms and legs to their longest length, and elongate every muscle in between. Let go one more time.
5. Return your attention to your breathing and your surroundings, opening your eyes.

Meditation

Meditation has traditionally been integral to religions from Roman Catholicism to Jewish mysticism to Tibetan Buddhism. It is as varied as these religions and cultures are themselves, and has many goals, techniques, and effects. Meditation was popularized in the United States in the 1960s and 1970s by the Maharishi Mahesh Yogi as Transcendental Meditation (TM). This form of meditation and others, some of which we describe below, are tools to help you develop a restful alertness. In TM the mind is focused on a mantra, or repeated phrase, and the typical mental chatter ceases, at first for moments, and then for minutes at a time with practice. During those moments, you experience the state of pure being, of oneness with the universe. Very interesting, you say—but what does this have to do with health?

In fact, hundreds of meditators have been studied and their physiological processes have been measured. At the very least, meditation has been shown to be deeply relaxing and rejuvenating. It lowers respiration, oxygen consumption, and metabolic rate. It reduces the blood levels of stress hormones, which are associated with poor health and aging. Some long-term meditators have been found to be 5–12 years younger biologically than they are chronologically, as indicated by their blood pressure, visual acuity, and hearing. New research shows that meditators have up to nearly 50 percent higher levels of a hormone called DHEA. Low levels of DHEA are considered to be a marker for exposure to chronic stress and a mirror for aging. High levels of DHEA are associated with reduced incidence of heart disease, breast cancer, and osteoporosis.

There are many schools of meditation, but what they all have in common is the effort to focus the attention inward by concentrating on (meditating upon) rhythmic breathing, an object, a word, or a thought, or a mantra such as the word *Om.* Or you focus outward on something such as a candle, a picture, God, or a space four feet in front of your nose. Meditation is a different experience for each person and each

session is different as well. The following exercise will help you get a
glimpse of what meditation feels like. If you want to know more or
explore this practice more deeply, there are many books and schools
available.

1. Sit in a comfortable position which you can hold for as many as
   10–15 minutes, in a quiet place where you won't be disturbed by
   the phone or other people.
2. Close your eyes; you may prepare yourself by doing the deep
   abdominal breathing described on page 92. If you are very tense,
   work toward total body muscle relaxation.
3. Choose a word or phrase to focus your mind on, such as the
   ancient Sanskrit mantra *Ham Sah,* meaning "I am that"; or repeat "5-4-3-2-1" to yourself, or "I am love, I am joy, I am
   one." Let your eyes roll upward and inward a bit so you focus on
   the spot on your forehead between your eyes, tongue resting behind your upper teeth, and all muscles as relaxed as possible.
   Smile inwardly to very subtly raise the corners of your mouth. As
   you repeat the focus word(s) silently, thoughts will enter your
   head. When you catch yourself on a random thought chase, be
   grateful to your "observer self" for its observance, and then let
   the seductiveness of your mental chatter recede. It is normal—no
   matter how many years of practice—for the mind to be caught
   chasing its own tail. Smile inwardly and let them drift by as you
   breathe deeply and rhythmically.
4. You can time your words or phrases with your breath, inhaling
   through your nose and keeping the inhale broad, deep, and easy
   and the exhale silent and effortless.
5. You can easily lose track of time in deep relaxation, so you may
   need to set a timer or stopwatch if you don't have unlimited time.
6. After the 10 or 15 minutes are up, remain seated for a minute or
   two with your eyes closed, and then open them.

As simple as it sounds, some people find sitting still "doing nothing" is a very difficult assignment. So if you're the kind of person
that usually buzzes around, doing twelve things at once, don't be
surprised if you can't sit quietly and or if your minds wanders madly.
Let that amuse you and congratulate yourself every time you see
yourself worrying, planning, rehearsing, or just plain old day-

dreaming. Keep with it, and don't be too harsh on yourself if you feel you aren't "doing it." *Everyone* feels unguided—there are no chartered waters for your own internal space.

According to mind-body expert Joan Boryshenko, the meditation session itself is the goal; even if you think you're not doing it "right," the relaxation response is still most likely to be occurring. She says that even beginners soon notice that they feel more peaceful and feel relief from their symptoms. And the more they practice, the more adept they get and the better they feel. Aim to meditate once a day; twice if possible. The best times are the first thing upon arising, when your mind is the most uncluttered and "suggestible." It's also nice to meditate again at the end of your workday, after exercising and before a meal.

Visualization or Guided Imagery

Visualization is a way of translating positive thoughts into mental images in order to achieve a specific result. It involves using your imagination—your "mind's eye"—to create internal visual images. Long used by competitive athletes to visualize their victory and give them a winning edge, this technique is now being used by medical patients to visualize health and wellness. For example, cancer patients mentally travel inside their bodies and picture the cells of their immune systems attacking cancer cells and the tumor gradually shrinking. It has also been used by many women to lose weight, stop smoking, and help heal a variety of gynecological problems.

How can a figment of your imagination possibly be linked to a concrete physical change—outside of scary science fiction movies? Visualization has always had its skeptics, but now science offers a plausible explanation. We know that there's a direct neurological link from the brain to the thymus gland, and that mental imaging can increase the secretion of the gland. There's also a neurological bridge between the front part of the brain to the limbic system, which is known as the seat of the emotions. From there, the nerves proceed to the hypothalamus gland—the gland that regulates other glands and the immune system, and affects sleeping, eating, temperature, and sexual function. The hypothalamus in turn influences the pituitary gland, whose hormones affect your ovaries, adrenals, thyroid, and parathyroid. So we all have an extensive network potentially connecting our brain and emotions to every organ and cell in our bodies.

If you'd like to try visualization to reduce symptoms of menopause, first put yourself in a state of deep relaxation using one of the techniques described above. Then, depending on your symptom, create an image that embodies the state you want to be in. We provide ideas for images in several of the conditions in the A-to-Z listings for common conditions. You might want to start with the image ideas we provide, but bear in mind that certain images may work for most women, but not all images will work for all women. Allow your own creativity to add details and engage as many of your senses as possible—sight, hearing, smell, taste, and touch. It's okay to change the image; feel free to experiment until you find images that feel right for you.

For chronic conditions, such as certain aches and pains, you need to practice visualization regularly, a few minutes each day, two or three times a week. For sudden, acute symptoms, practice visualization whenever they occur. Sometimes you may be able to visualize an image with crystal clarity; other times you may just have an overall "sense" of an image. Visualization is often used along with positive suggestions, or "affirmations," such as "I am becoming more relaxed and comfortable."

Visualization is not easy for most people, at least at first. Some people never get the hang of it, but for others, practice and persistence pay off. A professional imagery counselor certainly helps, and so can drawing on paper the images you are trying to imagine.

Yoga

Yoga derives from the Hindu religion and can be a spiritual practice that incorporates meditation and other mental exercises. There are many schools of yoga, but *hatha yoga,* which emphasizes physical postures called *asanas* and integrates them with breathing techniques, is the form most commonly practiced in Western countries, where it is available in health clubs, dance centers, and community centers.

Inactivity alone is responsible for much of the physical and mental deterioration we equate with aging and "feeling old." Practicing hatha yoga regularly not only builds strength, flexibility, balance, and grace, but helps you reach a state of awareness, tranquility, and well-being. During the menopause years, you'll especially appreciate the benefits of yoga because they include balancing and energizing the entire reproductive system and endocrine system. Yoga also restores health to your digestive tract, nervous system, and circulatory system.

The calmness achieved during the practice carries over into the rest of your life. Yoga students and teachers tend to look and act younger than their chronological years, and new students of the practice say they feel more energetic after only a few weeks' time. Although it can be strenuous, yoga is highly adaptable to your abilities and is suitable for people of all ages. You can learn yoga from books and videotapes, but it's best to participate in yoga classes (or get individual instruction), especially if you're new to the practice.

Precautions

These mind-body techniques are very safe, but some people experience the bubbling up of bottled emotion such as anger, sadness, or extreme happiness. Let the feeling wash through you. Does it help to move your arms? Shiver? If you moan or cry, let the waves come through an open chest and throat. Breathe into the center of your experience with your heart full of acceptance and your mind full of wonder. Maintain a childlike lack of judgment. As long as you breathe deeply, keep your heart loving, and feel you are in a safe place, the emotions should not be overpowering. If unpleasant or even traumatic old memories come to you, repeat "That was then, this is now" or "I'm safe now." Bear in mind that it's usually easier to feel the strong emotions of fear, anger, shame, or guilt in the presence of a strong, nonjudgmental, loving person who respects that part of you until you can be nonjudgmental and loving yourself. Another precaution involves the possibility that exaggerated claims of simply thinking positive thoughts will delay or prevent people from seeking medical treatment; these techniques complement but do not take the place of appropriate medical care, and we need actions as well to make real our intentions.

CHAPTER 4

Replacing Your Dwindling Hormones

Most women don't realize it, but today they have a choice among many types of hormone replacement. Often their doctors aren't aware of all the options, either. The question is not only whether you have hormone replacement therapy (HRT) but also what type, how much, and for how long?

Hormones may be prescription or nonprescription; synthetic or natural; estrogen alone, progesterone alone, or a combination. Other hormones such as testosterone or DHEA may be added to the mix. Hormones may be derived from horse urine or plants, and be taken by mouth (as pills, oil, herbs, or food), by injection, as suppositories, intranasally, or applied as creams or adhesive patches.

Touted as a miracle cure and fountain of youth in the recent past, today HRT is recommended primarily as a *preventive* measure to stave off osteoporosis, reduce risk of heart disease, and as a *treatment* to minimize hot flashes, vaginal atrophy, and a handful of other menopause-related problems.

HRT is clearly not for everyone. Statistics vary, but it is estimated that only 15–20 percent of all postmenopausal women in the United States are on prescription hormone replacement therapy. In Europe, it's even less: only 3–4 percent of all postmenopausal women are estimated to use HRT. This may indicate that most women are not bothered enough by menopause to take hormones. Or it may also be because HRT isn't always effective and it has many possible side effects, some of which are potentially serious. According to a 1994 report, 30 percent of the women who receive a prescription for post-menopausal HRT never fill it; 20 percent stop taking it within nine months after starting, and 10 percent use it only intermittently.

Clearly, hormone replacement therapy can improve the quality of life for some women after menopause; some argue that it may even extend their lives. We feel it is best used as part of an integrated, holistic approach. Hormones are no substitute for good, healthy living; they only add to it. If you take hormones of any sort, we recommend that you also follow our Balanced Life Plan (Chapter 2) of good nutrition, exercise, and stress management. In addition, natural therapies (Chapter 3) can also help reduce the dosage and duration of hormone therapy, and hence the side effects.

If you are undergoing hormone replacement therapy and are experiencing adverse effects, or are concerned about cancer risks, bring this book with you to your doctor and discuss the pros and cons of using other prescription or nonprescription hormones, as well as nonhormone natural alternatives to HRT.

In this chapter we describe the more popular hormone therapies prescribed by physicians: estrogen (such as Premarin) and progestins (such as Provera), which have been the most thoroughly studied. Then we'll also take a look at some of the other hormones and preparations now coming into use, such as natural progesterone, testosterone, and DHEA. Finally, we provide you with the most current information about estrogenlike substances found in beans, fruits, vegetables, and other plants which may be able to partially replace other forms of hormone therapy—and allow some women to avoid hormone therapy completely.

Forms of HRT

Prescription estrogen and progestin therapy is most often available in three forms. The dosage and scheduling vary depending on many factors, and may be adjusted until the woman and her doctor find the right program for her. Most women take hormone therapy *orally,* in the form of pills. Estrogen is also available as a *transdermal skin patch,* which delivers estrogen through the skin (transdermally). This method allows the estrogen to be released at a relatively constant rate and to bypass the liver—and so have less interaction on liver-mediated problems, such as gallbladder disease, and blood clots, as well as tax our busy livers less. Estrogen is also available as a *vaginal cream,* which is most useful for women whose primary concern is vaginal dryness and uncomfortable intercourse. Applied directly to the vagina, the cream restores tone and lubrication; it can also tone the urethra and bladder and prevent or treat incontinence and infections. There is some systemic absorption of the cream from the vagina, so it may increase the risk of breast cancer (*see* Chapter 6). Estrogens are also available in gels, and sublingual and injectable pellets. *Natural progesterone* is available in several forms: a cream that is rubbed into the skin, pills, an oil taken by mouth, suppositories, and subcutaneous (under the skin) implants.

Estrogen Therapy

Estrogens were first introduced as drugs in 1933, DES (diethylstilbestrol) being one of the first estrogen drugs. Subsequently a combination estrogen-progestin birth control pill was developed and by the mid-1960s the first wave of postmenopausal estrogen replacement use was gaining momentum. In 1966, gynecologist Robert Wilson passionately declared that the pharmaceutical industry now offered "Womankind a precious gift . . . the elimination of menopause, women's physical, mental, and final emancipation." Put that way, who wouldn't jump at the chance? And jump is what women did—by the 1970s estrogen became one of the top five prescription drugs. Women taking estrogen found that they had fewer hot flashes and no vaginal atrophy; their moods were better, their breasts firmer, and they had more energy.

However, studies soon showed that taking estrogen for longer than one year increased the risk of endometrial cancer. Estrogen's popularity plummeted when the Food and Drug Administration issued a warning that the dose should be one-quarter of the amount used at that time, but admitted that this still might not be protective enough to negate the increased risk of cancer. Estrogen has many other side effects, as listed on page 108. For a complete account of this fascinating period we recommend you read the book *Women and the Crisis in Sex Hormones* (*see* the bibliography in Appendix D).

Estrogen Plus Progestin/Progesterone Therapy

Today, physicians generally prescribe some form of progesterone along with estrogen in women who still have a uterus. Synthetic progesterone is called *progestin* and is the typical prescription hormone commonly referred to as "progesterone," such as Provera; but semi-synthetic and natural progesterone are also available and are being used with increasing frequency.

Progestins are added to estrogen therapy most frequently to avoid higher risk of uterine cancer. Estrogen stimulates the growth of endometrial cells, and when cells grow at a faster rate, the chance goes up that they will mutate into cancer cells. So giving estrogen alone— that is, "unopposed" by progesterone—builds up the endometrial layers without allowing the tissue to slough off every month. These thick growing layers are more likely to turn cancerous in some women if they remain unshed due to lack of a progesterone effect.

Studies showed that high doses of estrogen increase the chance of endometrial cancer by as much as thirteen-fold, depending on the length of therapy. So, in order to reduce the risk of cancer, two things happened: The pharmaceutical industry lowered the amount of estrogen and most doctors prescribe estrogen in combination with progestin. Studies prove that both natural progesterone and synthetic progestins protect against uterine cancer in most cases.

Many doctors prescribe estrogen and progestins to be taken *cyclically,* to mimic the body's own rhythm. Women on this program continue to menstruate—or begin again—as the progesterone triggers the shedding of the endometrial lining. The cyclic form of HRT is the type most often given in the United States today. The alternative is *continuous* therapy—daily estrogen with small amounts of progestins. This form has recently become popular because it doesn't bring on regular periods; some women still experience breakthrough bleeding, but this disappears with balancing of the hormone levels. However, we have no studies to show us the long-term effects of continuous progestins.

While adding progestin to estrogen therapy seemed to help solve one problem, physicians were initially worried about the side effects and that giving progestins would lower the benefits of estrogen therapy, particularly its ability to lower cholesterol. As we'll discuss later in this chapter, subsequent studies seem to indicate that the commonly prescribed synthetic progestins don't necessarily negate the cardiovascular benefits of estrogen. Interestingly, the less commonly prescribed natural or semisynthetic progesterone is the best in this regard—and may have fewer side effects and have beneficial effects beyond preventing endometrial cancer.

It was hoped that progesterone would also protect against breast cancer. Progestins, which are most often prescribed, have not shown to be protective. In fact, 1995 data from the Nurses' Health Study involving over 120,000 women revealed that breast cancer risk was significantly increased among women who were currently using estrogen alone (32% increase), or estrogen plus progestins (41% increase) as compared with postmenopausal women who had never used hormones. It's still too soon to tell whether natural progesterone offers some protection against any breast cancer stimulated by estrogen therapy.

Synthetic Progestins

Synthetic forms of progesterone (progestins) contained in conventional prescription HRT products such as Provera have many side effects (*see* page 109). Synthetic progestins mimic the action of progesterone, but they are not exactly the same. Since they don't match your body's chemistry, your body doesn't respond in the same way as it does to natural progesterone and the synthetics may actually aggravate your symptoms. Synthetic progestins may prevent you from ovulating and suppress your body's production of its own hormone, progesterone.

"Natural" Progesterone

We feel that synthetic progestin is the least desirable form, and for women who take estrogen and have a uterus, we recommend the natural form of progesterone instead. Unlike synthetic progestins, natural progesterone matches your own progesterone exactly; it appears to be gentler on the system and may actually be more beneficial than synthetic progestin. Some women are taking natural progesterone alone, without estrogen, because it may have benefits beyond endometrial cancer prevention; as explained later, natural progesterone may be a safer alternative for women who cannot (or will not) take estrogen.

Progesterone products are usually made from plant precursor molecules found in soybeans or the wild Mexican yam. As such, even though the progesterone molecules match the progesterone molecules made in your body, some are more properly called "semisynthetic." A well-known British physician and book author, Katherine Dalton, M.D., has been using natural progesterone suppositories to treat PMS for decades. Obstetricians often use progesterone suppositories to prevent threatened miscarriage. An American physician, Joel Hargrove of Vanderbilt University, has been using oral capsules of micronized progesterone (without estrogen) and has published a small study (of fifteen women) that showed improvement in menopausal symptoms with minimal side effects. Micronized progesterone is widely used in Europe, and is becoming more popular in the United States. It will probably become more often prescribed because a 1995 study (called the "PEPI" study) found that micronized natural progesterone had better cardio-risk-lowering effects on fats in the blood than the synthetic progestins. Pharmaceutical-grade progesterone can be made into micronized pills, creams, suppositories, pellets, injectables, and gels. (*See* Appendix C for suppliers of this and other nonsynthetic hormones.)

Most American women take natural progesterone transdermally, in the form of an over-the-counter cream, or orally, in the form of an oil. Progesterone creams are applied to areas of the body where your skin is soft and thin: breasts, abdomen, inner arms or thighs, wrist, nape of the neck, or face. The most energetic promoter of the cream, John R. Lee, M.D., says that as the cream is rubbed into the body, the progesterone is absorbed through the skin and is stored in your fat cells, from which it is gradually released and sent through the blood circulation to progesterone receptor sites on your cells.

The usual dosage of one popular brand called Progest cream is $\frac{1}{4}$–$\frac{1}{2}$ teaspoon morning and evening, alternating the sites to which it is applied. However, the dosage for creams varies according to the reason for taking it, the severity of symptoms—and the particular cream you use. Progesterone products that contain the semisynthetic hormone are much more potent—up to thirty times—than those containing progesterone precursors from plants. To put this in perspective, synthetic progestins are about ten to one hundred times as potent as the progesterone made by your body! Some of the precursors in these products have estrogenic qualities as well. The stronger natural progesterone preparations, such as micronized progesterone pills, tend to be available only by prescription. The exact amounts of the hormones in some brands of natural progesterone are considered to be proprietary. However, a recent FDA regulation requires that companies put the word "progesterone" on the label if the compound includes the active hormone, so you can check to see if a product is more or less potent. Some manufacturers claim that the wild yam, or other botanical source, is converted to progesterone by normal intestinal bacteria. Others find this test-tube conversion an unlikely event in our guts, and attribute the hormonal effect of these botanicals to other than direct hormonal reactions, as described in the section on herbs. To sum up, products with the weakest progesterone effect (if any at all) are those containing plant precursors; semisynthetic progesterone is stronger; and synthetic progestins are stronger still. Aeron Biotechnology, Inc./ LifeCycles has evaluated a number of commercial cream products for their hormone content, and will send you a copy of the results (*see* Appendix C).

Natural Progesterone's Other Benefits?

Natural progesterone may have benefits beyond that of blocking estrogen's possible cancer-stimulating ability. In the words of Dr. Lee, it is useful for any woman who has symptoms of too much unopposed estrogen, "whether occurring endogenously [that is, produced by the body] before menopause or as a consequence of estrogen supplementation." Symptoms of too much estrogen include water retention, depression, breast swelling, PMS, loss of libido, heavy or irregular menstrual periods, craving for sweets, and weight gain especially around the hips and thighs. Restoring the proper estrogen-progesterone balance helps relieve these symptoms.

Natural progesterone might well help balance the effects of estrogen therapy and be beneficial for all women on estrogen, but this is unproven. There is scientific evidence that progesterone is needed for bone to remain thick and healthy and that it may be at least as important as estrogen in preventing and treating osteoporosis. Dr. Lee has reported that in his small study of 100 women, the natural progesterone cream he prescribes for his patients increased bone density in postmenopausal women and thus not only prevents osteoporosis but can *reverse* it as well. Dr. Lee uses progesterone along with nutritional therapy (diet and supplements) and exercise. It may be that the nutrient supplements and the exercise were also critical for improving bone density. He sometimes prescribes estrogen as well, but he found progesterone built bone with or without added estrogen, and it may therefore be preferable for women who cannot (or choose not to) take estrogen. It may also allow you to lower the dosage of estrogen. Restoring progesterone levels also usually causes hot flushes to subside, according to Dr. Lee. He believes natural progesterone also protects against breast and endometrial cancer and he also says that, according to his experience, natural progesterone helps reverse fibrocystic breasts, ovarian cysts, uterine fibroid tumors, and cervical dysplasia. While there are no studies documenting the safety of progesterone creams (aside from Dr. Lee's small study), there are few reports of significant side effects or health problems with natural progesterone. Both progestins and progesterone can have androgenic (masculinizing) side effects, causing pimples in women and even male-pattern hair growth. Some women experience spotting when using natural progesterone, but this is usually temporary; natural progesterone may also potentially increase thyroid activity. Some women experience lightheadedness or drowsiness, others have reported bloating, and some just don't feel well using it. The creams have also been found to accumulate to the point where women have high blood levels from the typical doses prescribed—twenty to thirty times the premenopausal level! Do have your levels checked after you have found a comfortable dose. You should work with a trusted and knowledgeable physician if you use natural progesterone, especially if you have any unusual or bothersome symptoms.

What Are the Benefits of HRT?
The effects vary from woman to woman and often depend on the dosage as well.

Menopausal symptoms. Studies have shown that estrogen alone usually reduces or eliminates hot flashes, night sweats, and vaginal dryness and atrophy. It appears that estrogen, alone and with progestins or progesterone, reduces hot flashes by about 85 percent. Clinically, Dr. Maas and others have found that estrogen reduces urinary incontinence, and it has also been shown to do so in meta-analysis of subjective symptoms. There is no proof that HRT reduces nervousness. However, researchers at McGill University in Montreal found that estrogen therapy improves learning ability and verbal memory; it may also enhance mood. Some researchers claim it can counter depression.

Some women say they feel more cheerful, relaxed, and self-confident while on HRT. Dr. Maas finds that most of her patients feel better on a balanced regimen of estrogen and progesterone, possibly along with testosterone and DHEA, depending on their individual needs.

Keep in mind that in various studies, placebos were often as effective as estrogen replacement in reducing many menopausal symptoms, the only exception being hot flashes. Some women report feeling worse on HRT: it makes them feel anxious or depressed, and if progestin is included, they notice PMS-like symptoms of irritability, mood changes, and anxiety. The natural progesterones do not cause these side effects—the only usual problem is a slight "wooziness" or sedation, which is corrected by lowering the dose.

Osteoporosis prevention: In most, but not all cases, estrogen does decrease the rate of bone breakdown, even though it does not rebuild lost bone. It may therefore slow the development of osteoporosis if taken over the long haul. Studies show that life-long estrogen therapy begun shortly after menopause can reduce the risk of hip fracture by 30 to 40 percent. As calculated by the American College of Physicians, this means that some 2 to 3 percent of all postmenopausal women will avoid a hip fracture by taking estrogen therapy. A somewhat higher percentage of women would avoid spinal fractures using estrogen. As we shall see, however, the problems with long-term estrogen are many and there exist several more life-supporting ways to halt, prevent, and even reverse osteoporosis. In addition, not all women are at risk for osteoporosis and even if they do develop this condition, many women never break a bone because of it.

What is clear, however, is that when one goes off estrogen, rapid bone loss begins again. A 1990 study by Boston University researchers found that only women who had taken estrogen for seven or more years after menopause enjoyed higher bone density up to age 75. In women 75 and older, there was no significant remaining beneficial effect of estrogen on bone density. Remember that with exercise, good nutrition, and supplements, you may still gain bone mass, whether you take estrogen for the rest of your life or for a few years.

Cardiovascular disease prevention: Some, but not all researchers, suggest that current estrogen use is associated with a 35 to 45 percent reduction in risk of heart disease and a 28 percent reduction in the death rate from coronary disease. However, there are questions as to whether women who decide to take estrogen are healthier to begin with, and whether the results would hold true for estrogen with progestins added. The long-awaited results of a 1995 study provided some answers regarding the latter question. The study, called the Postmenopausal Estrogen and Progestin Interventions Trial (PEPI) showed that a combination of the two hormones (estrogen and either progestins or natural progesterone) can help prevent any increased risk of uterine cancer without totally negating estrogen's beneficial effect on HDL cholesterol (the good cholesterol) and fibrinogin (another heart disease factor). Still, we don't know whether the hormones' beneficial effects on cardiac risk factors will ultimately translate into less cardiovascular disease or longer life. This study also showed that a natural micronized (finely ground) form of progesterone preserved the bulk of estrogen's favorable effects, causing fewer side effects than synthetic progestins.

We would also like to point out that natural approaches have been found to be as effective—if not more effective—as ERT in reducing risk of heart disease. For example, the same researcher who in a large retrospective study found ERT to reduce heart disease by 50 percent also found that taking 200 IU of vitamin E supplements for at least 2 years had the same effect. In another large study, frequent nut intake reduced heart attack by 50 percent, as did flavonoids found in certain foods in another study. And eating four or more servings of carrots per week lowered the risk of stroke in women by 68 percent. (For a comprehensive critique of the PEPI study and a thorough listing of ways to promote heart health, see *Estrogen Therapy for Osteoporosis and Heart Health: Is It Worth It?* by Dr. Brown.

Aging prevention: What few scientific studies exist offer us conflicting results, so the jury is still out on whether estrogen helps keep you feeling and looking young. However, a 1994 study from the University of California discovered that women who took estrogen actually had thinner skin than women who took no estrogen. The younger-looking skin produced by estrogen may be nothing more than plumpness produced by water retention—estrogen does not enhance the skin's elasticity. Many women report skin improvements with the use of progesterone also; however, following the Balanced Life Plan in Chapter 2 and taking in essential fatty acids (see Chapter 3) are even more effective. Since there is no convincing proof that estrogen delays aging of the skin, the Food and Drug Administration requires that the patient information material that accompanies estrogen replacement therapy say this. However, long-term studies may yet reveal that hormone therapy is the closest thing to a chemical fountain of youth. That's because estrogen is involved in the formation of collagen. One study, published in 1984, found that women treated with estrogen maintained premenopausal amounts of collagen in their skin. There is some very preliminary evidence that estrogen may have antioxidant and antiinflammatory effects and protect against arthritis. There's tantalizing—but inconclusive—new evidence that it may help prevent Alzheimer's disease.

Side Effects of HRT

Many women are fearful of taking hormones because of the risk of side effects—either in the short term or in the long term. For most women, short-term side effects of estrogen are slight and diminish in a few months; in some cases they may be individual reactions to horse estrogens (Premarin). Long-term effects such as increased risk of breast cancer or uterine cancer may remain hidden for years. A 1995 study suggests another long-term risk: a doubling of the risk for the autoimmune disease lupus erythematosus among postmenopausal women. The following represent what we know about the forms of estrogen and progestins that have been the most studied. The most commonly used forms of estrogen are Premarin and Estrace ("conjugated estrogens"), estradiol, and estrone; we do not yet know much about estriol. Estriol may be the safest form of estrogen, with some studies suggesting a possible anticancer effect. We'll be more confident with prescribing estriol when further studies become available. Adding progestins (Provera, etc.) to estrogen therapy seems to lower one risk of estrogen therapy: endometrial cancer. However, synthetic progestins add a whole slew of additional potential side effects, as detailed below. Natural progesterone seems to have far fewer side effects.

POSSIBLE SIDE EFFECTS OF ESTROGENS
• Increased risk of endometrial cancer
• Increased risk of breast cancer
• Increased risk of lupus erythematosus
• Increased risk of fatal ovarian cancer
• Weight gain

- Increased risk of gallbladder disease
- Fluid retention and bloating
- Breakthrough bleeding, spotting
- Changes in pattern of menstrual bleeding
- Increased susceptibility to vaginal yeast infections
- Increased vaginal secretions
- Breast tenderness and enlargement and fibrocystic breast disease
- Nausea, vomiting, abdominal cramping
- Changes in the cornea, intolerance of contact lenses
- Increased sensitivity to sunlight
- Headaches, migraine
- Dizziness
- Changes in libido
- Increased blood pressure
- Decreased sugar tolerance
- Interaction with other drugs such as anticoagulants, corticosteroids, alcohol, tobacco
- Skin rash
- Anxiety
- Sensitivity to synthetics and additives

POSSIBLE SIDE EFFECTS OF PROGESTINS (SYNTHETIC PROGESTERONE)
- Bloating
- Emotional upset
- Anxiety
- Depression
- General "PMS" symptoms
- Dizziness
- Headache
- Fatigue
- Allergic rash
- Liver toxicity, jaundice
- Thrombophlebitis (blood clot in leg)
- Pulmonary embolism (blood clot in lung)
- Stroke
- Interaction with other drugs such as steroids, antidepressants, antibiotics
- Decreased absorption of nutrients, including vitamin B-6

POSSIBLE SIDE EFFECTS OF NATURAL PROGESTERONE
* Lightheadedness or dizziness
* Sedation
* Breast tenderness
* Increased sensitivity of eyes
* Androgenic effects such as pimples

Testosterone

Some doctors have begun prescribing testosterone in addition to estrogen in women who complain they have lost their sex drive either because of natural menopause or hysterectomy. Testosterone is produced by the ovaries, and continues to be produced after menopause, but as with other sex hormones, the output dwindles with age. Testosterone is often considered to be a male hormone, but is important in women too because it increases their sex drive, stimulates a healthy appetite, strengthens muscles, and improves well-being. Testosterone therapy has been found to be helpful, but the risks of long-term use are still unknown, and there is little information on doses, absorption, and blood levels for this therapy. Side effects such as facial hair, enlarged clitoris, and voice changes may not be reversible when you stop taking the drug.

DHEA (Dehydroepiandrosterone)

DHEA is the single most prevalent hormone in our bloodstream. It is produced by our adrenals and ovaries in decreasing amounts as we age and has gained a reputation as a ''youth hormone.'' Deficiency is common in people under a lot of stress; studies have shown it may protect against cancer, especially breast cancer, as well as osteoporosis and heart disease; it may also benefit people with diabetes and those who are overweight because of its effect on enzymes that break down fat. DHEA is converted to testosterone or other hormones in the body.

Should You or Shouldn't You Take HRT?

There is no definite yes or no answer; it depends on your particular symptoms and risks, philosophy, and lifestyle. Most physicians believe that women who have had a hysterectomy should take replacement hormones to restore what the scalpel prematurely took away.

And based on the latest study results, which suggest that HRT lowers certain risk factors for cardiovascular disease, many physicians strongly advise women with coronary heart disease or who are at high risk for heart disease to take HRT also. However, as the authors of a 1992 review article of all the literature written in English on the effects of HRT conclude, ''For other women, the best course of action is unclear.''

As you consider, remember that hormones affect all cells in our bodies, and they have a complicated interaction with all body processes—involving nerves, immune system, metabolism, digestion and absorption of nutrients, and regeneration. At the MEND Clinic, we prescribe a variety of hormones, and each time it is with full respect of the power of these potent chemicals and the individuality of the woman.

Some women feel that any replacement of hormones is unnatural, and want only to use herbs, homeopathy, and lifestyle approaches. Others come to us having exhausted some of their reserves with work and home pressures, dietary indiscretions, or difficult medical problems. Many of these women need the help of a balanced hormonal regimen tailored specifically to them, according to blood, urine, or saliva tests, and clinical response. Unfortunately, hormone testing is in the primitive stages, and the accuracy depends on the timing of day and month, and blood tests still may not accurately tell us how much of a hormone is actually being used by your tissues.

Some physicians believe all women should be on hormones for the rest of their lives. Yes, they say, there may be an increased risk of breast cancer or endometrial cancer—but since cardiovascular disease and osteoporosis statistically represent far greater health risks than these two cancers, they feel the relative benefits are greater than are the risks. For example, they point out that 50 percent of all women die of cardiovascular disease while only about 10 percent die of breast cancer.

Whether to take HRT is *your* decision. Whatever you decide, we urge you strongly to do whatever feels right and natural for you and, if you can, find the support among your medical team to do what you want to do.

Who Shouldn't Take Hormone Replacement Therapy?

The reasons not to take hormone replacement therapy continue to be debated. Until recently, it was universally agreed that any woman who has had breast cancer should definitely stay away from estrogen because many studies show estrogen may cause or worsen risks for breast cancer. Roughly 50 percent of all breast cancers are sensitive to and stimulated by estrogen. But estrogen is only one factor in breast cancer—or else why would the risk jump in postmenopausal women? Now a growing number of physicians are offering HRT to breast cancer patients who they feel have been cured. Whether or not this is wise will take years to prove. In addition, women with gallbladder disease, liver disease, some types of hypertension, and clotting problems may be able to use transdermal estrogen cream or patch, or vaginal or sublingual or injected pellets with more safety than oral estrogen because the hormone bypasses the digestive system initially.

DEFINITE REASONS NOT TO TAKE ERT
- Current breast cancer
- Current endometrial cancer
- Active liver disease
- Active thrombophlebitis or thromboembolism
- Abnormal and/or unexplained vaginal bleeding
- Pregnancy
- Previous adverse reaction to hormone therapy

POSSIBLE REASONS NOT TO TAKE ERT
- History of breast cancer or at high risk for breast cancer
- History of endometrial cancer
- History of liver disease
- Large uterine fibroids
- Endometriosis
- History of thrombophlebitis or thromboembolism
- History of stroke or ischemic attack
- Recent heart attack
- Pancreatic disease
- Gallbladder disease

• Fibrocystic breast disease
• Hypertension aggravated by estrogen
• Migraine headache aggravated by estrogen

Individualized Treatment

As we have seen, not all hormone replacement therapy is alike. A survey of 283 gynecologists in Los Angeles revealed 84 different regimens—and this only included estrogen and progestins! The best therapy is one that is tailored to your specific needs. You may need to do a bit of experimenting with different forms and different doses to find the right regimen for you. Compounding pharmacies now can tailor hormone replacement in almost infinite ways so that each woman is getting just what she needs and no more.

When making your decision, discuss with your physician your risks of serious diseases, your health concerns, your symptoms, and your lifestyle and personal philosophy. Do the benefits outweigh the risks in your case? Most important to consider is whether you are at high risk for heart disease, osteoporosis, or breast cancer. Second, consider the symptoms of menopause—hot flashes are so easily managed by nonhormonal methods that, if this is your only consideration, HRT is overkill. However, if you're eating well and exercising enough and you still have symptoms such as hot flashes and vaginal dryness, this indicates a hormone imbalance; you may consider using prescription or nonprescription hormones for a few years to get you through the worst.

It's important for you to realize that while you take estrogen, your body will again adjust to premenopausal levels of the hormone. If you stop, you will likely experience menopausal symptoms again. Ask yourself: Will I want to relive menopause at age seventy-five? Alternatively, you could wean yourself off slowly and replace prescription estrogen with the natural estrogen-enhancing factors described above. Some experts recommend that women consider taking HRT for only the 3–5 years after menopause, during which the most bone loss occurs, especially if they are at high risk for osteoporosis; however, there are no studies that show this prevents broken bones in later years. On the contrary, rapid bone loss occurs after ERT is stopped (similar to the first menopause) and recent studies show that long-term estrogen therapy is necessary to reduce fracture risk—and that life-long therapy is necessary to reduce risk of hip fractures. (*See* Chapter 6 for self-assessments for cardiovascular disease, osteoporosis, and breast cancer.)

The type of estrogen is another factor to consider. The three types of active human estrogens, estradiol, estrone, and estriol, can be prescribed alone or in combination. Estriol, although little-studied to date, may be as effective and safer than standard ERT; however, it is less potent and must be given in higher doses than the other two estrogens. Some investigators have found that unopposed estriol (that is, without progesterone) does not cause endometrial hyperplasia (increase in the number of cells), but this has not been Dr. Maas's experience. She believes that estriol, as with other forms of estrogen, should be given along with progesterone in postmenopausal women with or without a uterus. The balancing effect of progesterone with estrogen likely affects other tissues besides the uterus. Because of the experience we have with estradiol and estrone, Dr. Maas often prescribes an estrogen formula developed by Jonathan Wright, M.D., a well-regarded expert in nutritional medicine. It consists of all three naturally occurring forms of estrogen: estradiol, estrone, and estriol. This "tri-estrogen" preparation includes these hormones in what he calculated to be the same proportion as they are found in premenopausal women and appears to minimize the risks of estrogen and maximize their benefits. It may be used along with natural progesterone and other hormones.

Dr. Maas and many other natural health advocates offer many alternative hormone combinations including the naturally occurring estrogens and progesterone, tailored to the needs and comfort of the individual woman. Natural hormones, as opposed to the semisynthetic or synthetic which are foreign to the body, have fewer side effects than the standard HRT offered. Christiane Northrup, M.D., a holistic physician, says that women with a lot of body fat continue to be exposed to plenty of endogenous estrogen and not enough progesterone—and these women may reach hormonal balance by taking natural progesterone only, or improving their eating patterns.

As Dr. Northrup writes in her book, *Women's Bodies, Women's Wisdom:* "The current 'medicalization' of menopause has been so successful that most women's own menopausal wisdom and trust in their bodies to remain healthy during this natural life-stage is almost nonexistent. . . . Women may feel better on ERT in part because they are doing the culturally approved 'right thing.' This can be comforting and health-enhancing in and of itself.''

We are concerned that the narrow focus on estrogen replacement as the solution to osteoporosis and cardiovascular disease encourages people to overlook other obvious and important approaches to building health. No matter what you decide about any prescription medication, we strongly suggest that you embrace an ever healthier lifestyle. That having been said, we realize it may be too difficult to undertake a healthier lifestyle at this particular time in your life. Or you may not have access to a health care professional prepared to help you develop and monitor a program of natural alternatives to HRT. For that and other reasons, HRT may be the most attractive option for personal reasons and may feel ''right'' to you and your doctor.

Our patients have felt strongly both ways—and we feel that this is a personal and ethical as well as medical decision. Some women refuse to take Premarin, a synthetic estrogen made from the urine of pregnant mares, because of allegations that the horses are kept penned up and transported under less than humane conditions. Remember: *Once you start HRT, you can always adjust your doses, try various preparations, and even stop* if you find this makes you physically or psychologically uncomfortable. We have taught many women how to successfully move from uncomfortable HRT regimens to prescription and nonprescription alternatives and lifestyle changes that are more comfortable while enabling them to reclaim natural menopause and well-being.

Plant Estrogens

Many cultures traditionally use specific plant foods and products to gently support women through menopause. We now are discovering that one reason for their effectiveness is that certain foods contain chemicals or nutrients that have an estrogen-enhancing or estrogenlike effect. Although this is a large and varied group of chemicals, and they are not true estrogens such as are produced by our bodies, for simplicity's sake we will call them ''plant estrogens.'' These chemicals are just beginning to be understood, but it seems that they act in many different ways to normalize or balance hormones. In this sense, plant estrogens (or phytoestrogens) are ''adaptogens'' like the herb ginseng, which helps your body adapt and find a healthy balance. Sometimes phytoestrogens act like weak estrogens; they lock onto the estrogen receptors of your cells and stimulate them only partially. Thus, if you have too much estrogen, plant estrogens block its stronger effects. If you have too little estrogen, high doses of some plant estrogens can themselves act as estrogens and counteract that imbalance as well. Another mechanism of effect seems to be to change the way our bodies react to the estrogen we have. Some change how the estrogen is broken down or excreted. And still other plant estrogens affect our body's ability to convert other hormones to estrogen.

Formal research on phytoestrogens is still in its infancy. Because these chemicals work in many different ways, they fall under many different chemical classes. A molecule can look totally different from estrogen except for two uniquely positioned chemical appendages, and still fit the lock as an estrogenlike key. Some of the most powerful of these look-alikes you may hear about include coumestrol, genistein and daidzen; the latter two are lignans, a component of fiber which our intestinal bacteria convert into compounds that have weak estrogenic and antiestrogenic effects.

There are unanswered questions about phytoestrogen dosage and safety. Theoretically, one might wonder if they could stimulate hormone-sensitive cancers such as breast cancer. On the other hand, these substances could help explain why Japanese women who eat a traditional diet high in soybean foods have a lower rate of breast cancer and nearly none of our common menopausal symptoms. The weak phytoestrogens could be blocking the cancer-promoting effects of strong estrogens, while being powerful enough to minimize menopausal symptoms.

Low-fat and high-fiber diets may be important, but they are not the only factors influencing hormone production and metabolism. Herman Adlercreutz, a renowned Finnish researcher in this field, suggests that the risk for many Western diseases, including breast and prostate cancers, might be reduced by changing our diets to increase plant estrogens. Studies suggest that the genistein blocks the enzyme that makes normal cells cancerous, and thus may affect non-hormone-related cancers as well.

FOODS HIGH IN PLANT ESTROGENS

Foods that are plentiful in phytoestrogens include:

* Soybeans and soy-based foods such as tofu, miso and soy milk.
* Fruits such as apples, figs, dates, and apricots.
* Plants and vegetables such as alfalfa (sprouts, powder, and plants), garlic, sprouted green peas, fennel and anise seeds, parsley, and celery.
* Nuts and legumes such as cashews, peanuts, almonds; flax seed is especially high in lignans.
* Whole grains such as wheat, oats, and corn.

Many women have reported relief of menopausal symptoms when they eat these foods, particularly soy foods; soybeans are excellent sources of genistein and daidzein, the two phytoestrogens that have been the most thoroughly studied. Soy foods are a good source of protein and it's becoming easier and more pleasant to eat some everyday, preferably in place of animal foods. There are now several types of tofu or soy burgers on the market, flavored and unflavored soy milks (they work in shakes, on cereals, in cooking, and even in hot beverages such as tea), in addition to low-fat versions of tofu in firm, regular, and soft consistencies. However, some soy foods may have more plant estrogens than others—it appears that the whole beans may be most beneficial. Michael Murray estimates that 1 cup of soybeans provides about 300 mg of plant estrogens called isoflavones—the equivalent of about .45 mg of conjugated estrogens, as potent as a low- to medium-dose of Premarin (based on a 1991 *Journal of the National Cancer Institute* paper by Mark Messina).

Unanswered Questions About Plant Hormones

Although phytoestrogens can be effective and safe in many women, we need to acknowledge that we don't fully understand how plant-derived hormones work, the scope of their efficacy, or the appropriate doses required for the desired effect. They vary by plant and by processing, and by the woman's metabolism, absorption, and existing hormonal balance. Therefore, we cannot at this point recommend plant estrogens to completely replace prescription hormones if they are needed for important medical problems such as heart disease and osteoporosis. We don't know whether they are safe in breast cancer patients. Tori Hudson, a prominent doctor of naturopathy in Portland, Oregon, is also cautious in her practice and advises that natural estrogens and progesterone in plants cannot "be liberally substituted for conventional HRT in all circumstances." She emphasizes the importance of prescribing appropriately, based on a woman's risk for osteoporosis and heart disease as well as the severity of her immediate menopausal symptoms.

There are also herbs and food supplements that contain plant hormones; *see* Chapter 3 for a general discussion and Chapter 5 to find out which herbs are used specifically for individual symptoms or conditions.

CHAPTER 5

A-to-Z of Natural Remedies for Common Conditions of Menopause and Aging

In this chapter we describe the most common non-life-threatening physical and emotional symptoms women experience as they age, starting around menopause. Although the list of possible complaints seems long, no woman ever has all of them and few women have most of them. Many physical symptoms due to menopause such as hot flashes can be merely annoying—they are sometimes debilitating, but they are not permanently harmful and they will pass. Others, such as urinary problems, hair changes, loss of muscle tone, and weight gain are here to stay unless you take some action.

How to Use This Chapter
Adopting the Balanced Life Plan in Chapter 2 is the first step in preventing and easing common complaints, and under each listing we first provide you with reminders of how changing your eating habits and lifestyle can affect your symptoms. These dietary and lifestyle changes may be all you need. However, some women still need additional support as their body strives to maintain and establish better health. That's where specific natural therapies come in.

In Chapter 3, we introduced you to the most popular natural therapies available in the United States and provided you with general background information on nutritional supplements, herbal therapy, homeopathy, traditional Chinese medicine, acupressure, aromatherapy, and mind-body and relaxation therapies such as massage and visualization. All these therapies are generally useful for alleviating or preventing synmptoms associated with menopause, and in this chapter we provide specific instructions for those natural self-care therapies that we have found particularly useful for treating specific symptoms. For example, if you are suffering from hot flashes, turn to the section in this chapter called "Hot Flashes." You'll find suggestions for using nutritional supplements, herbs, homeopathy, acupressure, aromatherapy, and natural hormone therapy. If you're interested in using herbs, select one or several of the herbs recommended here, and then turn to Chapter 3 for more detailed information on how to buy them, prepare them, take them, and store them. Remember, however, that if you have a specific medical condition, are taking prescription drugs or otherwise under the care of a physician, you should check with your doctor before taking any new remedy or therapy.

Emotional Ups and Downs

People once mistakenly thought depression and moodiness were to be expected of women going through their change of life. Although we now know it's a myth that women can "go mad" during menopause, most women do report emotional changes as their hormone levels fluctuate and readjust, even so far as describing their experience as an emotional rollercoaster. Long-standing emotional difficulties may worsen during menopause.

However, it does women an injustice simply to point the finger directly at their biochemistry. Research studies in the physiology and psychology of women as they proceed along the life span show that these conditions have varied causes. Emotions triggered by hormonal changes often are intensified by other changes in your life, and vice versa. You may experience stresses in your social world as children leave home, your parents die, or your marital status changes; you may feel out of place in our youth-oriented society; you may mourn the loss of your reproductive capacity; you may feel new pressures on the job. You may feel diminishing self-esteem and social power; as we noted in Chapter 2, our culture devalues older people, and older women most of all. Fortunately, natural therapies are effective tools in learning to cope successfully with the psychological and mental aspects associated with menopause, as well as the physical ones.

Precautions: When Professional Care Is Advisable

While menopause and aging are healthy life events, many of the symptoms we describe may be early warning signs of illness, so consult your health care practitioner about anything that bothers you, either mentally or physically. We want to make sure you don't write any troubling conditions off "just" to menopause or growing older without finding out whether a disease process is under way. Doctors are only now finding out how many conditions, such as Alzheimer's disease, once called "senility," can afflict older people, but are not necessary accompaniments of aging.

Professional Psychotherapy and Group Support

Sometimes individual counseling, group therapy, or support groups provide the talking therapy that can help a woman cope with the changes and challenges she faces at menopause and in the second half of her life. Psychotherapy is not just for "sick people" but for healthy people with problems. There are many, many different forms of therapy, but they all aim to modify the way you feel about yourself or other people, and often the way you behave. For example, psychotherapy may be supportive—you merely talk about your problems to someone who will not judge you or talk about them with other people. Or it may be exploratory—by asking questions and making suggestions, the therapist helps you explore and better understand yourself and your feelings, and perhaps guide you toward a solution.

Aches and Pains

Aches and pains are usually the body's way of indicating that something is wrong. But having said that, we must note that aches and pains grow more common in older people as muscles and joints age. (Have you ever heard a young child or adult give a little grunt as they got up out of a chair or stooped to pick up something?)

Aches and pains can mean lots of things. When there is inflammation, it indicates that the body is trying to repair injured tissue, which may have gotten that way by overuse or underuse. Inflammation in the joints is called arthritis; in the tendons, tendinitis; in the bursae (small sacs that cushion the movements of muscles), bursitis. Pain is a cardinal sign of inflammation for any number of reasons—nerves relay pain messages from almost all tissues in our bodies, the brain being a notable exception.

Backache is one of the most common complaints of modern civilization—80 percent of American adults suffer from back pain at some point in their lives, and it is the leading cause of worker disability. It is also one of the most difficult and frustrating conditions to treat with conventional medicine—which consists of painkillers, muscle relaxers, antidepressants, physical therapy, and surgery. Osteopaths often stand alone in the realm of conventional medicine to offer a holistic and scientifically rigorous compliment of regimens in the diagnosis and management of pain by working with muscles, bones, and fascial tissues (sheets of tissue enclosing the muscles). Back problems take many forms. Stiff (or ''wry'') neck (torticollis) often occurs spontaneously for unknown reasons; it may be related to holding your neck in an unnatural position for a long time such as cradling the phone between ear and shoulder, to emotional tension, or to a chill to an exposed neck. Low back and sacroiliac sprain are often related to overexertion, reaching, or bending in a twisted position, sitting on the ground for a long time, or sleeping on the ground or a soft bed, or sometimes to imbalanced posture, such as carrying a child on your hip. In a coccyx injury, the ''tailbone'' is bruised in a fall. In sciatica, the sciatic nerve is irritated—by a bulging vertebral disc, squeezed by a muscle, or inflamed by other local irritation—resulting in sharp pain shooting down the back of the leg. Injured or irritated ligaments, muscles, and other tissues can also cause shooting pain down the leg, which is not sciatica.

Repetitive stress injuries, another increasingly common source of aches and pains, are usually work- or sports-related. So can any repetitive movement, especially if you're not accustomed to it or if you do something with imbalanced body mechanics. Needlepoint and knitting can cause repetitive stress injuries if you don't seek regular respite. People who spend a lot of time on computers may experience symptoms of numbness in the first three fingers and sometimes pain in the forearm and wrist—this is often diagnosed as carpal tunnel syndrome. The problems may originate in the neck, upper chest, or upper arm, where a single or a combination of irritations may affect the nerve which serves those fingers. The problem may be metabolic, such as a magnesium or B_{12} deficiency, or hormonal such as a thyroid deficiency or too much estrogen which causes the nerve sheath to swell up in its tiny carpal tunnel. Most physicians and physical therapists treat this condition with splints; a knowledgeable osteopath, chiropractor, or physical therapist may provide specific manipulation which frequently brings rapid relief. Most computer makers also can help you find keyboards that are kinder to your wrists than the older models. At any rate, give yourself a break every hour (better for your eyes too) and do something different with your hands.

There are almost infinite ways to manage pain, many of which you can do on your own, with your own hands, your mind, and ingredients found in your kitchen or local health food store.

General Nutrition

Follow the Balanced Life Plan in Chapter 2 to make sure your joints and muscles have the nourishment they need. To prevent or slow the development of arthritic joints, make a special effort to eat plenty of natural sources of the antioxidant nutrients vitamins C and E, beta-carotene, and selenium. Bioflavonoids in cherries, blueberries, and blackberries may also protect joint and vessel deterioration, as may sulfur-rich foods such as garlic, onions, and cabbage, which are also antioxidant. There's evidence that avoiding foods in the nightshade family—tomatoes, potatoes, eggplant, and peppers—reduces joint inflammation in some people. Food allergies are a common cause of arthritis, as are the effects of sugar.

Try to lose any extra weight that you are carrying around. Overweight bodies cause considerable stress on our joints and bones, particularly those of the feet, knees, and back. Extra weight also discourages us from moving around enough so that our joints get even stiffer and sorer.

See also ''Weight Gain.''

General Considerations

There are several ways you can help to heal and/or minimize back problems and other aches and pains. In most cases, moist heat will ease the pain. Avoid dry heat directly on the skin as it can dehydrate and even burn tissues, especially if you fall asleep with the heat applied. You may need to rest the injury for a day or two, but prolonged bed rest is not advisable. A recent review of 4,000 studies by the federal Agency for Health Care Policy and Research recommended spinal manipulation (osteopathy or chiropractic) and low-stress exercise such as walking or swimming, begun within two weeks of an injury.

Stress and emotional upheaval can precipitate muscle and joint injury and worsen existing pain so be extra good to yourself and consider exploring ways to relax and manage stress.

To prevent future injuries and pain, keep a limbering exercise routine a part of your life. Begin a program of back loosening, lengthening, and strengthening exercises geared to your level of ability. Learn the proper way to use your back, especially when lifting heavy objects: Face the object squarely, let your low back flatten, bend from the knees, broaden your stance, and use your thigh muscles, predominantly. (If you have a back problem, it is especially important to lift wisely, if at all.) Consult with a physical therapist, chiropractor, or osteopath who can teach you how to move, stand, sit, sleep, bend, turn, and reach properly to reduce the stress on your body and help forestall future problems. There are also videotapes and "back schools" or "back clinics" that teach good body mechanics.

Exercise in general prevents many aches and pains because it builds fitness, balance, and flexibility, especially if you work out regularly. The best activities for older bodies are those that put minimal strain on legs, back, knees, and hips. Swimming and walking and cross-country skiing are great, and so are yoga, tai chi, and hiking. But as with all exercise, start gradually, building up to longer, more strenuous workouts as you get stronger. Varying your activities will also make injuries less likely.

Also remember to change physical positions as often as possible. If you have a sedentary job or life, sit less often—sitting puts a strain on your lower back. (However, spending long hours standing especially in high heels also stresses the back.) Shift positions and take frequent breaks (about every hour) to move your back. Use well designed chairs or a back support when sitting, such as a "lumbar roll" or pillow. When you're on a plane, get up and move around; you'll find plenty of company in the back of the plane as people of all ages and physical conditions stand up and do their stretching exercises. Some people spend most of the trip standing in the back of the plane!

Another good idea is to bring any little pillows you have that you use at home for sitting for long periods. Bucket-shaped seats are usually very uncomfortable for people with lower back problems;

straight-back chairs which allow you to place both feet on the ground are better because they support the spine.

Driving your car is a prime source of lower back pain, so remember to stop at regular intervals and get out and walk around or loosen up. Back specialists recommend that when driving, your knees should be fairly high and your seat drawn as close as comfortable. You should not have to stretch to reach the pedal since that puts a steady pressure on your lower back.

Women have found the following specific natural therapies to be particularly helpful for everyday aches and pains.

Nutritional Supplements

Your muscles and joints need optimum nourishment. It is especially important for women who are getting older to have enough of the antioxidant nutrients—vitamins C and E, beta-carotene, and selenium—plus nutrients needed to maintain and repair the joints (the B complex vitamins and zinc). A good multivitamin-mineral formula containing the doses recommended in Chapter 3, pages 61–64, usually supplies the nutrients you need to prevent or minimize aches and pains. You may increase the daily total dose of the following:

• *Vitamin B-6,* 100–200 mg per day. For nerve irritation and to decrease swelling associated with aches and pains and repetitive stress injuries. You may need to take B-vitamin complex in up to ten times the RDA to stay in balance and prevent deficiencies in the other B vitamins.

You may also take:

• *Essential fatty acids,* 240 mg of gammalinoleic acid (GLA), found in evening primrose oil or borage oil supplements several times a day; or 1–1½ teaspoons a day of fresh flax seeds or flax oil. This is helpful for aches and pains, especially when taken with vitamin E.

• *Bioflavonoids,* up to 300 mg of quercitin, or picnogenol, up to six times per day.

• *Glucosamine sulfate,* 500 mg three times a day. For arthritis. This natural substance is needed to repair joint cartilage and to protect joints from degenerating. Several studies demonstrated glucosamine's superior pain-relieving and anti-inflammatory ability over conventional anti-inflammatory drugs. Because this substance works not by blocking pain, but by helping the body heal itself, expect to wait a few weeks to see relief.

Herbal Remedies

Many women have found herbs helpful for everyday aches and pains. For instructions on using herbal remedies, *see* Chapter 3, pages 70–75. The herbs listed below are particularly effective for relieving aches and pains. Use them singly or in combination, or look for a commercially prepared herbal formula that contains them.

• *Bromelain* is an enzyme from pineapples—200 mg per day helps reduce swelling, bruising, healing time, and the pain of an injury or carpal tunnel syndrome.

• *Star anise* has been used in Chinese medicine for centuries for lower back pain.

• *Capsaicin* (red pepper extract) has proved remarkably effective at relieving certain types of severe chronic pain; it interferes with the pain message going to the brain.

• *Valerian* has been used for many painful conditions; it is a sedative and helps particularly when pain is related to nervous tension. Take 1 cup of infusion before bedtime, or 1 teaspoon of tincture of valerian up to three times a day.

• *Ginseng* has also traditionally been used as an adaptogen to rebalance the body and an antistress remedy, whether the source is physical or mental. Take 1 capsule up to three times a day; 1 cup of decoction up to three times a day; or $1/2$–1 teaspoon of tincture up to three times a day.

• *Tumeric* has been found useful for carpal tunnel syndrome. Take 250–500 mg between meals, or use as a poultice for sprains, muscle strains, and inflammation. When used in combination with bromelain, tumeric was found to be as effective as Motrin as an anti-inflammatory.

Homeopathic Remedies

Homeopathy is helpful for aches and pains. Following the instructions in Chapter 3, pages 75–81, use a combination remedy that contains the substances listed on page 127, or choose the single remedy that most closely matches your symptoms. Follow the instructions on the package; if your symptoms are severe, it is usually recommended that you take a dose as often as every 5 minutes; for milder symptoms, take every 3 hours. One dose equals 2–3 pills or 5–10 drops. The homeopathic remedies most often used for aches and pains are:

• *Arnica.* Arnica is especially useful as the first remedy after an injury of any kind. It takes the "shock" out of your system, relieves pain, and speeds healing.

• *Hypericum.* For nerve pain; for lower back pain due to a direct blow to the spine, or if there are shooting pains.

• *Rhus toxicodendron.* For pain in the neck or lower back that is accompanied by stiffness; symptoms are worse with initial motion or cold, wet weather, and better with continued motion, but worse with prolonged activity. One of the best sciatica remedies.

• *Bryonia.* For pain in the lower back; symptoms are better when lying still and worse with slight movement, and during the menstrual period. Also a good sciatica remedy.

• *Pulsatilla.* For shooting leg pains; symptoms are associated with the menstrual period or vaginal discharge infections, and symptoms that improve with gentle continuous exercise such as slow walking.

Massage and Spinal Manipulation

These therapies are discussed in Chapter 3, page 86. Massage in general helps loosen up tense muscles, and is particularly effective when combined with essential oils. Relaxation therapies such as deep breathing also help you let go of tension. Massage is often helpful as is chiropractic or osteopathic work. Arthritis also responds well to physical therapy.

Dr. Maas has a series of movement videos specifically for the release of pain and tension (*see* Resources section). They have brought relief to many of her patients with a variety of types of musculoskeletal pain.

Acupressure

Acupressure (*see* Chapter 3, page 81) works wonderfully for aches and pains. Press firmly on the acupressure points shown on the diagrams shown on page 128.

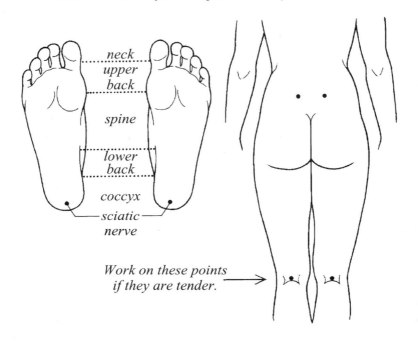

neck
upper
back

spine

lower
back

coccyx

sciatic
nerve

*Work on these points
if they are tender.*

Acupressure Points For Back Pain

Aromatherapy

Aromatherapy baths are a wonderfully soothing way to ease aches and pains caused by overwork, stress, and tension. Add to your bath water a few drops of *lavender,* which has a nurturing tonic affect on your nervous system, or *chamomile, bergamot, jasmine, marjoram, neroli,* or *rose.* Hot compresses are another way to get oils to the painful areas. The exception is acute inflammation—use cold chamomile or lavender oil compresses over the affected part to help relieve the pain.

Visualization/Guided Imagery

Creative imagery is useful for all types of pain. Begin with one of the relaxation techniques described in Chapter 3. Once you are in a relaxed state, draw your healing attention to the pain. Scan it closely, with an open, relaxed mind. Enter the sensation and feel it completely so that it can resolve itself and let you rest comfortably. Imagine the painful area in tangible detail—its temperature, color, size, shape. Does it pulsate, does it change as you perceive it? Let your mind settle on the very top of this area, as though a tiny traveler were passing through the middle of it, very slowly, with an open heart, very willing to feel and perceive. When you get to the bottom, turn around and come back up to the top, again moving slowly so you don't miss a single millimeter of the experience. Let the feeling wash through you, like a train ride through your most intimate places. Then start your journey from the front to the back, moving slowly, slowly, and then turn around and come back again.

You can also imagine the area as a particular color, which you can change and shift to a color that is soothing rather than painful; for example, many people find it helpful to imagine their pain as fiery red and gradually shift it through the colors of the rainbow to cool blue. Another possibility is to imagine the pain as a thermometer, with the level of pain slowing descending like mercury, until you relax and the pain goes away.

If you have low back pain, visualize your lower back lengthening, the muscles melting like butter so your pelvis drops down. If you are lying down, visualize your muscles melting into the surface. Put your hands on your sore muscles if you can comfortably reach them and imagine healing warmth emanating from them. For shoulder pain, picture your cares and woes literally rolling off your shoulders, your arms heavy, water running down your shoulders, arms, hands, and running out your fingertips, taking the pain and tension with it.

Precautions

If you can't find a position of relief, are awakened by pain, have difficulty moving or feeling your legs, or have a back problem that is accompanied by bowel or bladder trouble, you should consult your health care provider promptly. If your condition worsens or does not improve rapidly with the self-care methods described earlier, seek an osteopath specializing in the treatment of your problem. If a new pain anywhere in your body is accompanied by fever, swelling, redness, lumps under the skin, or faintness, a doctor should be consulted. Even with chronic pain that does not have any of the above components, you shouldn't accept a friend's assurance that this is "what you can expect if you're over forty.'' Bone, joint, or back pain may be an indication of serious health problems including fractures; in addition, pain from internal organs can radiate and feel just like a back ache. Unexplained aches and pains that are usually accompanied by fatigue and hair loss may be early indications of abnormally low thyroid activity, not unusual in older people and easily diagnosed by a simple blood test.

Anxiety

No aging woman should be surprised if she experiences some anxiety during and after menopause, when you consider the important physical and life changes that take place at that time. Anxiety can be expressed in both obvious and sneaky ways. Among the former are phobias (the intense and nonrational fear of some activity or place leading to complete avoidance of the offending stimulus), pounding heart, insomnia, high blood pressure, and overeating or loss of appetite. Some people are not really consciously aware of feeling anxiety and may express it covertly, such as by picking quarrels, heightened irritability, excessive use of alcohol, or "spacing out."

Many sources of anxiety in menopausal and older women have to do directly or indirectly with the low esteem in which aging women are held in our culture, which overvalues youth and beauty in females. Women may fear that with the signs of aging that accompany menopause and the encroaching years—i.e., wrinkles, a mature physique, graying hair—they will lose their social and economic power, and to a large extent, reality confirms these fears. Older women do have trouble finding jobs, in spite of the fact that they may be more reliable and healthier workers than younger people of either sex; older heterosexual single women do have more trouble than younger ones and more trouble than older men, heaven knows, in finding intimate partners; older women have more trouble in getting heard in meetings than younger people and older men. The poorest people in America are older women. So loss of power makes older women feel more helpless than when they were younger about changing their lives. They see their choices of where to live, where to work, and of intimate partners as severely limited, or likely to be limited. Thus they feel anxious.

Anxiety and depression are two ends of the same process, and the solution—like the cause—is multifactoral. Both psychotherapy and medications including antidepressants (such as the much-adored Prozac), tranquilizers, and sleeping pills can be combined with natural therapies for greater effect, or natural remedies may be effective alone, and without the side effects of prescription antidepressants.

General Considerations

Nutritionally speaking, following the Balanced Life Plan in Chapter 2 is a good place to start. Play down meat and emphasize whole foods and complex carbohydrates, which have a calming effect on some people. Emphasize foods high in the B vitamins, since these are considered to be good for the nerves and avoid aggravating foods containing sugar or caffeine such as sweets, chocolate, coffee, and tea. Exercise is a wonderful stress reliever; yoga, tai chi, and other forms of slow, rhythmic movements are excellent for centering the emotions.

Other than that, the best remedies for anxiety are social and economic: Find out what agencies help older people find work or explore with the help of social services all the income entitlements for which you're eligible; join support groups, become active politically in the service of causes that will inspire you, reorder your priorities. Are you really still putting a lot of energy into finding the right man? Trying to get your kids to pay attention to you? Maybe you should spend more time looking for helpful, kind, and smart women friends. They're all around you and they need you as much as you need them.

Finally, listen to your own needs: Do you feel better when you are left alone or in the company of others? Do you find comfort in talking to people who share similar experiences and feelings? Can you find ways to distract yourself until the anxiety or fear passes? By focusing on the positive, you will allow the negative to recede. Say ''I feel terrific'' twenty-five times every morning for a week as you first get out of bed and greet your friendly face in the mirror. Become conscious of any deprecating mental tapes you play. Instead of ''I can't do this,'' say ''I *can* do this.'' Instead of ''What a mess I made of this,'' say ''Okay, so what's the lesson and where do we go from here?'' When worries and pointless complaints encroach, invite some new thoughts. It works! Try it! You are in charge of your life.

Women have found the following specific natural therapies to be particularly helpful in treating anxiety.

Nutritional Supplements

A good multivitamin-mineral formula containing the doses recommended in Chapter 3, pages 61–64, usually supplies the nutrients you need to prevent or minimize feelings of anxiety. Stress is associated with deficiencies in vitamin B-12, potassium, vitamins C and B-6, zinc, pantothenate, and magnesium, so these are particularly important.

Herbal Remedies

Many women have found that certain herbs can gently ease feelings of anxiety. For instructions on using herbal remedies, *see* Chapter 3, page 70. The herbs listed below are particularly effective in treating anxiety. Use them singly or in combination, or look for a commercially prepared herbal formula that contains them.

• *Black cohosh* has been traditionally used to treat anxiety, and animal studies show that the herb does have a calming and sedative effect, especially if you are low in estrogen. Take 1 capsule up to three times a day; 1 teaspoon up to three times a day; or 10–30 drops of extract (in water or juice) daily.

• *St. Johnswort* is another traditional herbal folk remedy for anxiety. A small German study published in 1984 supports this use by demonstrating a significant improvement in people who took this herb, without any side effects.

• *Valerian* is a widely used herb that has antianxiety activity. Take 1 cup of infusion before bedtime; or 1 teaspoon of tincture up to three times a day. *Skullcap, chamomile,* and *aveena* are also traditional herbal remedies for anxiety.

• A good antianxiety combination is *valerian, hops, catnip, skullcap,* and *passion flower.*

Homeopathic Remedies

Homeopathy offers many remedies for anxiety. Following the instructions in Chapter 3, pages 75–81, use a combination remedy that contains the substances listed on page 134, or choose the single remedy that most closely matches your symptoms. Follow the instructions on the package; if your symptoms are severe, it is usually recommended that you take a dose as often as every 5 minutes; for milder symptoms, take every 3 hours. One dose equals 2–3 pills or 5–10 drops.

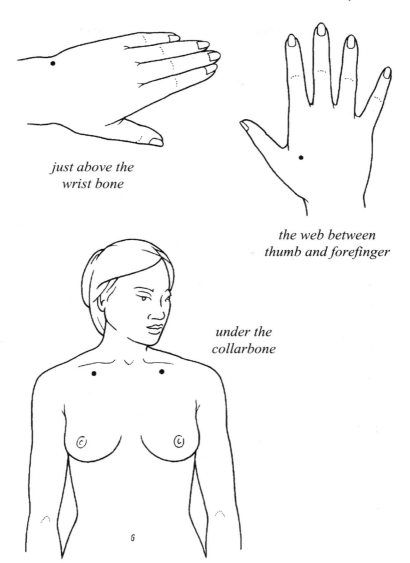

*just above the
wrist bone*

*the web between
thumb and forefinger*

*under the
collarbone*

Acupressure Points For Anxiety

Acupressure Points For Stress

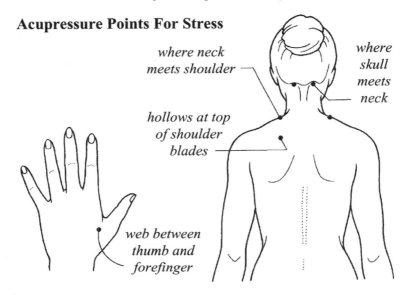

where neck
meets shoulder

where
skull
meets
neck

hollows at top
of shoulder
blades

web between
thumb and
forefinger

• *Gelsemium.* An often-used remedy for anticipatory fear before giving a speech or for pre-exam anxiety; useful when you become dull with fear, can't concentrate, and your mind goes blank.

• *Aconite.* When you are physically and mentally restless; you may have trouble sleeping and be hypersensitive to noise, light, and touch. You tremble, look pale, and are full of dread.

• *Ignatia.* For the ill effects of worrying, if your moods and symptoms are changeable and you are introspective, silent, and brooding; you may feel as though there is a lump in your throat.

• *Pulsatilla.* When the fear is accompanied by crying, or the anxiety causes trembling and flushing. Anxious or fearful thoughts prevent you from falling asleep or staying asleep, and you want company and support.

Acupressure

Massaging certain acupressure points can help lessen anxiety. Press firmly on the points shown in the drawings above and on page 133. Try using your fists to rub your back over your kidneys to stimulate and balance the adrenal release of fear hormones.

Aromatherapy

There are many essential oils that act as safe, nonaddictive sedatives; *see* Chapter 3, page 84, for suggestions on how to use essential oils. *Lavender* is very popular because of its nurturing, tonic effect on the nervous system. Other calming oils to choose from include *chamomile, marjoram, benzoin, bergamot, jasmine,* and *orange blossom.* Choose one or two that appeal to you and add to your bath, or sprinkle a few drops on your skin to gently soothe your psyche.

Relaxation and Mind-Body Therapies

The relaxation techniques described in Chapter 3 are tools that help us consciously relax for a short period every day and can help calm fears. Meditation, biofeedback, and massage (especially when combined with aromatherapy) are among the most popular and effective ways to reach a state of relaxation—they are like taking a minivacation. There are many books, tapes, courses, and one-on-one training opportunities for you to learn relaxation techniques. Or you might want to try progressive muscle relaxation, a simple, no-frills technique used to relax the body-mind by alternately tensing and relaxing the muscles, which is also described in Chapter 3.

Relaxation techniques are very effective when coupled with visualization or guided imagery. For example, if you feel tension in a particular part of your body, "breathe into" the area—imaging the lungs expanding into that place, or that the air you breathe includes a special calming energy that enters that place. When you breathe into a place, imagine you are breathing in light, love, or healing energy. Breathe out the dark smoke of tension, or that in focusing your attention on it, it melts away like butter in the sunshine. If you are anxious about a specific event, visualize it occurring successfully, going through it step-by-step, imaging people's favorable reactions, applause, or whatever you want the outcome to be.

We hope that you will promise yourself that you will take steps to deal with the underlying cause of your anxiety later, after the anxiety-provoking event—and approach this with real energy and feeling.

Natural Hormone Therapy

Hormone imbalance can affect this health problem. Should you suspect this to be the case, you would do well to discuss this possibility with a holistically minded physician.

Precautions

If anxiety is accompanied by a worsening of chest pain, abdominal pain, headache, difficulty breathing, or any other dramatic change in physical state, you should see your physician. Watch for these symptoms of anxiety that require a psychotherapy consultation: overeating or drinking more than you used to, or more often than you used to, in order to calm your nerves; developing true phobias that prevent you from enjoying your friends or earning a living—if, for example, you find it too frightening to go out of the house. Or if you're so fearful of failure that you're not able to take the first steps toward improving your social life or looking for work.

Back Pain

See "Aches and Pains."

Bloating

See "Digestive Problems" and "Menstrual Cramps and PMS."

Breast Lumps and Tender Breasts

Breast lumps are very common in women, and may appear to be more common or prominent as we grow older. That's because our breasts are made of fat and connective tissue, and as we age, the composition changes. Some areas of the breast start to feel denser because there is more connective tissue and less fat. This thickening of the tissue is common and usually not a problem. The medical term for this is fibrocystic breast disease, but we feel a better term is fibrocystic *changes*. Only rarely is it associated with an increased risk of breast cancer. However, lumpy breasts make it more difficult to feel cancers in the breast. Breasts feel swollen and tender, ebbing and flowing with the menstrual cycle. Breast tenderness that accompanies hormonal cycles may temporarily worsen during the perimenopause, when any hormone imbalance may become extended as the premenstrual period is longer in less frequent cycles. This eventually diminishes after menopause, and you should not be aware of breast tenderness in the absence of any trauma to the breast such as from an accident.

Although it may be alarming to feel a lump in your breast, 80–90 percent are benign and need no treatment at all once cancer is excluded from the diagnosis. (*See also* ''Breast Cancer'' in Chapter 6, and ''Menstrual Cramps and PMS'' in this chapter.)

General Nutrition and Other Considerations

Many women find that caffeine increases breast pain and lumpiness, and some studies confirm this, so begin by eliminating coffee (even decaffeinated, which still has some caffeine and may make a difference in sensitive women), tea (even green tea), colas, root beer, Dr Pepper and other caffeinated soft drinks, and chocolate. If you notice improvement after a few cycles, try reintroducing these items a little at a time to see if you can tolerate them. Some mammogram technicians recommend that before you come for your appointment you cut out caffeine for twenty-four hours because this helps reduce the pain when the x-ray machine squeezes the tender breast tissue. Some women also seem to respond well to eliminating meat and dairy products and eating a low-fat whole-foods diet such as the one recommended in the Balanced Life Plan provided in Chapter 2.

Another measure that helps some women is a castor oil pack made from a large soft cloth. Heat castor oil until it is warm and place the cloth in it until it becomes thoroughly soaked. Place the cloth over your breast and cover it with plastic to retain the heat and the oil. Leave on overnight. You need to repeat this for five nights, then skip two nights, then repeat for five nights, skip two nights, and repeat again.

Women have found the following specific natural therapies to be particularly helpful for reducing breast tenderness or lumpiness.

Nutritional Supplements

A good multivitamin-mineral formula containing the doses recommended in Chapter 3, pages 61–64, supplies the nutrients most women need to prevent or minimize lumpy, tender breasts. You may increase the daily total dose of the following:

• *Vitamin E,* up to 1,000 IU per day. Many women seem to respond to this vitamin, possibly because it decreases LH and FSH, the hormones secreted by the pituitary.

• *Vitamin B-6,* up to 300 mg per day. This vitamin acts like a diuretic. Take with B-complex, since the B vitamins work together.

You may also wish to take:

• *Essential fatty acids,* 240 mg of gammalinoleic acid (GLA), found in evening primrose oil or borage oil supplements several times a day; or 1 tablespoon a day of fresh flax seeds or flax oil. This is very helpful for decreasing inflammation.

• *Iodine supplements* may help when the other approaches have not; they appear to change the way breast tissue receptors bind to estrogen. Sea vegetables such as seaweed, or kelp tablets also provide iodine. If you eat iodized salt, or take iodine for a long time, get your iodine levels checked—you may be getting too much.

Herbal Remedies

Many women find that herbs help with lumpy, tender breasts. For instructions on herbal remedies, *see* Chapter 3, pages 70–75. Use an all-purpose menopausal herbal remedy, or choose one or more of the following herbs, which are particularly effective in treating this condition.

• *Red clover* is estrogenic and diuretic and helps balance stressed adrenal glands; Take 1 cup of infusion or ½–1 teaspoon up to three times a day for at least 10 days, especially if you are premenstrual.

• *Dandelion leaf* (3–4 cups a day of infusion or decoction daily, or 1 teaspoon of tincture three times a day) and *licorice* (up to 2 cups a day of decoction; ½–1 teaspoon of tincture up to twice daily; or 1 capsule up to three times a day) are diuretics that may help reduce swelling.

• *Dong quai* is an antiestrogen; take 1 capsule up to three times a day, 1 teaspoon of tincture up to three times a day. *Vitex agnus* balances female hormones and may relieve lumpy, tender breasts; take 1 capsule or 1 teaspoon of tincture up to three times a day.

Natural Hormone Therapy

You can assume there is a hormone imbalance if your breasts are painful and lumpy mostly during the premenstrual time. If the above approaches are not effective enough, before considering taking conventional hormone replacement therapy, you may want to try some of the OTC creams containing Mexican yam to see if you get relief. You don't need to rub progesterone cream on your breasts to be effective. You can also decrease the estrogen/progesterone ratio with plant estrogens or with liver herbs which promote the breakdown of excess estrogen.

Precautions

You'll be relieved to know that breast lumpiness only rarely increases the risk of breast cancer. However, don't try to diagnose a new lump yourself. Because lumpiness is related most often to hormone changes, you should see your doctor if you notice any new lump or breast tenderness after menopause. Be particularly alert to any redness, leakage, swelling, or puckering in the breast or nipple. It's also best to report any injury to the breast that becomes black and blue, raises a lump, or is still tender after twenty-four hours. Remember, sometimes doctors make mistakes. Plenty of women have been told without a biopsy or a mammogram that a lump is harmless. If you don't feel well, or if you have any misgivings at all about a lump that's still there especially if it is growing and doesn't go away after your period. Ask your doctor about having it aspirated, biopsied or viewed on a mammogram. Don't wait—get yourself another opinion now.

Confusion, Forgetfulness, and Poor Concentration

It's happened to everyone: Midsentence, you completely lose your train of thought; you meet someone for the first time and immediately forget her name; having just entered a room, you can't for the life of you figure out why you went there; balancing your checkbook is becoming more of a challenge. If it feels as if your brain has simply stopped working the way it used to, you may simply be overstimulated. In a effort to stay caught up, many women are simply trying to do too much and stuff too many pieces of information into their gray matter. While animal experiments have demonstrated that too little stimulation causes the brain to shrink, and an appropriate amount of stimulation causes new brain cells to grow, too much stimulation causes stress and appears to cause the brain to shut down and possibly deteriorate. It's as if it hangs out a sign that reads SORRY, FULL.

Although fear usually sharpens the mind, poor concentration often accompanies anxiety. We all have times when we're so worried we ''can't think.'' Most of us know that we have to write down even familiar phone numbers and keep them near us since, if we're faced with an emergency situation, we can't recall them—sometimes when we're stressed, we can't recall even our own number or the names of our best friends!

Confusion, forgetfulness, and poor concentration may also occur when your brain isn't getting enough oxygen or nutrients. Or they may be due to conditions that are either self-correcting or have relatively simple solutions. For example, confusion and forgetfulness are common for many months after a surgery that required a general anesthetic. These symptoms may also occur because of poor sleep patterns or depression (*see* "Insomnia" and "Depression"). Many commonly prescribed drugs and nonprescription drugs affect the concentration as well.

The widespread fear that aging women just can't cut it mentally is simply unfounded. A long-term study at Duke University found that people sixty-five to seventy-five years old experienced no general decline in intelligence. However, if you find you're not the brilliant, witty, clear-thinking genius you used to be, the following natural approaches offer safe ways to help you bounce back.

General Nutrition

Your brain's metabolism requires every vitamin and mineral to do its job well. Confusion and poor concentration may be the result of poor nutrition, so if you are not eating well, be sure to begin your campaign to smarten up by following the eating guidelines in the Balanced Life Plan provided in Chapter 2. Make a special effort to eat foods high in the antioxidant nutrients vitamins C and E, beta-carotene, and selenium. There's evidence that antioxidants minimize the accumulation of *lipofuscin,* the "aging pigment" that appears to slow brain function. Antioxidants also may help reduce atherosclerosis, which could slow the blood supply to your brain. If better nutrition, including more antioxidants, does not help, you may want to consider blood sugar abnormalities, or sensitivities or allergies to food or common environmental agents (particularly volatile organic compounds from carpets and other human-made materials, such as perfume or gasoline) as the root of a thinking problem. Systemic yeast infections are a common cause of "brain fog." There are several self-help books on the subject, or consult with a health care professional who is well versed in the subject.

Other Lifestyle Considerations

There are many methods and tricks used to improve memory and concentration. Jogging your memory is like jogging your body—you need to exercise it in order to develop it fully. So if you're bored and understimulated, read new books; get out and meet new people; attend lectures, museums, and group discussions. But remember, too much stimulation is stressful, so if you fall into this category, think of ways you can streamline your life. Just as you can overexercise your body, so can you overtax your brain; give both the rest they need so they can recharge. Speaking of which, regular exercise helps relieve stress, clear the mind, and sends oxygen and nutrients to your brain.

Women have found the following specific natural therapies to be particularly helpful for confusion, poor concentration, and forgetfulness.

Nutritional Supplements

A good multivitamin-mineral formula containing the doses recommended in Chapter 3, pages 61–64, usually supplies the nutrients you need to keep your brain and nervous system in tip-top form. You may also take:

• *Ginkgo biloba,* a plant substance that is often recommended to improve blood flow specifically to the brain. The extract of this tree is very popular in Europe, but is catching on here in the United States, too, thanks to over 300 scientific studies to evaluate its effect on mental functioning. Many of these studies demonstrated its benefits: enhancing blood flow, enhancing the utilization of glucose in the brain, improving the transmission of nerve messages. The standard dose is 40 mg of a standardized 24% ginkgo flavonglycodide product, three times a day. You may notice a difference in your mental ability in as few as two or three weeks, but usually three months' time is needed to adequately gauge how much ginkgo is helping you. Adverse effects are rare, and include gastrointestinal upset and headache.

Mind-Body Therapies

You may be able to quiet your overly busy and confused mind through relaxation and meditation (*see* Chapter 3). Meditation helps disperse thoughts, leaving a clean slate for clearer thinking. Visualization may help, too; some possible images you may use include clouds of different thoughts dissolving and clearing away, leaving crystalline blue skies in their wake; or image yourself floating in a stream that is gurgling with life's challenges, and then coming up out of the water into an open sky.

Aromatherapy

Several essential oils are known for their ability to stimulate, clear, and rejuvenate the mind. These include *basil, peppermint, lemon, tangerine,* and *rosemary. See* Chapter 3, page 84, for more information about how to use aromatherapy.

Natural Hormone Therapy

Hormone imbalance can be related to mental symptoms. For example, excess progesterone can cause foggy thinking. If you suspect hormone imbalance could be related to this problem, we advise you to discuss this possibility with a holistically minded physician.

Precautions

Only 10 percent of all people over age sixty-five show any signs of Alzheimer's disease, a figure that grows higher with each passing decade. There is a common joke that has some truth to it—if you're alert enough to think you have Alzheimer's, you don't. Confusion, forgetfulness, and poor concentration can be signs of a serious mental condition such as Alzheimer's disease or other brain damage such as that due to small, undetected strokes caused by high blood pressure. They can also signal the presence of a previously undiagnosed low thyroid condition (hypothyroidism) or low blood sugar (hypoglycemia). If the symptoms are new, came on suddenly, or seem to be getting worse, contact your physician, who may do some simple tests in the office (questions and puzzles). Or he or she may want to refer you to a neurologist or cardiologist for a consultation.

Cramping

Cramps or spasms are sudden contractions that may occur in any muscle and at any age. They occur most often in the calves of your legs, feet, and fingers and are usually due to a mineral deficiency—calcium, magnesium, or potassium. Hormone imbalances also cause leg cramps. Women are more likely to have muscle cramps during and after menopause. This is because the circulatory system which, in youth, is adequate enough to carry off the blood chemicals that are generated by fatigue no longer does its job as well as we age. Cramps in the legs and feet seem to occur most often at night, in bed, and can usually be alleviated if you stand up flat on the floor. Gently stretch the area during a cramp—and to prevent future cramps, stretch before going to bed. For cramps in the legs, you may have to rub vigorously to soften the muscles. Cramps in the hands and fingers can occur any time you use your hand in an awkward position. Again, stretching your hand out flat against a surface usually takes care of the cramp. Be sure that before you walk, run, or do any strenuous exercise, you do some mild stretching exercises to loosen up those muscles.

Conventional medical treatment usually consists of quinine, muscle relaxers, and pain relievers, which may have undesirable side effects or be ineffective. Natural therapies offer a side-effect-free approach to relieving and preventing cramping pains and are frequently very effective.

For abdominal cramps, *see* "Digestive Problems"; for pelvic cramps, *see* "Heavy Periods" or "Menstrual Cramping and PMS"; *see also* "Aches and Pains."

General Nutrition and Other Considerations

As you follow the Balanced Life Plan provided in Chapter 2, make a special effort to eat plenty of natural sources of foods rich in calcium, magnesium, and potassium because deficiencies in these minerals are associated with muscle cramps. Remember, smoking and caffeine tend to worsen all menopausal symptoms, including muscle cramps, so make a strong effort to quit. Stress and emotional upheaval worsen muscle tension and may contribute to muscle spasms, so be extra nice to yourself and considering exploring ways to relax and handle stress better. Regular exercise—yoga and tai chi in particular—helps keep muscles strong, flexible, and supplied with oxygen- and nutrient-rich blood, while carrying away waste products—all of which help forestall cramping. Regular strenuous exercise is also one of the best antidotes to stress. Hot showers and baths, saunas, and steam baths may be deliciously relaxing for you at this time, and daily self-massage of the muscle areas prone to cramping helps relax muscles and increase healing blood flow.

Women have found the following specific natural therapies to be particularly helpful for muscle cramps.

Nutritional Supplements

For many women, a good multivitamin-mineral formula containing the doses recommended in Chapter 3, pages 61–64, supplies the nutrients they need to keep their muscles from going into spasm. Some women may need to increase their daily total dose of the following:

• *Calcium,* up to 2,000 mg per day, along with magnesium, in equal doses. Both of these minerals are needed because they work together to minimize cramps.
• *Vitamin E,* up to 800–1,200 IU per day. Vitamin E has been shown to relieve leg cramps that occur while standing or walking.

Herbal Remedies

Many women find that herbs help with muscle cramps. For instructions on herbal remedies, *see* Chapter 3, pages 70–75. Use an all-purpose menopausal herbal remedy that contains the following herbs, or choose one or more of the following herbs, which are particularly effective in treating this condition.

• Herbs that help prevent muscle spasms in general include *valerian* (1 cup of infusion before bedtime; 1 teaspoon of tincture up to three times a day), and *scullcap.*
• You may take *ginger* orally or apply ginger compresses; *peppermint oil* rubbed on a muscle stimulates the blood flow and breaks the spasm.
• *Black cohosh* and *passiflora* are excellent smooth muscle relaxants. Take 1 capsule or 1 teaspoon of tincture up to three times a day.

Homeopathic Remedies

Homeopathy offers several helpful remedies. Following the instructions in Chapter 3, pages 75–81, use a combination remedy that includes the following substances, or choose the single remedy that most closely matches your symptoms. Follow the instructions on the package; if your symptoms are severe, it is usually recommended that you take a dose as often as every 5 minutes; for milder symptoms, take every 3 hours. One dose equals 2–3 pills or 5–10 drops.

• *Calcaria carbonica.* For cramps in your calf or hand, especially if they occur when stretching in bed.
• *Calcaria phosphorica.* For cramps in your leg that occur when walking.
• *Magnesia phosphorica.* For cramps in your calves, or ones in your arm or hand that are caused by prolonged use such as writing or playing the piano or violin; especially if the muscle twitches or is stiff or numb.

Acupressure
Massaging acupressure points often releases muscle cramps. During a cramp or spasm, apply strong pressure to the point in the foot shown in the drawing on page 146. At the same time, also press into the heart of the muscle that is cramping; begin with light pressure and gradually press harder, maintaining the pressure for up to three minutes. We also show specific acupressure points for relieving leg cramps, which are the most common. You may also prevent future muscle cramps and spasms by pressing on the foot point.

Precautions
Consult your physician if you repeatedly suffer from muscle cramps even after trying the above approaches. Remember that if you take an anti-inflammatory drug such as ibuprofin or aspirin to ameliorate cramping, you can expect to see bleeding increase. Therefore, if you're having heavy periods, you might want to take an analgesic, such as acetaminophen, that is not associated with increased bleeding.

Depression

Almost everybody gets the blues at certain times, but it would be a mistake to confuse being temporarily down in the dumps with true, major depression. Changing hormones change your moods—we know that a drop in estrogen is associated with depression and restoring levels to normal frequently lifts depression. It should come as no surprise, then, that women are twice as likely to suffer a bout of major depression than are men, and premenstrual syndrome includes depression among its long list of symptoms. There are receptors for sex hormones in the brain, so it's easy to understand how a hormone imbalance could affect your nervous system.

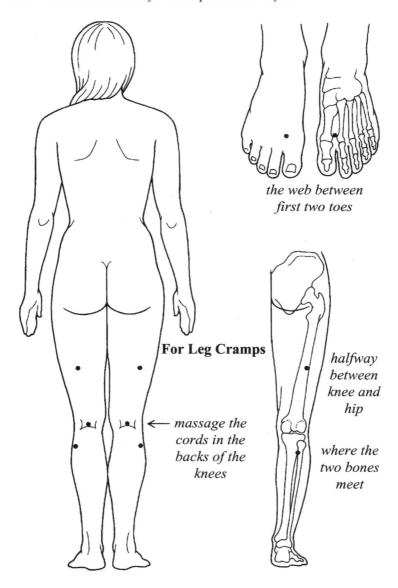

the web between
first two toes

For Leg Cramps

← *massage the cords in the backs of the knees*

halfway between knee and hip

where the two bones meet

Acupressure Points For Cramps and Spasms

Depression has many faces: loss of appetite or compulsive overeating; eyes filling with tears often at what you read or see on TV; insomnia or sleeping more than 10 hours a day or staying in bed during the day when you aren't physically sick. Most people know when they're depressed, but not all. There is a condition known as "masked depression" that tends to be chronic and may have afflicted you for most of your life, if not all of it. (Depression occurs in children, too.) Masked depression is shown by cynicism and pessimism—the feeling that nothing is ever going to turn out well for you or your loved ones or the world in general. While you may not recognize your own masked depression, others in your life may know that they avoid you because they know you won't support their successes, their optimistic hopes and fantasies. People with masked depression love to hear about everyone's failures, illnesses, and troubles of all kinds. They hate to get excited about anything and find it hard to acknowledge the silver lining in any cloud. Another sign of masked depression is agitation. If you or a relative seems hyper most of the time, this may not be because you or they feel so good, but because the symptom being expressed, agitation, is a common defensive reaction to depression.

Depression can be a result of dysfunction on several levels: psychological, social, spiritual, and biochemical. The spiritual roots of depression are often overlooked, but it's important to believe that life has meaning, to have faith in yourself, or love, or God, or *something*. We need to feel all of the human feelings—including the reverence, unity, and security which comes with faith—to be truly content.

As is the case with anxiety, the losses in self-esteem and social clout experienced by middle-aged and aging women in this society make it likely that almost any woman may experience depression as she gets older. This doesn't mean, however, that you should accept depression as a natural state; far from it. Whether it's some aspect of your inner self or our society that is setting you up for these bad feelings about yourself, you should seek some real support, preferably from a counselor who is aware of the social pressures most women face in middle age and older. These include loss of economic and sexual power, loss of attention from family and possible or actual lovers, indifference by many of the powers-that-be to our fates.

Biochemical approaches generally rely on conventional antidepressant drugs. These are used because they appear to correct or minimize imbalances in brain chemicals such as serotonin, melatonin, dopamine, and adrenaline. Some botanicals such as herbs also work on the biochemistry of the brain, but frequently in a gentler way, without the side effects of powerful drugs. Mild to moderate depression may respond to natural approaches, and may also be used along with psychotherapy for optimum effectiveness.

The most important thing about depression is that it responds so well to treatment. No one should go around feeling depressed just because they always have, or because they think all menopausal women get depressed. On the contrary, depression is a disease that has effective treatments, and sometimes it goes away by itself. Treatment, however, whether the natural approaches suggested here, or psychotherapy or medication, or a combination of both, can make it go away sooner.

See also ''Moodiness, Mood Swings, and Irritability'' and ''Menstrual Cramps and PMS.''

General Nutrition

Be sure you follow the eating guidelines provided in the Balanced Life Plan in Chapter 2 and emphasize whole grains and fresh fruits and vegetables. Many nutritional deficiencies are linked with depression, particularly vitamins B-12 and C, folic acid, niacin, pantothenic acid, pyridoxine, thiamin, and biotin. Failure to diagnose a B-12 deficiency in a depressed patient caused a landmark lawsuit. B-12 deficiency is common in vegetarians—especially in vegans—so be sure to eat plenty of seaweeds and blue-green algae and have your B-12 level checked. Other nutritional causes of depression include caffeine, sucrose; hypoglycemia, deficiencies in calcium, iron, copper; and excesses of magnesium.

You should be aware that depression is a possible side effect of caffeine and aspartame, so eliminate or reduce coffee and other caffeinated beverages as well as this artificial sweetener. In addition, some people are allergic or sensitive to certain foods, and depression is one symptom of food sensitivity.

Other Lifestyle Considerations

Alcohol is a depressant physically and emotionally. Depression may be caused by certain drugs such as the progestin in birth control pills or hormone replacement therapy, and by corticosteroids, so if you are on any regular medication, speak to your doctor about modifying your treatment. Cigarettes are also linked with depression, providing you with yet another reason you should try to quit. Since stress is a known depressant, try to be extra good to yourself and consider exploring ways to relax daily and manage stress better. Regular strenuous physical activity is the cornerstone of any effort to overcome depression. Studies show it's a superb mood elevator and stress buster in addition to its many other health-improving benefits. We especially recommend activities that get you out there, such as dancing and aerobics classes.

If your depression seems seasonal, and is better or nonexistent during the time of the year when days are longer, you might have seasonal affective disorder (SAD). Particularly common in wintertime in cold climates, SAD is a form of depression due to lack of sunlight; it is treated successfully with exposure to bright artificial light that mimics natural sunlight. So if you suspect you might have a mild form of SAD, try to spend more time in sunlight—indoors and out. Consider taking winter vacations to sunny climates, rise early in the morning and go outdoors, sit near an open window or skylight, and replace fluorescent or incandescent bulbs with full-spectrum fluorescent bulbs. Melatonin, a natural brain hormone, is a promising treatment for SAD. If you experiment on your own, try 2 to 3 mg at first and take on a regular basis at 8 P.M. and go to bed at 9 P.M.

Psychosocial remedies for depression include: seeing your friends, getting out and going to parties, perhaps attending or forming support groups, and a determined refusal to accept anyone's low regard for *any* reason, especially your age, which should be a sign of social status. Stand up for yourself—make sure you get the respect, the recognition, the money, and the good medical care you deserve. The very act of bestirring yourself to action could help chase the black clouds away.

Women have found the following specific natural therapies to be particularly helpful for treating mild depression.

Nutritional Supplements
A good multivitamin-mineral formula containing the doses recommended in Chapter 3, pages 61–64, supplies the nutrients most women need to keep their nervous systems functioning optimally. Due to the increased demand for, poor absorption of, or altered metabo-

lism of certain vitamins and minerals, some individuals may need more than others. In the case of depression, you will feel the difference within a few days. You may increase the daily total dose of the following:

• *Vitamin B complex,* up to 50 times the RDA for some of the B-vitamins. Have your doctor check your B-12 blood level. Low levels can decrease mental alertness; you may need B-12 shots initially, 1,200 mcg per day. Folate may be taken as well, up to 400 mcg per day.
• *Vitamin C,* up to 3,000 mg per day.

You may also wish to take:

• *Ginkgo biloba,* a plant-based product that has been shown to be somewhat helpful in treating depression. (*See* "Confusion, Forgetfulness, and Poor Concentration" for more information about this supplement.)
• Amino acid supplements powerfully affect the way our bodies use and synthesize the brain chemicals described earlier. *Tryptophan* is a precursor for serotonin and some women have gotten good results with supplementation. However, tryptophan supplements are available only by prescription in the United States at this time. You can get your supply from food but you need to eat quite a bit to get the same effect as a supplement. Tryptophan is found in soy foods, pumpkin seeds, turkey, and tuna; however, other high protein foods have other amino acids which compete with tryptophan absorption, so in general, keep protein intake low. *Methionine* also appears to affect serotonin levels; *phenylalanine,* found to be high in chocolate, and *tyrosine* are also critical amino acids for relief of depression. Studies of these amino acids (building blocks for the body's protein) have sometimes shown them to be as effective as some antidepressant drugs and electroconvulsive (shock) therapy.
• *Norival* is a combination nutritional formula containing N-acetyl-L-tyrosine, biopterin, and pyridoxal 5-phosphate that Dr. Maas has seen excellent results with in many of her patients alone and in combination with the herbal remedies on page 151. (Available from Cardiovascular Research, listed in Appendix C.) Take two first thing

in the morning, and two early in the afternoon—you should feel better right away, and even more so after a few weeks.

Herbal Remedies

Many women find that certain herbs help them with depression. For instructions on herbal remedies, *see* Chapter 3, pages 70–75. You might try an all-purpose menopausal herbal remedy if you are having menopausal difficulties. Or choose from among the following herbs, which are particularly effective in treating depression; use them singly or in combination, or look for a commercially prepared herbal formula that contains them.

• *St. Johnswort* has been extensively studied in Europe and has been found to influence brain chemicals and improve mood. Specifically, the extract of this herb helped symptoms of anxiety and depression and feelings of worthlessness. In a study it was shown to be more effective than several conventional antidepressant drugs such as Elavil and Tofranil. These drugs have troublesome side effects, but St. Johnswort has no known significant side effects. The dose used in most studies is 300 to 500 mg of 0.125 percent extract three times a day. You may also take capsules of 300 mg three times a day.

• Other herbs that may help are those that ease stress, including *skullcap, valerian,* and *passion flower* (*see* "Anxiety").

Homeopathic Remedies

Homeopathy offers several remedies for acute, temporary depression. Following the instructions in Chapter 3, pages 75–81, use a combination menopausal remedy containing the remedies listed below if you have other menopausal difficulties, or choose the single remedy that most closely matches your symptoms. Follow the instructions on the package; if your symptoms are severe, it is usually recommended that you take a dose as often as every 5 minutes; for milder symptoms, take every 3 hours. One dose equals 2–3 pills or 5–10 drops.

• *Lachesis* is used in women who are generally lively and cheerful but are depressed and sluggish in the morning upon awakening.

• *Sepia* is another commonly prescribed remedy for women during menopause who are depressed because they are worn down by too many responsibilities, who feel depleted and deflated, indifferent to life, but dislike sympathy.

• *Gelsemium* is useful for women who are depressed but cannot cry, who prefer to be alone, and who may also feel anxious.

• *Ignatia* is best suited for treating depression that grows out of suppressed grief, for women who are generally moody and don't want company.

• *Pulsatilla* is appropriate for women who are depressed and anxious but are also sensitive, gentle, and feel affectionate and dependent on other people.

Aromatherapy

Many essential oils have antidepressant effects, providing a safe, nonaddictive alternative to antidepressant drugs. Aromatic oils are often used by professional massage therapists, but you may also find that adding oils your bath to be uplifting. If your depression is accompanied by restlessness, irritability, and insomnia, choose one or more of the following: *chamomile, clary sage, lavender, jasmine,* or *sandalwood.* If you need uplifting, but not sedating, choose among *bergamot, geranium, melissa,* or *rose.*

Visualization/Guided Imagery

Visualization can temporarily help you get through a rough day. Put yourself in a relaxed state using one of the relaxation techniques described in Chapter 3. Then try one or more of the following visualizations: Visualize and feel a smile on the edges of your lips, your eyebrows slightly raised, and your heart opening up like a bright pink rosebud unfolding, and love vibrating from your chest. Visualize yourself as beautiful, adored, strong; with people treating you kindly and telling you that everything will be all right. You may want to hold a pillow to your chest, and visualize that the pillow is you as a child, and that you are lovingly and tenderly embracing her, cradling her, and telling her everything will be all right.

Precautions

Depression can be a serious illness—it can affect your whole life and even produce thoughts of suicide. Depression has detrimental affects on the immune system and, most interestingly, has recently been linked with accelerated bone loss in women. If natural approaches haven't helped and you are "down" for more than four months after a difficult event, such as a death in the family—or if sadness lasts more than a couple of weeks and you can't pinpoint the cause of your blues, you should seek advice, counseling, and perhaps medication, from a mental health professional. There are established criteria for diagnosing major depression—the presence of a depressed, irritable mood, with a loss of interest or pleasure in usual activities, including sex, plus at least four other of these symptoms over a 2-week period:

1. Poor appetite and weight loss; increased appetite with weight gain.
2. Disturbed sleep (too much, too little).
3. Excess physical activity or inactivity—agitation or lethargy.
4. Fatigue and loss of energy.
5. Feelings of worthlessness, self-reproach, excessive guilt.
6. Thoughts or attempts of suicide.
7. Difficulty thinking, concentrating, or making decisions; forgetfulness.

Depression can be readily diagnosed by a professional experienced in mental health and controlled by a combination of supportive counseling and medication with any one of a number of products. For psychotherapy, you may see a psychiatrist or a social worker trained in psychotherapy; a marriage, family, and child counselor; a clinical or counseling psychologist. You can expect that your therapist and your psychiatrist will work closely together to discuss your progress.

Digestive Problems

The digestive system, as most of us know only too well, is remarkably reactive to emotional and physical distress. As if that wasn't bad enough, as we age, some of its functions slow down, and we find that we're not able to eat as much as we used to without gastric discomfort, or we become constipated, as waste products move more slowly through the colon. Sluggish bowels, it appears, are more than uncomfortable—they increase the risk of diverticulosis and possibly colon cancer, a leading cause of death among both men and women of middle age and beyond.

While most of us won't get cancer in the digestive system, all of us have felt some dysfunction at one time or another; in this section we talk about the most common ones: constipation, intestinal gas, indigestion, heartburn, diarrhea, abdominal cramps, and nausea. All of these are likely to be more frequent in late middle age and older, and all respond to natural therapies.

Constipation is characterized by difficult, incomplete, or infrequent bowel movements. It is normal among all mammals, including us humans, to have at least one bowel movement per day. Faulty diet is the main culprit among all ages, and increased estrogen and prescription progestins cause bloating and edema, which pulls fluid from the gut, causing hard stools.

Intestinal gas is also related to the slowing down of the digestive system as we get older. Some of the effects of an accumulation of gas are burping, swelling and bloating of the abdomen, and flatulence. A major source of gas is the artificial sweetener sorbitol and the fermentation of food by bacteria that inhabit the large intestine, and some of the foods that produce the most gas are poorly digested beans, nuts, cauliflower, radishes, broccoli, turnips, and raw fruits and vegetables. Swallowing air also produces gas, as may food sensitivities and antibiotics.

Indigestion in older people is often caused by insufficient digestive juices in the intestines. This causes discomfort following meals. Stress, eating quickly, and eating rich foods can also wreak digestive havoc.

Heartburn is more common as people age because the sphincter that prevents acid from backing up into the esophagus may not work entirely properly, causing the bitter taste and burning that we call heartburn. Many people also have a condition known as hiatus hernia, where a part of the stomach goes above the diaphragm. Overeating and tight clothes around your waist can cause your stomach to be pushed up through the sphincter and even go into spasm.

Diarrhea is not a normal concomitant of aging, and should never be taken lightly. Sometimes you know perfectly well what caused a day of diarrhea: for example too many fruits, rich foods, or alcohol. Some women report that diarrhea accompanies their periods or regularly occurs just before a period. This condition hasn't been shown to relate to hormonal changes, but it's possible that if you eat more sweets than usual at this time, you may get diarrhea! Diarrhea may also be a sign of malabsorption—failure of the pancreas to produce the enzymes needed to digest carbohydrates or fats and other nutrients. This is a condition which is more often found in older than younger people because the exhaustion of this gland is more common in aging individuals. Fortunately, once the diagnosis has been made, most of these enzymes can be supplied through oral supplements and better diet can reverse the problem.

Nausea may be caused by viruses, food poisoning, motion sickness, or emotional shock.

General Nutrition

As you follow the Balanced Life Plan provided in Chapter 2, make a special effort to avoid foods that are notorious for causing digestive problems: fried or rich fatty foods, very spicy foods, and foods made with white flour and sugar. Avoid overeating, especially close to bedtime. Being careful not to swallow air (Don't talk while you eat! And don't argue!) will help most digestive problems such as indigestion and gas. So will eating small meals, perhaps six times a day, and eating slowly and chewing thoroughly.

The best cure for *constipation* is a balanced diet and exercise. Also drink 8–16 cups of water a day and don't substitute soft drinks or fruit juice for more than 3 of those cups because even fruit juice is very high in sugar. Artificially sweetened drinks may cause bladder cancer or diarrhea. Caffeinated drinks, by the way, are dehydrating, not hydrating, because they stimulate your kidneys, so if you're constipated, the last thing you need is caffeine, such as is found in coffee, tea, and colas. Caffeine is a bowel stimulant and one cause of constipation is caffeine or tobacco withdrawal. Your constipation should go away after a couple of days of the water treatment. But keep it up. Work it into your regular routine and don't forget to add more if you exercise. If you have *diarrhea,* you should drink water to replace the water you've lost from the loose stools, but eat binding, easily digested foods such as rice, toast, and bananas.

Fiber is also a wonderful substance for promoting regular, satisfying bowel activity. Add as many vegetables, fruits, whole grains, and nuts as you can to your diet. Be cautious with *raw* vegetables such as carrots, cabbage, cauliflower, and broccoli, and with concentrated fiber, such as bran. Add them to your diet gradually, because introducing them in large amounts can bind your stool and can cause cramps, constipation, or diarrhea. Foods that inhibit bowel movements and may add to constipation are: cheese, meat, dairy products, white flour, sugar, and white rice. Eat these in moderation, if at all, while you're trying to cure your constipation.

Although beans are a wonderfully health-building food and their fiber helps prevent constipation, they can cause *intestinal gas.* To reduce this tendency, prepare them by first boiling the dried beans for one minute; remove them from the heat and soak them overnight. Change the cooking water and then cook them completely until tender. You may also want to try taking digestive enzymes to aid digestion generally, or use a product called Bean-O, which works on the hard-to-digest starches in beans. There are also products that restore healthy intestinal flora (bacteria), such as lactobacillus, that many women find helpful in preventing gas. Cooking with certain herbs and spices may also prevent gas; these include cinnamon bark, nutmeg seed, lavender flower essential oil, cloves, rosemary, and cumin. Sprouting beans before cooking them can also eliminate the gas problem.

Finally, if none of the above measures is effective, consider that you may have developed a food allergy or food intolerance; common offenders that cause diarrhea are milk and dairy products, wheat, eggs, corn and corn products, and meat.

Other Lifestyle Considerations

Tension, anxiety, and other stress can cause situational intestinal cramps, gas, and diarrhea; chronic stress can also cause chronic diarrhea, stomach pains, and heartburn. So try to find ways to relax more often and manage the stress in your life. Stress and emotional upheaval can cause digestive upset during and between meals, so try to eat when you are relaxed and not under stress. Slowly sipping a warm beverage usually helps ease the spasm of heartburn, as does deep breathing.

You should get to the bathroom as soon as you ''feel the urge,'' since delaying bowel movements seems to promote constipation. Most gastrointestinal experts suggest that you try to ''go'' at the same time every day. According to traditional Chinese medicine, the ''hour of the bowel'' is early morning, and this is when we have the natural urge for a bowel movement. The brain, which rules the digestive system, is particularly responsive to habit, as you know from getting hunger pangs at the time you usually eat, even if you recently snacked. Remember, smoking tends to worsen heartburn and indigestion, and all that some people need to do to remedy digestive problems is to quit smoking. Although strenuous exercise may not be appealing during times of digestive distress, regular strenuous exercise improves circulation, strengthens muscles, and is a potent antidote to stress—all of which are a boon to healthy digestion. Exercise, even walking, stimulates proper bowel function. A moderately paced walk through pleasant surroundings helps digestion and is particularly helpful in passing painful intestinal gas.

Herbal Remedies

Many women find that herbs help ease digestive problems. For instructions on herbal remedies, *see* Chapter 3, pages 70–75. The herbs listed below are particularly effective in treating this condition; use them singly or in combination, or look for a commercially prepared herbal formula that contains them.

For indigestion or heartburn, an alternative to antacids is licorice. If you have high blood pressure, get pills or powder which is "deglycorrhized" so the licorice doesn't affect your blood pressure. Take ¼–½ teaspoon of licorice powder 15 minutes before meals. An alternative to digestive enzymes is herbal "bitters," which are believed to work by stimulating the taste receptors for bitterness on your tongue, and then the digestive juices. You can buy Angostura Bitters in the liquor section of most grocery stores.

Teas made of *chamomile, ginger, dandelion leaf,* and *gentian* are also useful for indigestion.

Homeopathic Remedies

Following the instructions in Chapter 3, pages 75–81, use a combination remedy or choose the single remedy from the list on page 158 which most closely matches your symptoms. Follow the instructions on the package; if your symptoms are severe, it is usually recommended that you take a dose as often as every 5 minutes; for milder symptoms, take every 3 hours. One dose equals 2–3 pills or 5–10 drops. The most commonly used homeopathic remedies for digestive problems are:

• *Nux vomica.* For heartburn, nausea, and burping after indulging in alcohol, tobacco, coffee, food, or mental stimulation; you feel headachy and irritability and cannot bear noise, odor, or light.

• *Pulsatilla.* When indigestion follows the overeating of rich, fatty foods and symptoms include bloating and a heavy feeling; you are not thirsty and crave open air.

• *Calcarea carbonica.* If you experience no urge to move the bowels, and the stool just sits in the rectum. Calcarea helps the body digest and assimilate food.

• *Lycopodium.* For hard stools that are difficult to pass, or that feel as though much remains behind; when there is a lot of flatus.

• *Natrum muriaticum.* For small round stools that are difficult to pass; when there is an unfinished feeling after a bowel movement; natrum helps by correcting water imbalance during a menstrual period.

• *Sepia.* When you have a weak feeling in the rectum; the stool is hard and large, the abdomen feels full and bloated, and straining to pass stool is unsuccessful; for constipation during menstrual periods.

Acupressure

There are several acupressure points that can help relieve digestive problems. Following the directions in Chapter 3, page 81, apply firm pressure to the points shown in the drawing on pages 159–60.

You may also use acupressure massage, performed either by yourself or by another person. Lie on your back with knees up and feet flat on the floor. Following the diagram, and starting at the top of your abdomen, press your hand gently into the points as shown, working slowing in a clockwise circle. Repeat the circle two or three times, increasing the pressure a bit with each repetition. Breathe deeply during the massage. Then, pressing your knees into your chest, press the heels of the hands firmly into the point below the knee on the outside of your leg. Breathe deeply for a few minutes in this position. Then stretch your legs out on the floor and relax.

When stress causes the abdominal muscles to spasm or bloat, digestion may be impaired regardless of what, how, or how much you eat. You may relieve the resulting indigestion, belching, and gas by practicing the yoga pose known as The Bow as shown in the drawing. Lie on your stomach, bend your knees, and grasp your feet. Inhale and pull on your feet, arching your back. Breathe deeply for half a minute, then release and relax for a few minutes.

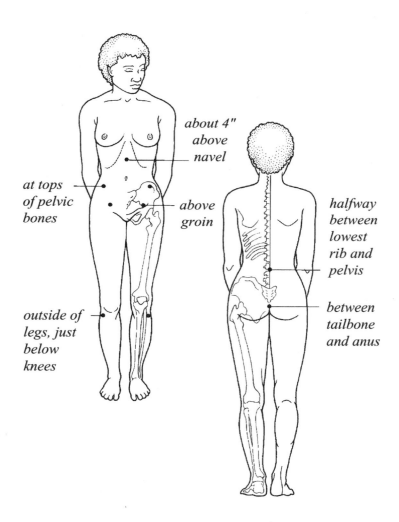

Acupressure Points For Indigestion

Acupressure Points For Constipation

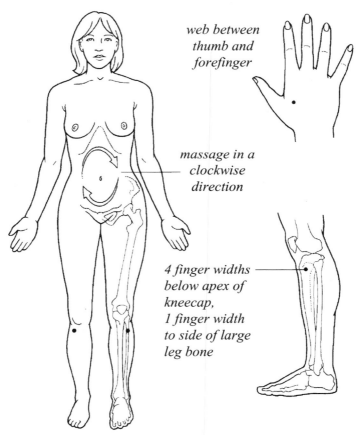

*web between
thumb and
forefinger*

*massage in a
clockwise
direction*

*4 finger widths
below apex of
kneecap,
1 finger width
to side of large
leg bone*

The Bow Pose For Constipation

*Lie facedown on the floor and
grasp your feet. Arch up and
hold for as long as is comfortable,
rocking back and forth gently.
Release down slowly.*

Aromatherapy

There are many ways to use essential oils to correct digestive problems and the tension that precipitates them, as described in Chapter 3, page 84. One way to use aromatherapy to relieve constipation is to apply oil of *marjoram* or *rosemary* (or both) to your abdomen and massage yourself in a clockwise direction. If tension is a contributing factor, a full-body aromatherapy massage will relieve the anxiety, although this may take a few months to resolve. Aromatherapy baths using sedative oils such as *lavender* or *chamomile* will also help relax you and your bowels.

For intestinal gas, apply a calming oil such as *chamomile, marjoram, lavender,* or *orange blossom* to your abdomen and gently massage in a clockwise direction to expel gas and relieve pressure from eating gassy foods.

For diarrhea related to fear, emotional stress or anxiety, try *lavender* or *chamomile;* if your cramps are severe, massage *ginger* or *fennel oil* over your abdomen to ease the gripping pain.

Precautions

Constipation can have serious effects, as you may have already discovered. For example, hard stools can cause hemorrhoids and tearing of the anus. Long-term constipation can lead to impacted stools, which are so hard they can't slide out at all. If you feel pain when you try to defecate, see your doctor.

Indigestion can occur either during or after a large or spicy meal, and can be confused with a heart attack. So watch carefully the course of an attack of indigestion, especially if shortness of breath, sweating, or pain in the chest or arms is present. Better to have it checked out in an emergency room than to deny yourself measures that can save your life. Frequent indigestion should always be mentioned to your health care professional since there are many digestive diseases that cause what we call "indigestion": gastritis, hiatial hernia, gallbladder problems, tumors, or various stones, liver and biliary, among them. Often the symptoms of indigestion are relieved when an osteopath or chiropractor manipulates the vertebrae or ribs.

Heartburn can be caused by ulcers, so if you have constant pain, particularly when your stomach is empty, or if there is nausea, vomitting, or black/bloody stools.

If *diarrhea* continues longer than twenty-four hours, a call to your health care provider is in order. If you have fever, you probably have a viral or bacterial infection or food poisoning. Diarrhea that goes on for more than a couple of days or has blood in it can be a symptom of many serious conditions that need to be ruled out by your physician. Diarrhea may also be a sign of colitis or growths in the colon. These must be assessed, of course.

While nausea and vomiting can occur at any age, their effects are likely to be most severe in the very young and the elderly. This is because of the danger of dehydration. Body fluids must be replaced, so don't go for more than a couple of hours without trying to take sips of ginger tea or ginger ale or sucking on ice. Take sweetened broth to get the salt, sugar, and minerals—we recommend an amino acid broth with honey and ginger. If you're vomiting and on any kind of blood pressure, heart, antipsychotic, antidepressant, or diabetic medication—particularly insulin, it's vital that you check in with your doctor for recommendations about taking your medication while you're not eating—and or not keeping anything down.

Dizziness

Some women report that they experience light-headedness or dizziness when they have a hot flash and when hormone changes occur just before or after a period. This is probably due to vasodilation which diverts blood to the skin surface, or to changes in the central nervous system brought about by hormone imbalance.

However, dizziness has many causes. Low blood pressure, or a poorly responsive sympathic nervous system causes light-headedness when you rise quickly from a lying or sitting position. This causes a momentary decrease of blood flow to the brain, and is called *postural (or "orthostatic") hypotension.* Other causes of dizziness are stroke, medications and drugs, hormone imbalance, inner ear problems, and other medical conditions.

General Considerations
Starvation dieting or sometimes just skipping a meal can sometimes cause dizziness in women. Make sure that, if you're trying to lose weight, you follow the recommendations in the Balanced Life Plan provided in Chapter 2.

Sometimes dizziness accompanies hot flashes or menstrual periods; *see* ''Hot Flashes'' and ''Irregular Periods.''
The following natural remedies are particularly helpful for dizziness.

Homeopathic Remedies

Following the instructions in Chapter 3, pagess 75–81, choose the single remedy that most closely matches your symptoms. Follow the instructions on the package; if your symptoms are severe, it is usually recommended that you take a dose as often as every 5 minutes; for milder symptoms, take every 3 hours. One dose usually equals 2–3 pills or 5–10 drops.

• *Pulsatilla* helps women who feel dizzy before or during their periods; they may also feel faint, nauseated, have vomiting or diarrhea, back pain, and headache at this time; heat usually makes them feel worse, but being in fresh air helps.

• *Lachesis* is a remedy that helps women whose dizziness occurs before their periods but disappears when the flow begins; it may be accompanied by pelvic pain, back pain, headache, and diarrhea. As a general rule, their symptoms are worse upon awakening and may have begun while asleep.

Precautions

If you don't get relief from your dizziness in a few days or by changing positions more slowly, or if the dizziness is associated with a spinning sensation, pain, fever, nausea, vomiting, weight loss, or nervous system changes, you should see your health care provider for a diagnosis.

Dry Eyes

Dry eyes can be common as we age. The signs of dry eyes are itching, a scratchy feeling, redness, tearing, tingling, and irritation. Paradoxically, dry eyes can cause excessive tearing. Eyelashes fall out more easily as we get older, and if the eyes are dry, eyelashes or other foreign bodies may stay in the eye and cause tearing and scratches. To remove an object safely, dampen a cotton swab with salt solution and gently dab the object. If you can't get the object out easily, go to your health care giver, who can do so for you. Dry eyes will tire more easily as you read, particularly at the end of the day. Dry winter air and wind, the dry air in airplanes, and certain medications that cause dry mouth and skin may also cause or aggravate dry eyes. Allergies and sensitivity to environmental toxins such as fumes, smoke, dust, and pollution may also irritate your eyes.

General Considerations

To keep all your tissues strong and as hydrated as possible, make sure to follow the recommendations in the Balanced Life Plan provided in Chapter 2. Women have found the following specific approaches to be particularly helpful for dry eyes.

Herbal Remedies

• *Eyebright.* Make an herbal eyewash by boiling 1 ounce of eyebright in 1 cup of water. Let cool and use as an eyewash to wash and freshen your eyes. This will keep for only 2 days in the refrigerator, so make fresh batches frequently.

Homeopathic Remedies

Homeopathy offers several remedies for dry eyes. Following the instructions in Chapter 3, pages 75–81, choose the single remedy that most closely matches your symptoms. Follow the instructions on the package; if your symptoms are severe, it is usually recommended that you take a dose as often as every 5 minutes; for milder symptoms, take every 3 hours. One dose equals 2–3 pills or 5–10 drops.

• *Belladonna* is useful when your eyes are dry, and bloodshot, and if they burn and are sensitive to light.
• *Bryonia* is useful if eyes are dry and sore and feel worse when you move them.
• There are also homeopathic eye drops that last much longer than artificial tears and can sometimes be curative. We recommend the Similasen brand.

Precautions

Artificial tears are a real boon as we get older. Two or more applications a day may take care of your problem but you should never put anything in your eyes without first consulting with a health care provider. Products that are advertised to "brighten" your eyes, for example, often cause "rebound" redness, or an allergic reaction, and can actually cause damage. They are vasoconstrictors and can even cause high blood pressure if you're susceptible. These are not the same thing as artificial tears. If you have pain, see an ophthalmologist—you may have a scratch on your cornea.

Dry Mouth and Bad Breath

Although our mouths are constantly bathed in it, we don't even give the flow of our saliva a thought until it starts to dry up. A common short-term consequence of anxiety (such as public speaking or going for a job interview), dry mouth is a daily occurrence for 30–50 percent of adults over fifty-five. We're not sure whether aging itself is a contributing factor; we do know that a major identifiable cause is long-term use of medications and drugs of many sorts including medications used to treat depression and high blood pressure. Another reason for dry mouth is Sjögren's syndrome, an autoimmune disorder of the lubricating glands in the mouth and eyes; it affects mostly middle-aged and older women, and may also be linked with silicone breast implants. Other causes of dry mouth are radiation therapy, alcoholism, depression, and diabetes.

Dry mouth not only is annoying, but may lead to yeast infections, tooth decay, mouth ulcers, and bad breath because saliva washes away mouth debris, plaque, sugars and carbohydrates, and helps prevent plaque buildup. Saliva remineralizes teeth and helps combat viruses and bacteria; it makes talking, kissing, and eating comfortable and enjoyable.

If you're bothered by bad breath, dry mouth is not the only cause. BO of the mouth is also caused by digestive problems such as constipation and tooth decay, both of which afflict older people more than younger. (*See* "Digestive Problems.") Tooth decay is more common in older people because of gum disease, which causes loosening of teeth and more room for bacteria to enter. Bad breath and unusual taste may also be due to bowel problems, and indigestion, yeast overgrowth, sinusitis, and tobacco use.

General Nutrition and Other Considerations

To keep all your tissues strong and as hydrated as possible, make sure to follow the recommendations in the Balanced Life Plan provided in Chapter 2.

If you notice your mouth is feeling drier than usual on a regular basis, avoid antihistamines, diuretics, caffeine, alcohol, and cigarettes. Munch on high-water-content raw vegetables such as carrots and celery to stimulate your salivary glands; rinsing your mouth with salt water accomplishes the same thing, as does sugar-free gum or hard candy. Be sure to brush and floss daily and thoroughly.

Women have found the following specific approaches to be particularly helpful for dry mouth and bad breath.

Nutritional Supplements

A good multivitamin-mineral formula containing the doses recommended in Chapter 3, pages 61–64, supplies the nutrients most women need to keep their mouths and digestive systems healthy. If you have or are at high risk for gum disease, you may increase the daily total dose of the following:

• *Vitamin C,* 3,000 mg per day. Take along with *bioflavonoids,* 900 mg per day.

Homeopathic Remedies

Homeopathy is helpful for symptoms of menopause and aging including dry mouth and bad breath. Following the instructions in Chapter 3, pages 75–81, you may find a combination menopause remedy that contains the following remedies, or choose a single remedy that most closely matches your symptoms. Follow the instructions on the package; if your symptoms are severe, it is usually recommended that you take a dose as often as every 5 minutes; for milder symptoms, take every 3 hours. One dose equals 2–3 pills or 5–10 drops.

• *Lachesis* is one of the most often used remedies for women in menopause and perimenopause. It is appropriate for women suffering from bad breath as well as hot flashes, fatigue not helped by sleeping, and symptoms that feel worse before a period and better when the flow starts.

• *Pulsatilla* is useful for many menopausal symptoms and is particularly effective in women with dry mouths and lips and bad breath, who have changeable moods and are clingy, excitable, and sensitive.

• *Sulphur* helps women bothered with bad breath and dry cracked lips, accompanied by a coated tongue; if you are usually very thirsty, sensitive to heat, dislike hot stuffy rooms, and have hot flashes, this remedy may help you.

Precautions

Saliva is necessary for a healthy mouth, so it's important to consult with your health care provider to find out the cause of your dry mouth. If necessary, he or she may prescribe artificial saliva, or 5% glycerine. Consult your dentist for recommendations that can slow down gum disease and tooth decay, such as flossing and brushing routinely.

Fatigue and Low Energy

Although low energy and fatigue are often viewed as inevitable signs of aging, a healthy body at any age supports a healthy, active mind. Fatigue and low energy are often signs of our bodies crying out for help and are frequently helped by nutritional support and botanical agents such as herbs. Let's start with some of the physical reasons for low energy and fatigue:

Insomnia is a prime suspect. Many women report sleep disturbances around the time of menopause triggered by hormonal changes that affect the sleep center of the brain. Other reasons for frequent waking in the menopausal years are the need to urinate more often, and the night sweats. For natural ways to combat these energy drainers, see "Incontinence," "Insomnia," and "Night Sweats" in this chapter.

Much fatigue and low energy in middle-aged and aging people comes from mental stress, overstimulation, overwork, depression, or understimulation. Just as our bodies can get too much or little nourishment, we can think of these factors as malnourishment of the spirit. We need to feel nourished and emotionally rewarded for the efforts we make in our daily lives. There are many reasons why middle-aged women may not feel this satisfaction; we can only mention a few of them here. One reason is that so much of what we do as middle-aged women is take care of others. Our jobs are by no means done just because our kids may be out of the house (indeed, they may be home again, given the expense these days of maintaining their own households and the difficulty of finding well-paying jobs). We may also be caring for our elderly or infirm parents. Even if not physically taking care of them, we have a great many decisions to make about their welfare. It still seems to be true that the daughters and daughters-in-law, not the sons and sons-in-law, take over these responsibilities. Of course, physically caring for elderly relatives would make you physically tired, but it's more than that. It could be emotionally draining if you are worrying again about someone else's well-being and neglecting your own needs, just as you probably did when your kids were young. The difference is that now you feel it's your turn to get something back for those earlier years of self-sacrifice and physical labor, but it seems not to be happening. Making matters worse, many midlife women are joining the "sandwich generation"— taking care of *both* elderly parents and their adult children.

There are so many other things that also might cause stress in the middle years. Maybe you're worrying about a deteriorating relationship with a spouse or partner after many years together. Maybe money worries and lack of employment opportunities or underemployment are getting you down. Perhaps health worries or fears of possible future ill-health bother you. Loss of self-esteem is another significant cause of low energy at this time of life. It hardly seems worthwhile to drag yourself around if you feel no one cares about you or appreciates who you are and what you stand for.

Another tragic and insidious cause of low energy is lack of stimulation. Because they have to care for an ill spouse or aged parents, some women simply take themselves out of circulation. Or they may drop out because they're afraid to meet new people or take on the additional responsibilities that might be a part of joining a new organization or social group. Unfortunately some people move to a new town for their retirement years, only to discover they're bored out of their minds in this new low-stress place. (Boredom can be a sign of depression; *see also* "Depression.") Or they may find that they don't much like the new crowd and miss their old pals more than they dreamed they would. The effects of all this may be that you just don't do enough and can't get excited by your life. Your energy runs low because none of us outgrows the need for stimulation and excitement. We can't thrive and our brains won't maintain its synapses if we're just sitting there in front of the TV or keeping ourselves out of the loop.

Fatigue is one of the most common complaints in a doctor's office and there are many causes for fatigue—some of them serious. Metabolic and hormonal disorders produce fatigue, as do almost all disease, so don't put up with feeling dragged down for longer than a week or two; certainly if your fatigue is severe, seek a professional diagnosis.

Since depression or anemia (for example, from loss of too much blood) may lead to fatigue and low energy, *see also* "Depression" and "Heavy Periods."

General Nutrition

One of the first things we do to combat fatigue is to give ourselves an artificial lift by reaching for the coffee, tea, colas, or other caffeinated beverages. Not only are these health-busters if you rely on them too regularly, but they actually set you up for a late-in-the-day letdown. If taken too late at night, they'll ruin your sleep, tempting you to perk up in the morning with another couple of cups, and setting you up for a vicious cycle. Better to start the day by splashing some cold water on your face. When you first wake up, make your first words "I feel terrific" and repeat them twenty-five times.

Eat a light lunch—large midday meals often lead to a midafternoon slump. Eating too much, especially of fatty foods or refined carbohydrates, can make you feel lethargic, as can inadequate vitamins and minerals, particularly the B vitamins, iron, manganese, phosphorus, and potassium. As you follow the Balanced Life Plan provided in Chapter 2, make a special effort to emphasize fresh whole foods and whole grains that are rich in B vitamins, and foods rich in iron and other minerals such as green leafy vegetables. There's anecdotal evidence that garlic may give you extra energy and endurance, so if you like the flavor, by all means indulge.

Other Lifestyle Considerations

If your get up and go "got up and went," you'll be amazed at the energizing powers of regular vigorous exercise. Lying around like a couch potato or desk potato doesn't conserve energy as some people think—it actually makes you more tired and lethargic. It may seem difficult to bestir yourself if you've been in a low-energy slump for some time, but once they start, many people have just as much trouble stopping as they did starting because they feel so much peppier.

Smoking and caffeine ultimately sap energy, so if you want more zing in your life, go ahead and quit them both.

If understimulation could be a root cause of your lack of energy, the answer is to get involved and don't wait for your partner to go with you or share your activities. It's your responsibility to take care of your own needs for more stimulation so get out there and mingle, or join, or take a class in computers and learn how to get on-line, or start politicking for better schools, or better government, or whatever. If your life isn't any good to you, that doesn't mean it isn't any good to somebody else, and when you make yourself valuable to someone else, whether through political action or personal contact, you'll begin to feel more valuable to yourself!

While that sounds familiar and you may know it's the right philosophy, if you're really depressed, you may not feel up to making the first move. If that's your situation, you need counseling, and group counseling may be just the ticket. It's cheaper than individual therapy, and research shows that it's just as effective. Better yet, a self-help or support group of your peers, with no paid leader, is effective, too. Self-help groups of all kinds are listed in the Resources section in the back of the book.

Women have found the following specific approaches to be particularly helpful for this complaint.

Nutritional Supplements

A good multivitamin-mineral formula containing the doses recommended in Chapter 3, pages 61–64, usually supplies the basic nutrients women need to keep their metabolism humming and their energy levels high. You may increase the total daily dose of the following:

• *Vitamin B complex,* up to fifty times the RDA for some B vitamins. Have your doctor check your B-12 blood level; you may need B-12 shots initially, to get your levels up. Folate may be taken as well, up to 400–800 mcg per day. Pantothenic acid is often recommended for low energy, too—the usual dose is a 500 mcg tablet once or twice a day.

• *Vitamin C,* 3,000 mg per day, to support the adrenal glands.

• *Chromium,* up to 200 mcg per day, to help stabilize blood sugar and raise your energy level.

You may also wish to take:

• *Bee pollen,* 1–2 tablespoons per day.
• *Adrenal glandular supplements,* 1 or 2 capsules with every meal.

Herbal Remedies
Many women find that herbs help elevate energy levels. For instructions on herbal remedies, *see* Chapter 3, pages 70–75. An all-purpose menopausal herbal remedy may help. Or choose from among the herbs listed below, which are particularly effective in treating fatigue; use them singly or in combination, or look for a commercially prepared herbal formula that contains them.

• *Ginseng,* particularly in combination with *licorice,* is often the first line of offense in combating fatigue, increasing energy, and boosting endurance and stamina. Take 1 capsule or 1 cup of decoction up to three times daily.
• *Rosemary,* either 1 cup of infusion or ¼–½ teaspoon of tincture taken in the morning and at night.
• *Peppermint,* taken as an infusion (drink as much as you want) two to three times a day.

Homeopathic Remedies
Homeopathy offers several remedies for fatigue and low energy. Following the instructions in Chapter 3, pages 75–81, use a combination remedy for general menopausal symptoms that contains the following remedies, or choose the single remedy that most closely matches your symptoms. Follow the instructions on the package; if your symptoms are severe, it is usually recommended that you take a dose as often as every 5 minutes; for milder symptoms, take every 3 hours. One dose equals 2–3 pills or 5–10 drops.

• *Lachesis* is often used by women who are menopausal and suffer from fatigue; this remedy is indicated if your exhaustion is worse in the morning, from the heat of the sun, or after physical or mental exertion. Women who benefit from lachesis are talkative and lively and very sensitive to touch.
• *Sepia* is another commonly prescribed remedy for women during menopause. This remedy is indicated if you are generally sluggish,

irritable, depressed, feel "worn out," and want to be left alone; if your fatigue is worse in the morning and during your periods or after exercise.

• *Pulsatilla* is called for if you have "nervous" exhaustion and if you are a gentle, emotional person who wilts in the sun or feels worse in a stuffy room or in the heat.

Acupressure

Acupressure massage (*see* Chapter 3, page 81) is a quick and pleasurable way to restore energy. Foot massage is generally stimulating; work from your ankle to the arch, sole, and then toes. Use firm pressure and enjoy the rejuvenating effects of massaging the many energy meridians that run through your feet and toes. The drawing on page 173 shows a first-aid revival point on the foot that reportedly energizes the whole body. Another pick-me-up is to rock on your back; this stimulates the acupressure points all long your spine, providing a whole-body treatment. If you rock onto your upper shoulders, you'll help release muscle tension which contributes to fatigue. As you rock, press your thumb or finger on the point shown in the other diagram, on the outside of your knees; this is another traditional energizing point.

Aromatherapy

There are many essential oils that are known for their invigorating properties. Add 6 drops of *geranium, rosemary, thyme,* or *marjoram* to your bath, or 2 drops of *clove* or *nutmeg* to 4 drops of the former. *Rosemary* and *basil* are particularly effective at combatting mental burnout. Alternatively, use calming oils to enhance sleep (*see* "Insomnia") to help you recharge your batteries naturally.

Natural Hormone Therapy

Fatigue may be due to a hormone imbalance. Replacing thyroid, DHEA, and testosterone as well as estrogen and even progesterone can improve energy. If you suspect hormone imbalance could be related to this problem, we advise you to discuss this possibility with a holistically minded physician.

Acupressure Points For Fatigue

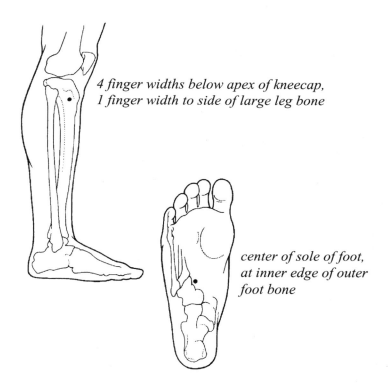

4 finger widths below apex of kneecap, 1 finger width to side of large leg bone

center of sole of foot, at inner edge of outer foot bone

Rocking Motion For Fatigue

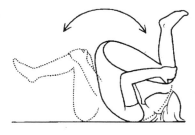

Lie on your back and grasp the sides of your knees. Roll back until your shoulders touch the ground, then roll forward; repeat as often as you like, until you feel invigorated.

Precautions

Mild fatigue is best treated with natural methods. Chronic or overwhelming fatigue that doesn't respond to the self-care approaches suggested here may signal any number of underlying serious conditions, including anemia, hypoglycemia, diabetes, cancer, fibromyalgia, infection with bacteria, fungi, or viruses. If you or your doctor believe you have chronic fatigue syndrome, be aware there may be an underlying cause—anything from parasites to a toxic exposure can be a cause of fatigue. However, your doctor may not be prepared to hunt down and treat the less threatening causes of vague symptoms such as fatigue. These include exhaustion of your adrenal glands (for example, from too much stress), environmental or food allergies, sensitivities, a burned-out immune system, and problems with assimilating food. Immune dysfunctions may allow systemic infection such as yeast infection and the flourishing of common viruses which often include fatigue as the initial overwhelming symptom.

Hair Loss and Excess Hair

Changes in hair are common as people age. Scalp and pubic hair gets thinner and loses body; simultaneously, hair may sprout and thicken in unaccustomed and undesirable places such as the chin, the upper lip, and the abdomen!

Excess hair in women is usually due to a higher proportion of the sex hormone testosterone as compared to the hormone estrogen. Both men and women have a small amount of the other sex's primary sex hormone. As women age, their estrogen loss raises the testosterone-to-estrogen ratio in their bodies, and because of the hair-growing effects of testosterone, hair pops up in new places and may thicken in the armpits and groin.

Thinning hair, on the other hand, is usually due to a decreased thyroid effect or other hormone imbalance. Estrogen treatments to try to reverse or prevent hair loss, however, seem to be ineffective. Anorexia also can result in hair loss, as can anemia and vitamin and mineral deprivation, emotional stress, and disturbed estrogen production. Temporary and reversible hair loss can also result from chemotherapy, anesthesia, oral contraception, and other medications such as cortisone, blood thinners, and drugs or treatments meant to reduce thyroid output. Amphetamines (speed or "uppers"), chemical toxicities and sensitivities, and autoimmune problems have also been associated with hair loss.

General Nutrition

Although sometimes very ill or malnourished people have gorgeous heads of hair, generally hair is a reflection of overall health (as is skin). So if you care about your hair, follow the Balanced Life Plan outlined in Chapter 2, making a special effort to get adequate protein and foods high in vitamin B and essential fatty acids.

Other Lifestyle Considerations

Stress and emotional upheaval can contribute to hormonal imbalance and hair loss so be extra good to yourself and consider exploring ways to relax and manage stress (*see* ''Anxiety''). Regular strenuous exercise is a terrific stress-buster and can improve the blood circulation to your scalp. But be sure to shampoo after each workout that makes you sweat, to keep your scalp clean and healthy.

Avoid practices that increase hair loss. Swimming in chlorinated water, and chemical treatments such as permanents or body waves, straightening, and/or excessive bleaching, damage the hair and can promote breakage or damage to the follicles from which hair grows. Even henna is drying to your hair; try mixing it with coconut oil instead of water.

Tight hair styles such as pulled-back ponytails or braids may cause the hair in the front of the scalp to fall out by damaging the follicles; backcombing also damages hair. Rollers and clips pull follicles out when you wind the hair tightly around them; foam rubber rollers may be gentler—be sure to wind the hair very loosely. Use a wide-toothed comb to gently unsnarl any knots, beginning from the ends and working your way to the roots; a good conditioner also forestalls tangles. Excessive heat from hair dryers can cause the hair to become brittle by removing the natural oils that keep your hair flexible and stretchy. If your hair is brittle, obviously it will break easily when you want to pin it or during brush and combing sessions. Some hair experts believe that because gentle daily scalp massage stimulates the blood circulation to scalp and rids the hair follicles of debris, it may also minimize hair loss as we get older. Use gentle motions similar to those used when you shampoo. Try to wear a hairstyle that doesn't require that you sit under a dryer for a half-hour or so. The best way to dry your hair is by gentle toweling followed by air-drying; if you must, use an electric dryer on medium-heat, held at least 6 inches from your head. If you swim regularly, use a snug-fitting bathing cap and also wash your hair with shampoo specially formulated to remove chlorine deposits.

You can compensate for hair loss by a number of measures. For instance, you can choose a hairstyle that makes your hair look fuller. Short hair is better than long; gentle curls better than straight, unless to get your hair curly you'd have to use too-strong chemicals; hair that frames or hugs your face is better than hair that hangs below your chin. Hair-thickening shampoos and products really do make a difference—after several weeks' use, they coat the hair shaft, making it feel and appear to have more body and thickness. Mousses also add bulk and body to fine, limp hair.

Women have found the following specific natural approaches to be particularly helpful for hair changes.

Herbal Remedies

Many women find that herbs help with hair problems. For instructions on taking herbs internally, as teas, tinctures, and infusions, *see* Chapter 3, pages 70–75. Use an all-purpose menopausal herbal remedy to balance your hormones. You may also find the following herbal hair rinse helpful: Add 1 tablespoon each of *rosemary, dried nettles,* and *yarrow* to 2 cups of water. Bring to a boil; then shut off the flame and let the mixture cool. Strain the herbs and add 1 cup of plain water; use as a leave-in rinse after every shampoo. This is reputed to stimulate regrowth of hair and add shine.

Homeopathic Remedies

Homeopathy offers several remedies for problem hair. Following the instructions in Chapter 3, pages 75–81, use a combination menopausal remedy or choose the single remedy that most closely matches your symptoms. Follow the instructions on the package; if your symptoms are severe, it is usually recommended that you take a dose as often as every 5 minutes; for milder symptoms, take every 3 hours. One dose equals 2–3 pills or 5–10 drops.

- *Kali carbonica* for hair that falls out and is dry.
- *Bryonia* for hair that falls out and is oily.

• *Sepia* for hair loss associated with PMS, and for women who cry and feel irritable and chilly.

Aromatherapy

The essential oil of *sage* may help balance hormones, which is important whether your hair is thinning or sprouting where you'd rather it didn't. Stress, which can contribute to hair problems, may be relieved by aromatherapy with *bergamot, clary sage, neroli, rose, jasmine, sandalwood,* and *ylang-ylang.* Try adding *rosemary, lavender,* or *thyme* to a base of warm coconut oil or jojoba or almond oil, and rub into your hair follicles gently twice a week. Leave on for 2 hours and then shampoo gently.

Precautions

See your health care provider if your hair loss is sudden or your hair is coming out in clumps. Sudden or dramatic hair loss can be a sign of illness, stress, or an abnormal physical condition such as anemia or hypothyroidism, which can, when treated, reverse the hair loss. Excess hair is a cause for concern if it is accompanied by a deepening of your voice, acne, and an enlarged clitoris. Your doctor needs to rule out pituitary or adrenal problems.

Headaches

While almost everyone gets a headache at one time or another, some women are more prone to headaches, and if you are one of them, this may indicate that the symptom is your way of reacting to some form of stress. While some women report increases in the number and severity of headaches around the menopausal years, even more say that the headaches that plagued them just before, during, or just after their periods for years nearly disappeared once their periods stopped for good. Headaches that appear for the first time or intensify around menopause seem to be related to different hormone balances. The estrogen in hormone replacement therapy (HRT) may cause headaches.

There are two main categories of common headaches: muscle contraction or tension headache; and vascular or migraine headache. Sinus headaches and headaches due to eyestrain are also very common. Very often headaches are a mixed variety.

Muscle contraction ("tension") headaches. The most common type of headache, this usually feels like a dull ache with some tightness and tenderness at the temples, around the forehead, or where the skull meets the neck. It may be due to mental stress from, for example, overwork, or the mundane stress of everyday life such as being stuck in traffic. A tension headache may also be the result of physical stress, such as too little sleep, a long tedious drive, or poor posture. Sometimes both mental and physical stress are involved, as when sitting at a desk or straining at a computer for long periods of time in order to meet a deadline. Under stress conditions, the body reacts by tightening the muscles in the scalp, jaw, neck, shoulders, and back; eventually the muscles protest from the constant contraction. They stay sore and tight, and squeeze the nerves and blood vessels that feed muscles and other soft tissues, causing radiating pain that you can feel anywhere in your face and neck.

Vascular headaches (migraine). Migraine is a French word derived from the Latin word *hemicrania,* which means "pain in half of the head." This type of headache usually affects only one side of the head, bringing severe throbbing pain. Before the headache begins, there may be visual disturbances such as visions of lights, bright or geometric shapes and lines, and "tunnel" vision, or sensations of a strange taste or odor, tingling, dizziness, slurred speech, ringing in the ears, and weakness in a part of the body. As the headache progresses, there may be nausea, vomiting, chills, and extreme fatigue. This type of headache is associated with the spasm of blood vessels; however, what actually causes the pain is unknown. We do know there is an inflammatory response involving many biochemicals. A migraine may last for hours or days, and may be triggered by hypersensitivity or allergic reactions to foods, alcohol, bright lights, some medications, or loud noises. Some women also experience migraines due to hormonal fluctuations such as occur with the menstrual cycle or menopause; the culprit seems to be too much estrogen in relation to progesterone, and progesterone therapy sometimes helps these women.

General Considerations

For tension headache, try to determine and relieve the source of physical or emotional stress that is causing the headache. Examples are: poor posture at work, noise, holding the telephone between the ear and shoulder, eyestrain or ill-fitting eyeglasses, and various emotional and social conflicts. Take frequent breaks, periodically look into the distance if you do close work, and get proper work equipment. Rest if the headache makes you tired, or is severe. Wet, hot compresses or a hot bath reduces the muscle spasms and relaxes you all over.

Headaches may also accompany constipation (*see* page 154) or dehydration, both of which are often prevented and relieved by drinking plenty of water throughout the day. Also make sure your diet emphasizes high-fiber foods such as fruits, vegetables, and whole grains to keep your system unclogged.

Headache Triggers

Keep a food headache diary and look for foods and beverages that may be associated with your headaches. Some people are sensitive to certain foods or combinations; some people get headaches when they skip a meal, or do not drink enough fluids. Many people have headaches as a withdrawal symptom when they suddenly cut out all coffee—it's better to taper off gradually. Several foods are known to trigger migraine, including chocolate, nuts, coffee, cheese, citrus fruits, and alcohol. However, any food can be a trigger if you're sensitive to it, as can cigarette smoke, perfumes, lights, outgassing from building materials and gasoline. We find that 85 percent of all headache problems resolve by uncovering and dealing with food and environmental allergies or by treating osteopathic bone or muscle causes in the neck or jaw. Stress is another possible trigger, so think about stressful situations that you could avoid.

Women have found the following specific natural approaches to be particularly helpful in treating headaches.

Herbal Remedies

Many women find that herbs help relieve mild headaches. For instructions on herbal remedies, *see* Chapter 3, pages 70–75. An all-purpose menopausal herbal remedy may relieve the headache that accompanies other menopausal symptoms; or choose from among the following herbs, which are particularly effective in treating this condition:

• *Feverfew* is a popular herbal headache remedy for headaches arising from stress. It inhibits the secretion of serotonin, decreases blood vessel constriction, and inhibits the production of inflammatory chemicals. Take 1 capsule up to three times a day.

• *Black cohosh* is used for headaches related to muscle spasm and anxiety; this herb can make women feel sleepy, especially the elderly. The dose is 1 capsule or 1 teaspoon of the tincture, up to three times a day.

• *Valerian* is a useful herb if your headache is related to nervous tension. Take 1 cup of the infusion before bedtime, or 1 teaspoon of tincture up to three times a day.

• *Avena sativa* helps if your headache is from overwork or depression.

Homeopathic Remedies

Homeopathic remedies are helpful for mild to moderate headaches. Following the instructions in Chapter 3, pages 75–81, use a combination remedy containing the following substances or choose the single remedy that most closely matches your symptoms from the list below of commonly used remedies. Follow the instructions on the package; if your symptoms are severe, it is usually recommended that you take a dose as often as every 5 minutes; for milder symptoms, take every 3 hours. One dose equals 2–3 pills or 5–10 drops.

• *Belladonna.* For burning, throbbing, violent headaches that start suddenly; when the symptoms are worse from light, noise, and bending down, cold or heat, exposure to sun, or during the menstrual period, when symptoms are better with lying down in a darkened room, pressure or wrapping the head in a warm covering, or sitting down.

• *Nux vomica.* For a "splitting headache" brought on by too much food, alcohol, coffee or mental strain, or too little sleep; for headaches that are worse in the morning, after eating, and upon shaking the head and better at night, with excitement, and after getting up.

• *Bryonia.* For dull, steady, or heavy headaches that last all day and are located mostly behind the eyeballs (particularly the left one) and in the forehead; when symptoms are worse with coughing, after getting up, and with even slight motion of the head or eyes; and when the headache is better with pressure and cold compresses.

• *Pulsatilla.* For throbbing, "nervous" headaches that may affect just the forehead, or be one-sided; they may be related to the men-

strual period, or come about as the result of nervousness or excitement. The headache is worse in a hot stuffy room, or after eating,
bending or lying down, blowing the nose, or a vigorous activity such
as running. It is better with walking in the fresh air and with pressure.

 • *Gelsemium.* For heavy, aching, sore pain that begins in the back of
the head and may spread to the forehead, or is felt over the right eye or
temple. There may be visual disturbances or other accompanying
symptoms common in migraine; the head feels as though a tight band
were encircling it and the eyes feel heavy lidded. The symptoms are
worse with motion, light, and noise.

Acupressure

Several acupressure points are used to relieve headache pain (*see*
Chapter 3, page 81). Apply firm pressure directly to the painful areas
on your scalp, face, and neck (use the drawing below as a guide to the
most common painful spots). Maintain the pressure for a few minutes.
You can also try pressing the points on your hand, in the web between
your index finger and thumb—this often provides instant relief for all

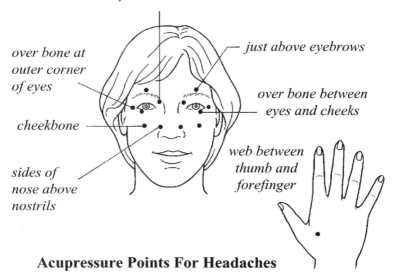

over the bone between
inner eye corners and brows

over bone at
outer corner
of eyes

just above eyebrows

over bone between
eyes and cheeks

cheekbone

sides of
nose above
nostrils

web between
thumb and
forefinger

Acupressure Points For Headaches

kinds of pain. Finally, if your headache is one-sided, you can press the thumb of the affected side as shown.

Aromatherapy

The essential oils of *lavender* and *peppermint,* used singly or together, work wonders for painful headaches. Inhale or rub a few drops of the lavender on your temples, forehead, or back of the neck; or apply a cold aromatic compress. *Rosemary* helps clear your head and relieve pain, particularly after mental exertion. If your headache stems from sinus congestion, inhale any of these oils, plus *eucalyptus,* to clear the sinuses and relieve the pain. Tiger balm, available at most health food stores, is a classic Asian headache reliever.

Relaxation and Mind-Body Techniques

The relaxation techniques for reducing and managing stress can work wonders in relieving and preventing chronic tension headaches (*see* Chapter 3, page 86). If you experience frequent headaches, regularly scheduled massages or body work may help prevent them; self-massaging the scalp, face, neck, shoulders, and back may also help. In addition, migraine sufferers report relief with biofeedback, which teaches you how to warm your hands by increasing the blood flow to them. Dr. Maas produced a series of video and audiotapes for the release of tension and pain that have helped many women get relief from tension headaches (*see* Resources section).

Natural Hormone Therapy

There are reports that *natural progesterone* relieves premenstrual migraines. (*See* Chapter 4 for more information on natural progesterone.) The suggested dose is ¼–½ teaspoon of progesterone cream applied to the back of your neck and across your forehead and temples, along with ¼ teaspoon (4 drops) of natural progesterone oil held under your tongue and repeated every half hour as necessary.

Balancing hormones can relieve premenstrual migraines. Natural progesterone, which balances the water-retention effect of estrogen, has been helpful in relieving headaches. Have your hormone levels checked and appropriately replaced if low.

Precautions

A severe, sudden headache that is not accompanied by any uterine cramping, or headaches that go on for days, should be investigated by your health care professional—especially if blurred vision, numbness in the face or limbs, or dizziness are present. Medical care should also be sought when a headache is unusually severe; lasts more than three days; occurs frequently; is steadily worsening; is accompanied by a stiff neck or fever; or occurs after a head injury or after taking a medicine (including birth control pills). Also see a doctor if you have a headache that for the first time is accompanied by migraine symptoms. You may need treatment for sinus or other infection if the headache goes with fever, night sweats, putrid post-nasal drip, or unusual aches and pains anywhere.

Heart Palpitations

Some women experience heart palpitations during menopause. Although this can be frightening and uncomfortable, a racing heart does not usually indicate heart disease. The rapid or irregular heartbeat—up to 200 beats per minute—that some women experience during or after menopause can be related to the same vasal mechanisms that produce hot flashes. They can also accompany hot flashes. A hormone imbalance is implicated in both, since your endocrine system interacts with your nervous system and together they are sometimes referred to as the neuroendocrine system.

Nerves and muscles control the width of your blood vessels, and the fibers of the muscles surrounding your blood vessels contract, closing off the arteries, or relax, allowing them to open. This is controlled by the vasomotor center in your brain stem and by local hormonal factors which regulate blood pressure and heart function. Misread signals from the nerves to the brain may also be responsible for the sensations of itchy, crawly skin, and numbness and tingling in the extremities that some women experience during this time of life.

Heart palpitations may also indicate anxiety or stress; metabolic problems such as low calcium, magnesium, or potassium; caffeinism; thyroid or adrenal imbalance; or a surge of adrenaline due to toxicity, food allergy, or environmental sensitivity.

See also ''Hot Flashes'' and ''Night Sweats.''

General Considerations

Heavy smoking and lots of caffeine or alcohol increase the frequency and severity of heart palpitations during menopause. If you experience minor heart palpitations, close your eyes and place one hand on your heart, the other on your belly. Breathe slowly and deeply for several minutes or until your heartbeat slows down to normal.

Nutritional Supplements

A good multivitamin-mineral formula containing the doses recommended in Chapter 3, pages 61–64, supplies the nutrients most women need to prevent or minimize heart palpitations. You may increase the total daily dose of the following:

- *Vitamin E,* up to 1,200 IU, is a frequently used remedy for heart palpitations.
- *Magnesium,* up to 1,000 mg between meals, relaxes the muscles of the chest, heart, and lungs.
- *Calcium,* in equal doses to magnesium.
- *Potassium,* 99 mg three times a day.

You may also wish to take:

- *Gamma-oryzynol,* 20 to 300 mg per day. This component of rice oil is used in Japan because it rejuvenates and stabilizes the autonomic nervous system (ANS). The Japanese believe the ANS is involved in vasomotor menopausal symptoms such as hot flashes and those mentioned here. In one study using 75 mg per day, women experienced improvement in palpitations within one week of beginning the therapy.
- *Carnitine,* 500 mg three times a day.
- *Co-enzyme Q-10,* 25 mg three times a day. This vitaminlike substance increases the energy of the heart cells.
- *Ginkgo biloba,* 40 mg three times a day. This antioxidant aids oxygen supply to the blood and heart.

Herbal Remedies

For instructions on herbal remedies, *see* Chapter 3, pages 70–75. An all-purpose menopausal herbal remedy may alleviate heart palpitations and other vasomotor menopausal symptoms. Or choose from among the herbs listed below, which are particularly effective in treating this condition. Use them singly or in combination, or look for a commercially prepared herbal formula that contains them.

• *Hawthorne* is the preeminent herb for the heart. Take it as an infusion up to 2 cups daily, or ¹/₂–1 teaspoon of tincture of hawthorne up to three times a day. This herb requires 1 month to see results.

• *Motherwort* taken with meals and before bedtime tones the heart; take up to 2 cups of the infusion daily, or ¹/₂–1 teaspoon of the tincture up to twice daily. Or you may take 25–50 drops of the tincture for immediate relief of a wildly pounding heart.

• *Valerian* is used traditionally as a natural sedative and it helps slow a racing heart due to anxiety and probably affects the muscles of the heart, too. Take 1 cup of infusion before bedtime, or 1 teaspoon of the tincture up to three times a day.

• *An-Plex,* a formula containing a combination of vitamins, minerals, herbs, and other botanicals, is highly recommended by Dr. Maas.

Precautions
Palpitations can be a serious problem. It is wisest to have an EKG and a medical evaluation, especially if heart disease runs in your family. Heart disease is often overlooked in menopausal women. Minor heart valve prolapse (which is present in 10 percent of the population) may become suddenly noticeable at menopause. Go to an emergency room immediately if palpitations accompany dizziness, troubled breathing, sweating, chest pain or pressure, nausea, weakness, or unusual heaviness in your neck, jaw, or arm.

Heavy Periods (Menorrhagia)

Changes in your menstrual cycle are often the first sign of approaching menopause. The time between your menstrual periods may become longer or shorter. Some women's flow becomes lighter; others experience menorrhagia, the heavy, excessive menstrual bleeding which often occurs during the years preceding menopause (perimenopause).

Moderately heavy menstrual bleeding can prove both physically annoying and emotionally stressful to any woman. But you may find it particularly troublesome if you have had regular, mild periods during your twenties and thirties. As early as your late thirties or early forties, you may begin to have excessive bleeding for a day or two each month. Heavy bleeding may even be accompanied by other symptoms, such as dizziness, weakness, and cramping. Some women experience the symptoms of temporary anemia owing to the loss of oxygen-rich red blood cells.

The important thing to remember is that all this is part of your body's way of coping with natural hormonal changes. Irregular and somewhat heavy bleeding is a normal physiological reaction to the prolonged release of the hormone estrogen from your ovaries, without ovulation actually taking place. Ovulation is delayed because, as you grow older, the remaining follicles in your ovaries become resistant to FSH (the follicle-stimulating hormone) secreted by the hypothalamus gland in your brain. Either that, or they don't develop an egg, and thus no progesterone is produced. Without progesterone, the estrogen is "unopposed" and keeps building up the lining of the womb. The menstrual fluid which you normally shed during your period never gets the signal to stop thickening. It keeps growing and sheds irregularly. Because of the extra thickness, the bleeding is unusually heavy. Less frequently in this age group, the irregular bleeding is due to too little estrogen.

While most cases of menorrhagia are due to normal hormonal changes preceding menopause, you should see your doctor to rule out other underlying causes if the bleeding persists. There are many steps that you can take to make yourself as comfortable as possible as you pass through this natural change of life.

See also "Menstrual Cramps and PMS" and "Irregular Periods."

General Nutrition

As you follow the Balanced Life Plan provided in Chapter 2, make a special effort to eat plenty of natural sources of iron, such as legumes, kale, molasses, and yeast. Lean meat, poultry, and fish are other iron-rich foods, but some women who bleed heavily bleed less if they avoid meat; many of Dr. Maas's patients have decreased their bleeding during perimenopause by switching to a vegan diet. Vegetarian sources of iron should be eaten with vitamin C–rich foods (citrus fruits, tomatoes, and broccoli) to increase absorption. Also try to eat plenty of citrus fruits, which are rich in valuable bioflavonoids, and foods rich in beta-carotene (carrots, cantaloupe).

Other Lifestyle Considerations

Around the beginning of your period, avoid caffeine, spicy foods, alcohol, aspirin, ibuprofin, or other drugs that inhibit blood clotting. Remember, smoking tends to worsen menopausal symptoms, including menorrhagia, so now is the time to quit. Stress and emotional upheaval seem to worsen bleeding so be extra good to yourself and consider exploring ways to relax and manage stress. Although strenuous exercise may be the last thing on your mind *during* a heavy period, strenuous activity when you're not bleeding is one of the best antidotes to stress. In addition, an active life and regular exercise can help balance ovarian hormones. Finally, hot showers or baths may be relaxing, but are best avoided when you are bleeding heavily because this can increase blood flow.

Women have found the following specific natural therapies to be particularly helpful in treating heavy bleeding.

Nutritional Supplements

Studies have shown that nutritional deficiencies can worsen or even induce cases of menorrhagia. A good multivitamin-mineral formula containing the doses recommended in Chapter 3, pages 61–64, usually supplies the nutrients needed to prevent or minimize this condition. You may increase the total daily dose of the following:

• *Iron,* 30–300 mg. Women who experience heavy menstrual bleeding tend to lose excessive amounts of iron in their menstrual fluid. Some medical studies have shown that an inadequate amount of iron in a woman's body may actually *cause* menorrhagia. Get your blood iron level tested before you take iron supplements to determine how much supplementation you need. Iron overload is a serious health hazard and anything over 20 mg should be taken under medical supervision. Ferritin and iron chelated to amino acids and other carrier molecules are better absorbed and cause fewer digestive problems than elemental iron such as iron sulfate.
• *Beta-carotene,* 25,000–50,000 IU. Carotenes are critical to forming healthy new blood to replace the blood you are losing. Women with menorrhagia have low vitamin A more often than healthy women; supplementing with beta-carotene, the precursor to vitamin A, may alone decrease heavy bleeding.
• *Vitamin C,* 500–5,000 mg per day; take with an equal amount of

bioflavonoids. Bioflavonoids have had remarkable success in the relief of heavy bleeding because of their ability to strengthen capillary walls.

You may also wish to take:

• *Essential fatty acids,* 45 mg per day of gammalinoleic acid (GLA), found in evening primrose oil, black currant oil, or borage oil supplements, and 250 mg of EPA per day from fish oil help you maintain prostaglandin production and substantially reduces menorrhagia. Or take 1–1½ teaspoons of fresh, organic flax seeds or flax seed oil.

Herbal Remedies

Many women have found herbs reduce their bleeding and discomfort. For instructions on using herbal remedies, *see* Chapter 3, pages 70–75. Use an all-purpose menopausal herbal formula that helps menopausal symptoms generally, or choose from among the herbs listed below, which are particularly effective in treating heavy bleeding. You may use them either singly or in combination.

• *Dandelion leaves* (1 cup of infusion, 1 teaspoon of tincture, or 1 cup of decoction up to three times a day) or *yellow dock root* (1 cup of decoction or 1 teaspoon of tincture up to three times a day) are excellent herbal sources of extra iron. (However, if you are bleeding very heavily, these may not contain enough extra iron for you.)
• *Shepherd's purse* is the primary herb recommended for heavy uterine bleeding.
• *Lady's mantle* was recently studied in 300 women. When taken after their periods began, this herb controlled bleeding within 3–5 days; when taken 1–2 weeks before bleeding began, it prevented heavy bleeding. The usual dose is up to 3 cups a day of infusion, or ½–1 teaspoon of tincture up to three times a day.

Homeopathy

Homeopathy is sometimes helpful for this condition. Following the instructions in Chapter 3, pages 75–81, use a combination remedy or choose the single remedy that most closely matches your symptoms from the following list.

• *Lachesis* is one of the best remedies for this condition. Use this when your blood flow is very dark, thick, and strong-smelling; if you have pain that is more intense at the beginning of your period; and if you have feelings of rage during bleeding.

• *Sepia* is another commonly prescribed remedy for heavy bleeding. This is indicated if your periods are frequent, you bleed heavily, you feel pain, and if bleeding is accompanied by backache, constipation, and depression.

• *Belladonna* is useful when your bleeding is bright red and has clots; if you feel oversensitive; and if you have a headache.

Aromatherapy

Oil of *cypress* has helped reduce heavy menstrual bleeding as has *geranium, rose,* and *eucalyptus.* The essential oil of *sage* may help balance hormones, which is important during menorrhagia. Stress, which can aggravate bleeding problems, may be relieved by aromatherapy with *lavender,* which has a nurturing tonic effect on your nervous system. *Chamomile* can also calm the tensions which accompany menopause. See Chapter 3, page 84, for suggestions on how to use essential oils.

Precautions

Most cases of menorrhagia are temporary and due to hormonal changes in your body as you make your way through this natural change of life. However, heavy bleeding is sometimes due to more serious underlying causes. To be on the safe side, promptly report any unusually heavy bleeding to your doctor. If you feel tired all the time, you may be anemic; anemia has many causes besides menorrhagia, such as stomach ulcers or improper diet. A period that lasts twice as long as usual, pain or bleeding during intercourse, weight loss, palpitations, weakness, or other problems or persistent pain in your pelvic area or lower back also call for professional evaluation. Your physician must rule out other causes of menorrhagia, such as fibroid tumors. Heavy bleeding can also be a symptom of cancer of the cervix, uterus, or ovaries. Early detection is paramount to successful treatment in these cases. Diagnostic tests include Pap smear, endometrial biopsy, and pelvic ultrasound. Menorrhagia is usually treated medically with hormones, or surgically with a dilation and curretage

(D&C), and sometimes with hysterectomy, but this is rarely necessary.

Hot Flashes

Most women—up to 65–75 percent of those in the United States—experience hot flashes at some point during menopause. Hot flashes vary widely from woman to woman in their intensity, frequency, and duration. Some people make a distinction between a hot "flash" and a hot "flush." You may experience a hot flash as a passing feeling of warmth over your face or upper body, with perhaps a little perspiration forming on your upper lip which usually isn't noticeable by other people. Or you may experience a hot flush, during which you literally become drenched in sweat, followed by chills, after excessive perspiration has lowered your total body temperature. But often no distinction is made between the two extremes, making it difficult to truly understand the scope and depth of this menopausal symptom.

While a hot flash may simply cause one woman's face to turn rosy, in other women hot flashes are accompanied by distinct changes in heart rate and blood pressure. Some women become very uncomfortable and find hot flashes distressing and embarrassing, but others are able to ride the waves of sensation and even enjoy them.

Most women come to recognize the particular warning signs that precede their own hot flashes. Feelings of tension and anxiety are common, and there are also physical signs that a hot flash is imminent; these include nausea, dizziness, heart palpitations, and tingling in the fingers. Hot flashes typically last several minutes—although a few women may experience them for as long as an hour.

We think that hot flashes are brought on by changes in the hypothalamus, the gland in our brain that connects our nervous system to our endocrine system and regulates many body functions including body temperature and the release of sex hormones. Sudden changes in hormone levels most likely trigger a neurochemical response by the hypothalamus which temporarily affects its ability to regulate body temperature. A normal, comfortable room temperature suddenly feels like a tropical heat wave to your body, and your body temperature actually rises. Your system takes "appropriate" steps to combat this perceived situation: your blood vessels dilate and you perspire to cool your body, triggering a hot flash.

Women usually begin to experience hot flashes as monthly menstruation becomes irregular, and continue to experience them for about 2 years. However, in some women, hot flashes persist for up to 10 years. They are usually more pronounced at the beginning of menopause, and then taper off as your body adjusts to hormone changes.

It helps if you can acknowledge that hot flashes are often a normal part of going through menopause. Don't try to deny them; in fact, many women find relief simply through discussing hot flashes and other symptoms with friends who are going through the same process. Hot flashes are the single most identifiable symptom of the onset of menopause and they are also the most readily relieved by any number of appropriate approaches. Some women turn to hormone replacement therapy (HRT) to control hot flashes. HRT does indeed provide relief from hot flashes—but it is not right for every woman, and debate continues over its overall safety. Fortunately, there are many natural, holistic ways to cope with hot flashes. We have met very few women who couldn't correct their hot flashes naturally, without resorting to potentially hazardous hormone therapy.

Nutritional Considerations

As you follow the Balanced Life Plan described in Chapter 2, be sure to eat foods high in vitamin E, which helps relieve hot flashes for many women; such foods are primarily vegetable oils and whole grains. Also try to eat plenty of citrus fruits, which are rich in bioflavonoids, another natural weapon against hot flashes. Cut out refined sugar, sweets, chocolate, and caffeine—these can all worsen hot flashes. Most important, eat foods high in plant hormones every day—such as soybeans, grains, peas, yams, and alfalfa.

Other General Considerations

If you still smoke, now is the time to kick the habit! Smoking and drinking too much alcohol can intensify the effects of hot flashes. Although they may be relaxing, saunas, steam rooms, hot showers or hot baths are all known to trigger hot flashes, so avoid them if they bother you.

Regular exercise can help prevent hot flashes, perhaps by influencing the hypothalamus and leveling out hormone fluctuations in the blood. A study conducted in Sweden demonstrated that regular physical activity lowered the frequency and intensity of hot flashes; and women who got an average of 3.5 hours of exercise per week had *no hot flashes at all!* Deep breathing exercises (*see* page 91) have also been shown to reduce hot flashes by 50 percent.

Keep your room temperatures low, around 65 degrees Fahrenheit. Many women also find it helpful to keep a pitcher of ice water, fruit juice, or herbal iced tea handy. They take frequent cool showers, buy a good fan, and consider investing in an air conditioner. But you don't have to suffer—hot flashes are generally corrected with natural remedies.

Hot Flash Triggers

Many foods and beverages can bring on hot flashes. In order to determine whether a particular food or drink poses a problem for you, keep a journal of your hot flashes, being careful to include everything you have ingested before experiencing them. Watch to see if a pattern develops; if you consistently experience hot flashes after eating dairy products, for example, try to cut down on them or use nondairy substitutes.

The following foods are common triggers of hot flashes:

- Items which contain caffeine, such as coffee, tea, chocolate, and colas
- Alcohol
- Spicy dishes
- Salty foods
- Hot soups and drinks
- Sugar
- Dairy products
- Meat and poultry
- Fatty foods

Other possible triggers include:

- Stress
- Hot weather
- Anger and agitation

Women have found the following specific approaches to be particularly helpful for hot flashes.

Nutritional Supplements

Menopausal symptoms in general are associated with nutritional inadequacies, and studies have shown that hot flashes are associated with deficiencies in B complex and C vitamins, magnesium, and potassium in particular. A good multivitamin-mineral formula containing the doses recommended in Chapter 3, pages 61–64, generally supplies the nutrients you need to correct deficiencies and to prevent or minimize hot flashes in the first place. In addition, you may increase the total daily dose of:

• *Vitamin E,* up to 400–800 IU per day, until you see a decrease in the frequency, intensity, and duration of your hot flashes. Then maintain the effect by taking 400 IU per day. Many studies show that this important vitamin minimizes this symptom. As far back as the 1930s and 1940s, vitamin E was reported to bring relief to one-half to two-thirds of the women who used it. (If you have hypertension, chronic rheumatism, heart disease, or diabetes, start with 100 IU per day and increase the dosage slowly.) Take *selenium* along with vitamin E to enhance its effectiveness.

You may also wish to take:

• *Bioflavonoids,* 900 mg daily. In a clinical study, the bioflavonoid hesperidin was given along with 1,200 mg of vitamin C daily. After one month, 53 percent of the women found relief from hot flashes and in 34 percent hot flashes were reduced. Bioflavonoids may reduce hot flashes in many ways—for example, they strengthen the capillaries, are anti-inflammatory, and some have phytoestrogen activity.
• *Gamma-oryzanol:* 300 mg daily. Several studies reported that this substance, found in grains and extracted from rice bran oil, relieved hot flashes without side effects in 67–85 percent of the women taking it.
• *Bee pollen:* 500 mg per day, or royal jelly or propolis has helped some women reduce hot flashes and nervousness.

Herbal Remedies

Many women have found herbs reduce the frequency and intensity of their hot flashes. For instructions on using herbal remedies, *see* Chapter 3, pages 70–75. Use either an all-purpose menopausal herbal formula that helps menopausal symptoms generally, or choose from the herbs listed below, which are particularly effective in relieving hot flashes. You may use them either singly or in combination. A great combination formula for hot flashes is *Pulsatilla-Vitex Compound,* containing chaste tree berry, pulsatilla, motherwort, black cohosh, and licorice root.

• *Black or blue cohosh, false unicorn root,* and *licorice* are herbs rich in plant hormones and help normalize your system. Black cohosh was shown to be as effective as hormone replacement therapy in reducing menopausal problems. The usual dose is 1 capsule or 1 teaspoon of tincture up to three times daily. *Motherwort* is also rich in plant estrogens; the usual dose is up to 2 cups of infusion per day, or ¹/₂–1 teaspoon of tincture per day.

• The Chinese herb *dong quai* has excellent balancing properties for menopausal women, and is considered the female version of ginseng. Millions of women all over the world have safely and effectively use dong quai to promote menopausal well-being and avoid hot flashes. Take 1 capsule, or 1 teaspoon of tincture, up to three times a day.

• *Chickweed, elder,* and *violet* tend to cool the system. So do *hibiscus, oatstraw,* and *mint.*

• *Dandelion* and *yellow dock* nourish the liver and help your body metabolize excess hormones, which could be triggering your hot flashes. *Milk thistle, chicory, oatstraw,* and *burdock* also support your liver.

Homeopathic Remedies

Homeopathy is quite helpful for hot flashes. Following the instructions in Chapter 3, pages 75–81, use a combination remedy formulated for menopause; *BHI Mullinen* is an effective combination formula. Or choose the single remedy that most closely matches your symptoms from the list given below. Follow the instructions on the package; if your symptoms are severe, it is usually recommended that you take a dose as often as every 5 minutes; for milder symptoms, take every 3 hours. One dose equals 2–3 pills or 5–10 drops.

• *Lachesis* is one of the best remedies for hot flashes. Try it if your flushing emanates from the top of your head; if flashes are worse just before sleep and when you awaken; and if you also suffer from palpitations, sweating, headaches, and easily irritated skin.

• *Sepia* is another commonly prescribed remedy for hot flashes. This remedy works well in women whose flashes travel up the body and leave them feeling weak, nauseated, exhausted, and depressed.

• *Sulphur* is useful in women whose flashes are triggered by alcohol, are worsened by heat, and occur mostly during the evening or midmorning; in women who are irritable, moody, and exhausted.

Aromatherapy

Several essential oils can be used to relieve the discomfort and stress of hot flashes. Sprinkle a few drops of *calmus/sweet flag, basil,* or *thyme* essential oils on a cotton ball and inhale the fragrance as you feel a flash coming on. Stress, which can aggravate hot flashes, may be relieved by aromatherapy with *lavender* or *chamomile*. See page 84 for instructions on how to use aromatherapy.

Natural Hormone Therapy

If following the Balanced Life Plan and using natural therapies are not completely effective in reducing your hot flashes, you may want to try natural hormone therapy under a doctor's supervision (*see* Chapter 4). According to health professionals who recommend it and women who use it, natural progesterone, estriol, Tri-est (a combination of human hormones), and even DHEA can help. Remember, hormone treatment may be overkill for hot flashes if they are mild.

Precautions

A few women may experience hot flashes that defy self-help. Notify your physician if you experience any of the following: very frequent hot flashes; very intense, lengthy, or exhausting hot flashes; hot flashes that disrupt your sleep on a regular basis (hot flashes that occur at night are also known as night sweats).

Incontinence

As you make your way through menopause, you may find yourself going to the bathroom more frequently or even leaking small amounts of urine. As your estrogen level decreases, your bladder tissues begin to change; they may become thin, dry, or inelastic. Pelvic and abdominal muscles which help support the bladder often weaken, especially if you've had several children. Any one or a combination of these circumstances can result in incontinence: the sudden and involuntary release of small amounts of urine.

About a third of all women over forty experience stress incontinence, the most common type of incontinence, at some point in their lives. In this form, a physical reaction—such as coughing, sneezing, jumping, or laughing at a friend's joke—causes an involuntary release of urine. Another common type of incontinence in women is urge incontinence, in which you frequently feel the need to urinate, sometimes so strongly that you don't always make it to the bathroom in time.

Some women become extremely embarrassed and self-conscious about incontinence; it becomes an inconvenience and forces them to change their day-to-day lives to avoid circumstances which provoke it. Happily, there's a better alternative. There are a number of safe and natural ways by which you can prevent or reduce incontinence, and the disruptive effect that it can have on your lifestyle.

See also ''Urinary Tract and Bladder Problems.''

Trigger Foods

Although we're not always sure why, certain foods and liquids may worsen incontinence in some women, particularly urge incontinence. So as a first step, cut down or eliminate from your diet the following foods and beverages, which can irritate your bladder and add to incontinence:

- Alcoholic beverages
- Caffeine-containing beverages such as coffee, tea, and colas
- Acidic foods and juices such as citrus products including oranges, lemons, pineapples, strawberries, and tomatoes
- Spicy foods
- Dairy products
- Sugar

Other Lifestyle Considerations

Losing weight may help if you're overweight; the pressure of excess weight on your bladder may be causing or adding to your incontinence. So follow a sensible diet and exercise program, such as that provided in Chapter 2, to shed excess pounds.

Other simple measures you can take include stretching the bladder so it holds more urine by letting yourself experience the urge to urinate without releasing the urine. Hold it in through a round or two of urge spasms, unless ignoring the urge to urinate could lead to an imminent problem because you won't have access to a bathroom. Avoiding medications such as antihistamines and tranquilizers that can cause bladder trouble can also help. In addition, researchers now recommend that you follow your instinct of crossing your legs to avoid losing urine when you cough or laugh. Believe it or not, a scientific study was conducted involving 48 women with confirmed stress incontinence. Of various positions tried, the women who crossed their legs while coughing were most successful at minimizing leakage—and 73 percent remained completely dry. The researchers pointed out that this instinctive behavior is effective, socially acceptable, cost-free, and has no side effects.

As part of your daily whole-body exercise regimen, include Kegel exercises, which specifically strengthen the pubococcygeal (PC) muscle supporting your bladder and urethra. To isolate your PC muscle, imagine that you want to stop your urine in midstream; the muscle that you contract in order to do this is your PC muscle. To do a Kegel exercise, gradually tighten your PC muscle, hold, then relax. You need to do 50 to 100 Kegels in a row several times daily in order to strengthen the PC muscle enough to correct your problem. The advantage of this exercise is its complete privacy; only you will know if you are practicing your Kegels while sitting at your desk at work or at the movies, while waiting in line at the bank or for a bus.

Women have found the following specific self-help approaches to be particularly effective for incontinence.

Herbal Remedies

Herbal remedies may help you handle menopausal symptoms such as incontinence as smoothly and comfortably as possible. For information on using herbal remedies, *see* Chapter 3, pages 70–75, where we provide an all-purpose herbal formula that will generally help strengthen the pelvic region and act as a tonic for the entire female reproductive system. The following herbs are particularly effective in relieving incontinence in women during menopause and beyond. Use them singly or in combination, or look for a commercially prepared herbal formula that contains them.

• *Agnus castus, black cohosh, false unicorn root, St. Johnswort,* and *beth root.* These herbs seem to work best when taken in combination (choose three). They generally tone and help tighten your entire urogenital area, but work best if you are not overweight. The usual dose is 1 capsule, 1 cup decoction, or 1 teaspoon of tincture taken up to three times a day.

• Another combination to try is *corn silk, platina leaf, St. Johnswort, thuya leaf,* and *arnica root, leaf, and flower.*

Precautions
If incontinence persists, see your medical doctor. In some cases, incontinence may be the sign of a serious underlying disorder, such as diabetes or bladder cancer.

Insomnia

Almost everyone has trouble falling or staying asleep once in a while, or wakes up tired in spite of having spent "enough" hours in bed. However, insomnia often increases in women who are going through menopause. Nearly one-fourth of all midlife women report that they have trouble sleeping—twice as many as young women. You, too, may take longer to fall asleep, wake up one or more times during the night, or sleep lighter and more fitfully than when you were younger.

Sleep problems may be the result of hormonal changes, but may also relate to psychological stress. If stress and depression are accompanying this life change for you, your sleep patterns will probably be different. Other possible factors include physical changes such as night sweats, muscle cramps, and aches and pains. If you suspect any of these might be at the root of your sleep problem, turn to the sections of this book that deal with these problems.

And don't discount an unsatisfying sex life as a possible contributing factor. In addition, a lot of menopausal women live with men who are experiencing prostate problems at this time. These men need to get up to go to the bathroom many times a night and may disturb the sleep of their partners. If the guy you sleep with keeps you up at night by his disturbed sleep, try to move into another room or get him to move into one, or better yet, let him know that there are very successful natural treatments for benign prostate enlargement, and that he might consider a referral to a nutrition-oriented physician.

In natural medicine systems such as homeopathy, sleep is one of the important components a person needs to restore and maintain physical and mental health. New studies show that chronic sleep deprivation, which may be due to insomnia, affects your immune system, slows healing, and limits your ability to stay alert and concentrate. Inadequate sleep may be responsible for poor productivity, irritability, and a large portion of accidents on the road, on the job, and at work.

We are only now discovering how important healthy sleep is and how widely requirements vary from individual to individual. Some people can thrive on 4 or 5 hours (not to be confused with those who "get by" on a few hours but require 5, 6, or more cups of coffee to get going and keep going). Others need 9 or even more hours to feel and do their best.

Insomnia can become a chronic and infuriatingly vicious cycle. The less sleep you get, the less well you are able to deal with stress, and the more difficult it is to fall or stay asleep. If you need an alarm clock to wake up every day, or awaken exhausted rather than refreshed, don't delay in setting things straight.

(*See also* "Aches and Pains," "Anxiety," "Depression," and "Night Sweats"—all of which may disturb sleep and should be treated.)

General Nutrition

If you suffer from occasional, acute insomnia, or sleep fitfully and wake up tired, the Balanced Life Plan outlined in Chapter 2 supports good general health and may help to restore a normal sleep schedule. In addition, try to eat a light supper; you may find it relaxing to eat a snack such as toast or a small bowl of cereal an hour or so before bedtime. Some studies show eating a high protein meal late in the day is detrimental to sleep, while carbohydrates encourage drowsiness. There's some evidence that eating a diet rich in tryptophan, an amino acid (protein building block), encourages normal sleep patterns. (Tryptophan supplements were taken off the market in the United States because of toxicity problems, most likely owing to contamination during manufacture by one supplier.) You can still get this calming nutrient by eating tryptophan-rich foods including turkey, bananas, figs, dates, and yogurt, although you would have to eat quite a lot of them. Ask your doctor to prescribe tryptophan, available from compounding pharmacies. Dr. Brown finds that a woman who wakes between 3 and 5 A.M. and can't fall back asleep can frequently solve this problem by eating regular meals to stabilize the blood sugar; avoiding all stimulants, coffee, sugar, alcohol, nicotine, and colas; and reducing stress, for example, with meditation.

General Lifestyle Considerations

Although they may help you fall asleep initially, a few drinks before bedtime may actually awaken you in the middle of the night. Also avoid caffeine (in coffee, black tea, sodas, chocolate, and some conventional drugs) for several hours before bedtime. Some people are so sensitive to caffeine that even one morning cup of coffee keeps them up at night, and for some even decaffeinated coffee and green tea are too stimulating. Smokers also tend to have more trouble falling asleep.

Stress and emotional upheaval wreak havoc with restful sleep, so explore ways to relax and manage stress during the day and particularly at night before bed. Establish a regular bedtime and waking time that remains the same for weekends and vacations, and create your own bedtime ritual to cue your body that it's time to wind down and disengage from daytime problems and thoughts. Many women are able to relax by reading, taking a hot bath (especially with certain aromatic oils as explained later), or listening to music. Some relax with friends; others find even lively conversation too stimulating. Watching TV may be relaxing, but can also be stimulating. Exercise is one of the best antidotes to stress, but avoid aerobic-type exercise in the last two hours before bedtime because it is stimulating. Yoga and gentle tai chi may be just what you need to calm down before bed.

Following a few simple tips may make all the difference. Wear ear plugs if your bedroom is noisy. Use a sleep mask and cover windows with heavy blinds or drapes if too much light comes through. Make sure the room temperature is comfortable and that there is adequate air circulation. Some people find daytime naps help; others find they make it more difficult to sleep at night, so experiment to see to which group you belong.

And finally: Keep the bed for two things—sleep and sex. Using the bedroom for working overtime or paying bills signals the mind for activity, not relaxation. Some women find sex and self-pleasuring to be a pleasurable way to relax for sleep (although they could become habit forming!).

These approaches will probably take some time—two or three weeks—to establish a new sleeping routine; but they are worth a try because they are the safest, most natural way to deal with a chronic sleep problem. That having been said, all the natural therapies described in Chapter 3 are generally helpful for combatting stubborn sleep problems. Instead of "knocking you out" as habit-forming conventional sleeping pills tend to do, natural therapies encourage your mind and body to drift into a natural restful sleep. Even so, they should be used only occasionally, when the other lifestyle considerations aren't enough. Women have found the following specific approaches to be particularly helpful for insomnia.

Nutritional Supplements

A good multivitamin-mineral formula containing the doses recommended in Chapter 3, pages 61–64, usually supplies the nutrients you need to minimize sleep problems. Women who awaken between the hours of 3 and 5 A.M. may benefit from a multivitamin-mineral supplement because it will help stabilize blood sugar levels. You may also take the following:

• *Calcium* and *magnesium* can both be helpful when taken together. Divide your total daily supplements to include at least 500 mg of both calcium and magnesium before bedtime.

• *Melatonin* is a natural hormone made by your pineal gland deep inside your brain. Melatonin resets your inner clock, so it is important to take it at the same time every night—for most people that is an hour or so before bed. Melatonin is most useful for insomnia due to jet lag. Melatonin supplements are readily available in many health food stores; it is promoted as a safe, natural sleeping pill and many women swear by it. However, we caution against using it because the potency sold is high—ten times that naturally found in the body—and because some pills have been found to contain impurities that could be harmful. Melatonin drugs are being tested but have not yet been approved by the Food and Drug Administration. You may need up to 10 mg to fix your insomnia, but start with a low dose of 2 to 3 mg or less, as larger amounts may cause a hangover effect. Long-term effects are unknown, so use higher doses only as necessary.

Herbal Remedies

Many women find that herbs relax the mind and body and allow sleep to come naturally. For instructions on herbal remedies, *see* Chapter 3, pages 70–75. Use an all-purpose menopausal herbal remedy, or choose one or more of the following herbs which are particularly effective in relieving insomnia:

• *Valerian* is the most popular traditional herbal sedative, and is used widely in Europe. Studies have shown that this herb improves the quality of sleep and helps people fall asleep sooner. Although these studies indicate that instead of making you drowsy in the morning, as conventional sleeping pills do, valerian actually increases morning alertness, some of our patients notice that it does cause a hangover effect. The usual dose is 1 cup of infusion before bedtime or 1 teaspoon of tincture up to three times a day. While this dosage is safe, many people find that 20 drops of tincture at bedtime is sufficient to induce sleep.

• *Passiflora (passion flower)* has also been used traditionally as a sedative for its mind-calming properties; it elevates the level of serotonin, the brain chemical that initiates sleep.

• Other herbs that may help ease sleeping problems include *hops, skullcap, catnip.* These work very well in combination and are often taken as teas in the evening, before bedtime.

Homeopathic Remedies

There are many homeopathic remedies that gently help you fall asleep and stay asleep. Following the instructions in Chapter 3, pages 75–81, choose the single remedy from the list below that most closely matches your type of insomnia. Or use one of the many combination remedies specifically formulated for sleep problems. In a recent study, a product called Quietude was found to be as effective as Valium in enhancing sleep, and without side effects such as morning drowsiness. One dose usually equals 2–3 pills or 5–10 drops.

• *Nux vomica.* For sleeplessness resulting from too much coffee, alcohol, or any other drug; from overexertion of the mind; from excess studying or working; when you are sleepy and fall asleep in the evening, but sleep fitfully and awaken around 2 or 3 A.M. and are unable to fall asleep again for several hours.

• *Pulsatilla.* If you can't fall asleep until after midnight and wake up a few hours later; when a specific thought or memory keeps you awake and you weep over sleep difficulties; the problem is worse in a warm room, and improves in the open air; you may prefer to sleep with your arms thrown up over your head.

• *Arsenicum.* When the cause of sleeplessness is fear or anxiety; for people who are restless after midnight and cannot remain in bed, and who are chilly and want extra covers.

• *Coffea.* For insomnia due to sudden acute overactivity and overexcitement of body or mind, following either a good event or bad event; also useful for people who stay awake because of drinking coffee. Coffea is a good illustration of "like cures like"—small doses help cure what large doses cause.

Relaxation and Mind-Body Therapies

When insomnia is an outgrowth of stress and anxiety, some type of formal relaxation therapy is called for (*see* Chapter 3, page 89). Regular daily meditation reduces stress and promotes more restful sleep. If you're having trouble sleeping, we recommend you meditate twice a day—30 minutes before breakfast and 30 minutes before dinner. Getting a massage regularly (especially with aromatic oils), deep breathing, total body relaxation, yoga, and visualization can also help your mind and body release stress. *Spinal manipulation* by an osteopath or a chiropractor may also be helpful if musculoskeletal pain is preventing you from getting a good night's rest. Also, you might try a relaxation technique (*see* page 89), which you can use both during the day and at night before retiring. Soothing relaxation tapes and soft music can serve as lullabies for grown-ups. You may want to combine relaxation techniques with visualization. After putting yourself in a relaxed state, imagine a sense of sleepiness seeping into one part of your body after another, until your whole body and mind are able to drift off.

Aromatherapy

Women often report dramatic results when using aromatherapy for sleeping difficulties. The best ways to use essential oils for this purpose are either in your nighttime bath or on your pillow. The most effective oils are *lavender, chamomile,* and *neroli* because of their sedative properties. *Benzoin* is helpful when worries are keeping sleep at bay; *bergamot* is best when depression is the cause. *Marjoram, sandalwood, juniper,* and *ylang ylang* are other useful relaxants. Following the instructions in Chapter 3, page 84, experiment with these oils singly or in combination to find the blend that works best for you. After 2 weeks, switch to another oil or combination because your body will get used to the aroma and it will gradually become less effective.

Natural Hormone Therapy

If after following the Balanced Life Plan and using natural therapies you still can't sleep well, and you are experiencing other menopausal symptoms, you may want to have your hormone levels checked. High cortisol, imbalances of DHEA, or an imbalanced estrogen/progesterone ratio may be a marker for stress-related insomnia. If DHEA is low, for example, meditation, exercise, and even DHEA supplements may resolve the stress and the hormonal markers of your stress will also revert to normal. If progesterone is too low, supplements frequently reverse insomnia by balancing a woman's needs.

Precautions

Chronic insomnia due to physical illness or emotional imbalance requires professional evaluation and counseling. Seek medical care if you experience insomnia for more than seven consecutive days, or if you have a painful medical condition that is keeping you from getting a good night's rest. Sleeping too much or too little may be symptoms of depression. While there's no really clear evidence that depression occurs more often at menopause than at other times of life, there is a lot of anecdotal evidence that stress for women, due to society's low regard for middle-aged and older women, will affect some of us at this time. People with environmental sensitivities and allergies may suffer insomnia from contact with feathers, mold, dust, or fumes from carpeting, vinyl, or even gasoline fumes from outside the bedroom. If you suspect this is your problem, seek help from a health care giver knowledgeable about diagnosing and treating environmental sensitivities.

Irregular Periods

Irregular periods are, of course, a ubiquitous sign of approaching menopause. You'll probably begin having unpredictable periods and even skip some for as long as 2 or 3 years before you stop altogether, but remember that everyone is different. Some women's periods end quite suddenly, and others begin skipping periods 5 or 6 years before the last one.

Periods become irregular because you're ovulating irregularly. As we explained in Chapter 1 and in "Heavy Periods" in this chapter, when you don't release an egg, only estrogen (although perhaps in lower amounts) is stimulating the lining of your uterus; progesterone levels are way too low to cause the lining to shed. It may take several months for the lining to break down and create a menstrual flow.

The most common pattern is that of unusually heavy periods, in which you may see large clots of blood, accompanying some irregularity. Irregularity may mean that instead of having a period every 28–36 days (whatever your usual cycle), you'll start having them quite unpredictably, perhaps one time 40 days after the last, and another, 28 days, and the next, 52 days. Then you may skip a couple of cycles altogether, then go back to your regular pattern, and then skip three or four cycles. None of this is unusual or indicative of a problem, as your health care professional will probably tell you.

Annoying as irregular periods are in and of themselves, you should know that if you tend to experience PMS, symptoms may drag on for weeks or months at a time, because there is no menstrual flow to bring on relief. You should also know that even if your periods are still appearing at least once every 6 months, even if they are spotty and brown, and even if you're 55, you can still get pregnant. (Whether you will retain the fetus is another story since you may not be producing high enough levels of hormones to give the developing fetus a sufficiently nourishing uterine lining.) To prevent unwanted pregnancies, use serious birth control all the time until you have not had a period for a whole year. You can then assume that menopause has occurred, and you're no longer ovulating. Even so, birth control isn't guaranteed, and irregular periods can be quite nerve-racking. It may help if you keep these guidelines in mind: If you do skip a period and have unusual symptoms such as breast tenderness and nausea, it's quite possible you're pregnant, on the other hand, if you have menopausal symptoms such as hot flashes, it's a fairly safe bet that you're not pregnant.

(*See also* "Cramping" and "Heavy Periods.")

General Nutrition

Make sure you follow the Balanced Life Plan suggested in Chapter 2, to give your body the nutrients it needs to encourage hormonal balance. If you like the taste of cinnamon, you may want to use it liberally when flavoring food because this spice seems to help regulate menstrual cycles.

Other Lifestyle Considerations

It's a good idea to keep a menstrual calendar to track changes in your periods so you can accurately report this sign to your doctor, and monitor any improvement gleaned from any natural therapies you decide to try.

Smoking tends to worsen all menopausal symptoms including irregular menstrual cycles, so try now to quit. Stress and emotional upheaval also worsen erratic periods so be extra good to yourself right now and consider exploring ways to relax and manage stress on a daily basis. Regular strenuous activity is one of the best antidotes to stress, and can help regulate hormones and thus your monthly schedule. Exercising your pelvic organs helps keep them toned, which may help prevent or minimize irregular cycles. Regular sexual stimulation and orgasm are a pleasurable way to do the job.

Women have found the following specific natural therapies to be particularly helpful for this common sign of approaching menopause.

Herbal Remedies

Many women find that herbs help regulate their periods. For instructions on herbal remedies, *see* Chapter 3, pages 70–75. Use an all-purpose menopausal herbal remedy, or choose from these herbs, which are particularly effective in treating this condition; use them singly or in combination, or look for a commercially prepared herbal formula that contains them.

• *Agnus castus* is the primary herbal remedy to regulate irregular periods. It works on the brain to stimulate your ovaries, and as long as

they have eggs (in early or peri-menopause) this is the first remedy to try. Take 1 capsule or 1 teaspoon of tincture up to three times a day.
• *Raspberry leaf* tones and nourishes your ovaries and uterus. Take 1 cup of infusion or 1 teaspoon of tincture, up to three times a day.
• *Dong quai* balances every organ in your reproductive system and may be most useful for you if you also have PMS. The usual dose is 1 capsule or 1 teaspoon of tincture up to three times a day.

Homeopathic Remedies

Homeopathy offers several remedies for menopause and menstrual irregularities. Following the instructions in Chapter 3, pages 75–81, use a combination remedy that contains at least one of the following substances, or choose the single remedy that most closely matches your symptoms. Follow the instructions on the package. One dose usually equals 2–3 pills or 5–10 drops.

• *Lachesis* is one of the most common remedies for menstrual irregularities. Use this when your blood flow is very dark, thick, and strong-smelling; and if you have pain that is more intense at the beginning of your period and is relieved when your period starts.
• *Sepia* is another commonly prescribed remedy for irregular periods. This remedy is indicated if your periods are frequent, you bleed heavily, you feel pain, and if bleeding is accompanied by backache, constipation, and depression.

Aromatherapy

Some essential oils are classified as *emmenagogues*—they help stimulate the appearance of a late period or bolster scanty flow. These include *clary sage, myrrh,* and *sage,* and perhaps *basil, juniper, fennel,* and *rosemary. Rose oil* helps regulate the cycle without increasing or decreasing the flow.

Natural Hormone Therapy

If after following the Balanced Life Plan and using natural therapies, your periods are still irregular, you may want to try *natural hormone therapy* under a doctor's supervision (*see* Chapter 4). According to health professionals who recommend it and some women who use it, natural progesterone cream restores regular periods when the uterus is still responsive to this hormone, because there is enough estrogen to prime the uterus. To mimic the natural cycle you might take progesterone at a steady dose for two weeks straight, or increase the dose over the two weeks, and then stop for two weeks, during which you could expect a period to occur. It may take months to normalize periods. Many women bleed irregularly for months until the periods just diminish. If you have enough estrogen to prime the uterus, you will continue to have periods as long as you take cyclic progesterone. If this doesn't work, you might need estrogen supplements initially. We recommend that you have your hormone levels measured so you know what hormone(s) to take, if any.

Precautions

If, after you've not had a period for six months, you then start bleeding, you need to check out with your health care provider whether something other than normal menses is the cause. Many conditions, such as cancer or other pelvic disease, may cause bleeding from the uterus, and we urge you to check in if this is happening to you.

Loss of Sexual Desire

Although some women going through menopause find their libido takes an upswing, about half say they feel less lusty than they used to. Estrogen may be at least in part to blame. But our minds and bodies are not that simple. Another hormone, progesterone, may also be involved. A third hormone, testosterone, which is secreted by the ovaries and adrenal glands, is the principal agent influencing female sexual desire. Testosterone is considered a "male" hormone because men produce much higher levels. However, research shows that when levels of testosterone in women decrease after menopause, sexual drive also may decrease. (Testosterone is still produced in lesser amounts in aging and elderly women's ovaries and adrenal glands.)

After a hysterectomy, many women say they find sex is less pleasurable. There are psychological and physiological reasons for this. In total hysterectomy, removal of the ovaries also removes a woman's primary source of testosterone and estrogen. And with her uterus and cervix gone, she has lost a body organ that is a source of sexual pleasure when it is stroked and pressed against by, for instance, a penis or a finger.

There are many other reasons for a lack of sexual desire or arousal difficulties besides hormonal changes and hysterectomy. Loss of sexual desire may be a sign of a physical problem and should always be discussed with your health care professional. Fatigue is a frequent cause of decreased sexual drive, and fatigue is the end product of many physical problems and diseases. (*See* "Fatigue and Low Energy.") Unfortunately there are some physicians who believe that loss of desire (with or without fatigue) not only is "natural" in aging women, but confirms their notions that "randiness" isn't appropriate "at your age." If your physician is one of these, he or she isn't likely to take seriously the loss of a mature woman's sex drive. You may have to change physicians or be more assertive in your interest in exploring various treatment options, including testing hormone levels and or considering a hormone replacement regimen which may include a little testosterone (*see* Chapter 4).

The psychological conditions that negatively affect a woman's sex drive are primarily depression and anxiety. In the "Depression" section earlier in this chapter, we discussed masked depression. Loss of sexual desire may be one of the few symptoms that indicates a masked depression. Anxiety is much more overt and nearly everyone knows when they're anxious, but not everyone knows that one of the ramifications of anxiety can be a loss of libido.

See also "Anxiety," and Chapter 7: "Enjoying Sex During Menopause and Beyond."

General Considerations

Because poor nutrition, fatigue, and stress can affect hormone levels and douse the flames of sexual desire, be sure to follow the Balanced Life Plan in Chapter 2; pay special attention to getting enough rest and relaxation and to managing any extra stress you may be experiencing at this time. Remember that there's more to sex than intercourse, and explore other ways of expressing and enjoying yourself sexually. You may take longer to become aroused; so instead of giving up or settling for disappointing encounters, allow foreplay to expand to a greater role than it may have occupied in your youth.

Women have found the following specific natural approaches to be particularly helpful for low libido.

Herbal Remedies

Although traditionally several herbs have been touted as natural aphrodisiacs, including astragalus, burdock, damiana, dong quai, false unicorn, ginseng, and kava, today most reputable herbalists avoid making such claims. However, in theory at least, herbs that contain plant hormones could affect sex drive by influencing hormonal balance in the body. For information on using herbal remedies, *see* Chapter 3, pages 70–75, where we provide an all-purpose herbal formula that will generally help balance hormones and act as a tonic for the entire female reproductive system. The herbs listed below are particularly rich in plant hormones and thus may perk up a flagging libido. Use them singly or in combination, or look for a commercially prepared herbal formula that contains them.

• *Black cohosh, licorice,* and *red clover* are rich in plant estrogens; the usual dosage is 1 capsule or $1/2$–1 teaspoon of tincture, up to three times a day.

• *Agnus castus, sarsaparilla root, wild yam root,* and *yarrow flowers and leaves* are rich in plant progesterones; the usual dose is 1 capsule or 1 teaspoon of tincture up to three times a day.

Aromatherapy

Several essential oils are believed to be aphrodisiacs, but they probably achieve this benefit by virtue of their ability to relax and reduce anxiety in general. So why not pamper yourself with body oils and baths containing *neroli, ylang-ylang,* or *jasmine*? Better yet, ask a willing partner to give you a massage with one of these aromatic oils. Many women report good results with *rose oil,* though it is not known as a relaxant; rather it is tied closely to female sexuality as a uterine tonic and is considered the premier female aphrodisiac. Now you know why our lovers bring us bouquets of fresh roses!

If your male partner could also use some help, take a cue from recent research conducted by the Smell and Taste Treatment and Research Foundation. A neurologist set out to explore the effects of odors on penile blood flow, hoping to find a treatment for impotence. Among the odors found to increase blood flow to the penis the most were lavender and pumpkin pie, and doughnut and black licorice. Older men were most turned on by the scent of vanilla.

Natural Hormone Therapy

If after following the Balanced Life Plan and using natural therapies, your sex drive is still not where you'd like it to be, you may want to discuss *natural hormone therapy* with a holistically minded physician (*see* Chapter 4).

Precautions

Loss of libido may be due to a physical problem, so be sure to consult with your physician to rule out disease, or to get the right treatment. If loss of sexual desire is something that bothers you and your partner and you may be in a state of depression or high anxiety, it's a good idea to have a consultation with a mental health professional.

Menstrual Cramps and Premenstrual Syndrome (PMS)

Many women in our culture experience some form of discomfort 1–2 weeks before or during their menstrual period. As they get closer to menopause, both psychological and physical symptoms may intensify. Cramps, back pain, bloating, swollen and tender breasts, food cravings, acne, mood swings, irritability, crying spells, insomnia, and fatigue are some of the symptoms from which you may suffer each month.

Premenstrual syndrome (PMS) begins at or after ovulation (usually around the middle of the menstrual cycle) and may continue until the beginning of menstruation. Many women continue to experience symptoms such as cramps during menstruation. Some women experience a lessening of their symptoms as their periods gradually diminish. Others may experience stronger cramps because of heavy menstrual bleeding or PMS that drags on forever because their periods are farther apart.

While PMS has often been brushed off as being "all in our heads," there are clear hormonal, structural, and metabolic causes of PMS. Some estimate that PMS affects more than 90 percent of all American women at some point in their lives. In some women the condition is so severe that it disrupts work and social relationships. Most women with PMS have too much estrogen relative to progesterone. This can be due to too much estrogen, or too little progesterone, and there can be many causes of either. These hormones invariably affect almost all organ systems. The ratio of estrogen to progesterone governs emotions, electrolyte and water balance, vitamin B-6 metabolism, and blood glucose levels, triggering a cascade of related physical symptoms that are characteristic of PMS.

Most conventional medicines for PMS fall under the category of aspirin or ibuprofin-like substances called NSAIDS (nonsteroidal anti-inflammatory drugs), which interfere with prostaglandins, a natural substance produced by our bodies and which is associated with inflammation. Inflammatory chemicals increase the pain, local swelling, and cramping associated with PMS. Some doctors prescribe diuretics, which address the bloating by reducing excess water in the tissues through increased urination. Most of these medicines have potentially serious side effects. There are more natural substances, such as vitamins and herbs, which decrease inflammation and act as diuretics. You can build your own natural prescription based on your specific symptoms, and you will likely find that many of your symptoms disappear.

See also ''Breast Lumps and Tender Breasts,'' ''Heavy Periods,'' ''Insomnia,'' ''Irregular Periods,'' and ''Moodiness, Mood Swings, and Irritability.''

General Nutrition

Good nutrition is the first place to begin to treat menstrual discomfort and is often the only measure a women needs to take to get relief. As you follow the Balanced Life Plan suggested in Chapter 2, make a special effort to reduce or possibly eliminate all sugars and refined starches because these, combined with hormone changes, can trigger fatigue, irritability, and headache. You may crave sweets at this time, but try to satisfy them with fresh fruits and sweet vegetables like carrots and sweet potatoes instead. Eating small meals of vegetables, fruit, whole grains, nuts, seeds, sea vegetables, beans, and fish throughout the day helps stave off blood sugar dips and minimize sugar cravings.

Reducing salt discourages your tissues from retaining water and this helps reduce bloating and perhaps many other related PMS symptoms. Also cut out caffeine and alcohol. Coffee and other caffeine-containing beverages may act as diuretics and loosen stools, but caffeine adds to your nervous irritability, and worsens insomnia and pain. Many women have found that completely eliminating dairy products from their diets dramatically reduces their symptoms of PMS.

Emphasize foods high in calcium, magnesium, and potassium. Also try to eat foods high in omega-6 essential fatty acids such as flax seeds and pumpkin seeds, and their oils (up to 3 tablespoons per day).

Other Lifestyle Considerations

To help ease cramping, take a warm bath or curl up with a hot water bottle or ''Bed Buddy'' or heating pad on your belly, pelvis, or low back—wherever you feel discomfort. Or use a ''Bed Buddy,'' which you can make yourself by filling a sock with oat groats, tying off the end, and microwaving it about 30 seconds until warm and toasty. Drink hot herbal teas (*see* page 214), or just plain hot water. Warmth increases your blood flow, and can relax your cramped pelvic muscles. Some women find relief using castor oil packs (*see* ''Breast Lumps and Tender Breasts''); however, they can be messy.

Exercise—particularly gentle approaches such as yoga—can also help; swimming is gentle too and acts as a natural diuretic as well. Moderate activities such as walking and stretching also alleviate menstrual cramps in many women. Stopping smoking usually helps too.

Women have found the following specific approaches to be particularly helpful for minimizing or eliminating cramps and PMS.

Nutritional Supplements

In one study, women with PMS who were given a multivitamin-mineral supplement showed a reduction in premenstrual and menstrual symptoms. For good overall nutrition, begin with a good multivitamin-mineral formula containing the doses recommended in Chapter 3, pages 61–64, and take it every day. About 1 or 2 weeks before your period is due to begin (depending on the duration of your symptoms—experiment with what you need), you may increase the total daily dose of:

• *Calcium,* up to 1,000–1,500 mg. Calcium is anti-inflammatory and a muscle relaxant and can help relieve menstrual cramps. Take calcium with an equal amount of *magnesium,* which aids calcium absorption, relaxes muscles, and may reduce breast tenderness, nervousness, and weight gain.

• *Vitamin B complex,* up to 50–100 mg. We need to supplement all

214 / Natural Medicine for Menopause and Beyond

the B vitamins if we add one because they all work together; for water retention and uterine cramping, B-6 in particular is effective and it is safe to take up to 200 mg per day, as needed.

• *Vitamin E,* up to 600–1,000 IU. Studies have shown this vitamin reduces breast tenderness in some women, as well as nervousness, headache, fatigue, depression, and insomnia.

• *Essential fatty acids,* up to 9–30 grams of gammalinoleic acid (GLA); found in evening primrose oil, borage oil, or black currant oil supplements; or take 1–1½ teaspoons a day of fresh flax seeds or flax oil.

Herbal Remedies

Many women find that herbs help with menstrual cramps and PMS. For instructions on herbal remedies, *see* Chapter 3, pages 70–75. Use an all-purpose menopausal herbal remedy, or choose from these herbs, which are particularly effective in treating PMS and cramping. Use them singly or in combination, or look for a commercially prepared herbal formula that contains them.

• *Dong quai, black cohosh, raspberry leaf,* and *chamomile* are helpful for cramping and PMS symptoms. The usual dose is 1 capsule or 1 teaspoon of tincture, up to three times a day.

• *Valerian* is useful for menstrual pain or tension (take 1 teaspoon of tincture up to three times a day, or 1 cup of infusion before bedtime). So are *skullcap, hops, passiflora, feverfew,* and *cramp bark.*

• *Siberian ginseng* is useful for PMS during menopause. The usual dose is 1 capsule or ½–1 teaspoon of tincture up to three times a day.

• *Black haw* is an antispasmodic, and 1 teaspoon of the tincture taken up to three times daily helps relieve menstrual cramping.

• *Jamaican dogwood* is the best for strong cramps; take 500 mg as needed.

Homeopathic Remedies

Because PMS and severe menstrual cramping are related to hormonal function and reproduction, they are considered to be important and deep conditions by homeopaths. For a cure, you may need professional care. However, for short-term relief try a combination remedy specifically formulated for menstrual discomfort that contains at least one of the single remedies listed on page 215, or choose the single remedy that most closely matches your symptoms. Follow instructions on the package; if your symptoms are severe, it is usually recommended that you take a dose as often as every 5 minutes; for milder symptoms, take every 3 hours. One dose equals 2–3 pills or 5–10 drops. (*See* Chapter 3, pages 75–81, for more information about homeopathy.)

• *Belladonna.* For acute cramps that may feel like bearing-down labor pains; for menstrual cramps in which bending over aggravates the pain; when pain is aggravated by motion of any kind.

• *Pulsatilla.* For PMS symptoms which include moodiness, sensitivity, depressions, and a tendency to cry; also relieves dizziness, nausea, diarrhea, headaches, and back pain; for many types of menstrual pain especially if you moan or cry with the pain.

• *Magnesia phosphorica.* The best remedy for simple menstrual cramps which are relieved by warmth, pressure, or bending over, especially if the menses and pain are associated with lethargy.

• *Colocynthis.* For severe menstrual cramps which are relieved primarily by bending over, although warmth and pressure may also help; to relieve irritability or anger during your period.

Aromatherapy

Warm baths help relieve symptoms of bloating, cramps, muscle tension, emotional dips, breast pain, and insomnia even more effectively when you add a few drops of oil of *geranium, fennel,* and *rosemary* to the bath water. To gently soothe depression and irritability, use *chamomile, bergamot,* or *rose* essential oils.

Acupressure and Massage

Acupressure massage (*see* Chapter 3, page 81) may help lessen menstrual cramps and PMS. Press the points shown on the diagram on page 217 to ease cramps and emotional symptoms such as tension; you may also try massaging your feet and hands. Have someone apply pressure to each side of your sacrum (see the illustration on page 218). An easy way to do this is to curl up in a ball—the Yoga position called the ''child's pose''—and have a friend sit on these points. To do this correctly, your friend starts by straddling your bottom facing away from you. She squats down, slowly shifting most of her weight from her feet to your sacrum; guide her to settle into a position where your friend's *ischia,* or ''butt bones,'' fit nicely right on the base of your sacrum. *Do not sit on the lower back.* Breathe deeply into these points.

Lymphatic massage is designed to rid the body of excess water by physically moving the fluid from the tissues toward the heart, where it enters the circulatory system for elimination through the kidneys. Schedule your massage to coincide with your most bloated time of the month. You may do well with several massages at that time.

Natural Hormone Therapy

If after following the Balanced Life Plan and using natural therapies, you still suffer from PMS, you may want to investigate your hormone balance under a doctor's supervision (*see* Chapter 4). Many women who use natural progesterone in its several forms report relief of PMS symptoms. At the MEND Clinic, women have relieved almost 100 percent of menstrual cramping and PMS symptoms if adequate doses of progesterone are used for women who have documented low progesterone levels compared with their estrogen. There are over-the-counter creams and oils containing variable amounts of progesterone from plants.

Progesterone cream is usually applied twice a day to areas of your body where your skin is soft and thin and covers a layer of fat, particularly the breasts, abdomen, inner arms, and inner thighs. Most experts say you will need to determine your own dosage, by monitoring your symptoms, and be sure to check with your physician about how much progesterone cream you should use, if any. Dr. John Lee, who has extensive experience with Progest, one of the nonprescription progesterone creams, recommends that you use a 2-ounce jar over 14 days, from days 12 to 26 of the menstrual cycle, increasing the dose during the last 4–5 days. Another approach is to use ¼–½ teaspoon twice a day on arising and before going to bed.

If you have severe premenstrual symptoms, consult with your doctor about taking progesterone pills containing micronized progesterone made from soybeans; these are more potent than the creams. Or you may consider using natural progesterone cream *and* natural progesterone oil (also more potent than cream used alone) taken under the tongue for faster relief. One suggested regimen is to take ¼ teaspoon of the oil (4 drops) held under your tongue for 60 seconds every 10–15 minutes until symptoms are relieved. (You may need to do this as often as four to eight times at first, depending on the severity of

Acupressure Points for Menstrual Tension

Acupressure Points for Premenstrual Water Retention

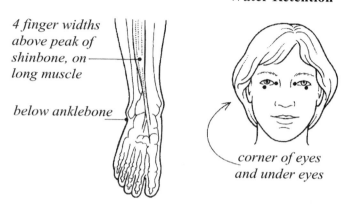

4 finger widths above peak of shinbone, on long muscle

below anklebone

corner of eyes and under eyes

Acupressure Points For Premenstrual Emotions

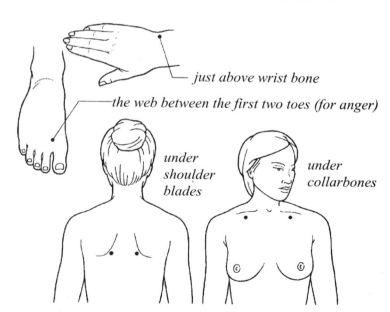

just above wrist bone

the web between the first two toes (for anger)

under shoulder blades

under collarbones

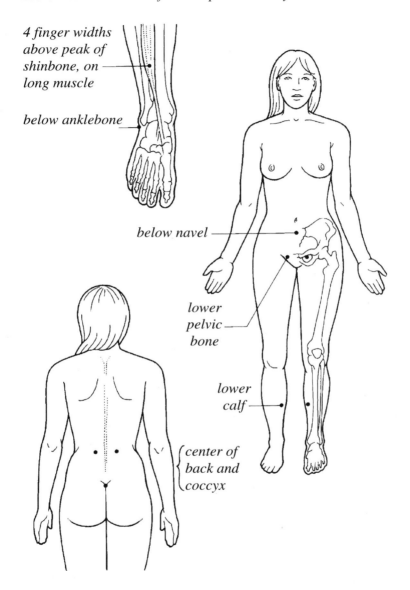

4 finger widths above peak of shinbone, on long muscle

below anklebone

below navel

lower pelvic bone

lower calf

center of back and coccyx

Acupressure Points For Premenstrual Pain and Tension

your symptoms.) In his book, *Natural Progesterone,* Dr. Lee cautions that the cream "does not preclude proper attention to other contributing factors such as diet, . . . supplements . . . relaxation techniques and good exercise."

Precautions

There are many possible causes and many possible treatments for severe menstrual cramping and PMS. So don't give up if the suggestions we offer here don't bring you complete relief. Seek the advice of a professional knowledgeable in natural therapies who will develop a plan to treat the underlying chronic illness. Medical care should also be sought if there is very severe pain or unusual pain in the pelvic area or abdomen, particularly if accompanied by fever or unusual vaginal bleeding (heavy, clotted, scanty, or none). One easily treated cause of PMS and cramps is misalignment of the pelvic bones. Dr. Maas treats many women who experience cramps and PMS after an injury or accident that has disrupted the normal alignment of the pelvic bone. Misalignment often worsens low back pain during the premenstrual phase, but it may exist even if you aren't bothered with back problems. You should consider an evaluation and treatment by an osteopath or chiropractor if you suspect misalignment.

Moodiness, Mood Swings, and Irritability

In spite of recent surveys and studies that suggest that mood swings or instability of moods are not demonstrably more frequent during menopause, some women report increased incidence of irritability, nervousness, and "bad moods" during the menopausal years. Changes in self-image, job pressures, family upheavals, sleeplessness due to hot flashes, hormonal fluctuations . . . is it any surprise that a woman might not feel like little Mary Sunshine?

Also, women often attribute feeling bad to being bad. They may feel guilty for not being able to care for others' needs while they feel lousy and may blame their physical limitations on themselves. For example, we might sometimes say, "Why can't I get over this stupid headache?" or "I can't do anything with myself," or "I just can't seem to get it right." Pay attention to your self-talk. When you use self-deprecatory expressions like these, immediately forgive yourself for your harsh words and undo the damage with affirmations: "I know exactly what to do about this headache—I'll take a bath as soon as I get home," or "I can do a lot with myself, I'm coping really well under the circumstances," or "I can get it right—I *can* do it!" This way of talking to yourself may seem awkward or even silly at first, but the power of positive thinking has been proven time and again to affect the way we feel and behave.

Guilt about being sick and needing something from others instead of the other way around causes some of us to deny ourselves care and comfort, even when it's freely offered. "Don't come near me" may be one expression of that feeling. It may sound like irritability, but it's really low self-esteem. If we're not able to take care of others, much less ourselves, we feel undeserving.

Therapists often attribute irritability to repressed anger. Women are discouraged from expressing anger overtly, and usually want to "be nice" all the time, even when challenged or insulted, or even abused. This pent-up tension may result in all kinds of irritability, from crying spells to bad tempers, and worsens the symptoms of hormonal imbalance, which leads to more physical problems. Another possibility is that any moodiness you experience is related to premenstrual syndrome, which may worsen in some women as they reach midlife.

See also "Anxiety," "Depression," and "Menstrual Cramps and PMS."

General Nutrition and Lifestyle Considerations

Sometimes physical conditions or symptoms such as hot flashes or insomnia are at the root of moodiness or irritability, so refer to our sections on whatever other symptoms you may be experiencing. Make sure you are optimally nourished, relaxed, and exercised by following our Balanced Life Plan in Chapter 2. Exercise is a great mood elevator. Sometimes food intolerances or allergies are a factor in our moods.

All the natural therapies provided in Chapter 3 are generally helpful for maintaining emotional equilibrium. However, women have found the following specific approaches to be particularly helpful for this complaint.

Herbal Remedies

Many women find that herbs help with these emotions. For instructions on herbal remedies, *see* Chapter 3, pages 70–75. Use an all-purpose menopausal herbal remedy, or choose one or more of the following herbs, all of which are particularly effective in treating negative moods and emotional symptoms such as nervousness, irritability, oversensitivity, and crying.

• *Valerian* is popular all over the world as a natural sedative. The usual dose is 1 teaspoon of tincture up to 3 times a day, or 1 cup of infusion before bed time.
• *Motherwort,* up to 3 cups of infusion daily; ½–1 teaspoon of tincture up to three times a day.
• *Lemon balm,* 3–4 cups of tea daily; ½–1 teaspoon of tincture up to three times a day.
• *Hops,* 5–10 capsules or ½–1 teaspoon of tincture up to three times a day.

Homeopathic Remedies

Following the instructions in Chapter 3, pages 75–81, use a combination homeopathic formula that contains at least one of the remedies listed below, or choose a single remedy that most closely matches your symptoms and personality. Follow the instructions on the package; if your symptoms are severe, it is usually recommended that you take a dose as often as every 5 minutes; for milder symptoms, take every 3 hours. One dose equals 2–3 pills or 5–10 drops.

• *Chamomilla.* Use this remedy when you have been in a very emotional state for some time, and are now highly sensitive and irritable, mentally or physically. You may rage violently and be difficult to please.
• *Nux vomica.* You may benefit from nux vomica if you tend to be quarrelsome, irritable, and aggressive and hate to be contradicted; you become angry when you are forced to reply to something you don't want to; your anger tends to be violent and you feel terrible if you hold it in.
• *Hepar sulphuricum.* This is useful when the slightest thing causes irritation and oversensitivity; when anger turns to violence; if you are touchy, chilly, and crave spices and strong-tasting foods.
• *Lycopodium.* When you are angry because you were contradicted, and are essentially low in self-confidence.
• *Natrum muriaticum.* If you suppress your emotions, but then fi-

nally explode; you do not cry easily, especially in public; if irritability is worse just before menstruation.

• *Sepia.* If you become irritable when contradicted; especially useful for women who may be irritable because they are worn out and exhausted from having too much to do.

Precautions

These changes in our lives that occur at or after menopause may intensify depression and other psychological conditions. For example, a phobic woman may become terrified, rather than just mildly anxious, as she was earlier in her life, about leaving home or going across bridges or riding to a high floor in an elevator. (Even mild phobias are not really "normal," however, and you might want to seek help for them. We discussed this in the "Anxiety" section.) Certain addictions or preoccupations may increase as well. If your life is becoming more circumscribed because of these problems; if you notice you're taking more substances to calm you down such as over-the-counter medications or alcohol or narcotics; or you're driving your family and friends crazy with your need to protect yourself from things that frighten or annoy you; if you're flying off the handle to the extent that people keep their distance or you cry whenever they're around you, better get some help. You'll feel better and so will your pals and intimates.

Nervousness

See "Anxiety" and "Moodiness."

Night Sweats

When hot flashes occur at night, they are called night sweats. Many women experience hot flashes both day and night, but in some women, hot flashes never occur in the day at all. There is tremendous variation among women in the intensity of night sweats, from needing to get up and change one's sleepwear and bedding, to just throwing off the bedcovers, to toweling off your neck and chest. Although women who experience hot flashes during the day may be annoyed and inconvenienced that they occur in public, night sweats can wake you several times a night, disturbing your sleep and leading to insomnia and all of its irritating accompanying symptoms.

See also "Hot Flashes" and "Insomnia."

General Considerations

Some women report some relief from night sweats by having sex twice or more weekly. Sexual stimulation, by pleasuring yourself or with a willing partner, stimulates hormones, redirects blood flow, and serves as a wonderful distraction. Some women keep a fan near the bed to cool them off when a hot flash occurs at night; a pitcher of cool water or a damp washcloth kept on your bedtable may also help provide cooling relief.

For natural therapies that may help night sweats, see the section on "Hot Flashes." Women have also found the following herbs to be particularly helpful for night sweats: *oatstraw, motherwort,* and *garden sage.* And the homeopathic remedy *sepia* is particularly useful for hot flashes that are worse or more frequent at night.

Precautions

Sometimes hot flashes that occur at night can be confused with night sweats due to other causes. Don't forget that night sweats may also be a symptom of metabolic problems, infectious and other sometimes serious diseases, so don't automatically write them off as just a menopausal symptom without investigating further. If your night sweats are accompanied by headache, an odorous or discolored nasal discharge, weight loss, pain, or other problems, you should seek medical care.

Painful Intercourse (Dyspareuna)

See "Vaginal Dryness."

Skin Changes

Certain skin changes are inevitable as we get older, so far as we know. Lowered hormones—both female and "male" hormones—play a role. As hormone levels diminish, our skin gradually gets thinner, drier, and secretes less oil. The aging process itself causes us to lose fat from under the layers of skin, allowing skin to become looser and for any wrinkles to become more apparent.

As with other body changes, the role of aging and hormones is heavily influenced by lifestyle and environmental factors. You may be surprised to learn that much of the wrinkling and sagging, the blotches, roughness, and "age spots" that accompany aging may put in an earlier appearance or are aggravated primarily by sun and cigarettes, two factors that are usually under our control.

Smoking literally starves your skin of oxygen and nutrients by constricting blood vessels. Recent research indicates that smoking ages skin two to three times faster than normal. Our bodies need sunlight to form vitamin D, but in excess, the sun's rays cause our skin's outer layers to become thick and leathery, and they damage the DNA in our skin cells, setting the stage for cancer. Too much sun also damages the under layers, causing them to lose their elasticity and allowing our skin to become lined and sag. Light-skinned women who freckle and burn easily have the highest risk for skin damage. Black women have less trouble with the sun than those who are fair because their skin contains more melanin. Melanin protects them from the worst effects of the sun's radiation, and tanning increases our skin's supply as a protective mechanism. But that doesn't mean dark-skinned women— or light-skinned women with tans—are completely safe from skin cancer. It's vital that all women of all ages avoid overexposure to the sun. If you don't believe in the power of the sun and other elements, just compare your face with the skin on other parts of your body that have been less exposed, such as your buttocks and undersides of your breasts.

General Nutrition

Your skin is a reflection of your general health, so be sure to follow the Balanced Life Plan provided in Chapter 2. Make a special effort to drink plenty of water and eat lots of fruits and vegetables to keep your skin young from the inside out. In addition, antioxidant vitamins and minerals may protect skin from environmental damage, so emphasize foods high in vitamins C and E, beta-carotene, selenium, and the B vitamins. Also try to eat plenty of vegetables and citrus and other fruits for their bioflavonoids, which strengthen capillaries and may avoid the spider-web look.

Remember that after crash dieting or yo-yo dieting, your skin probably won't bounce back the way it used too, especially as we get older. And being generally thin makes most women's faces look a bit more gaunt and possibly haggard than they would be if they had more body fat; this is particularly true as we age because our faces naturally lose their cushioning fat. As Zsa Zsa Gabor has sagely observed, "Dahlink, at a certain age a woman must choose between her face and her behind."

General Considerations

Unfortunately, by the time you've reached menopause, much of the damage to your skin has already been done. Tans that were beauty-enhancing at sixteen make you look like a mummy at sixty and may lead to a lot worse than wrinkles. There's plenty of evidence that skin cancers, too, begin in youth. Still, it's never too late—or too early—to do what you can to protect your skin from further damage.

Remind your teenage daughters or nieces that life-long beautiful skin depends on avoiding prolonged sun exposure. Avoid sunburn at all costs, no matter what your age or color. If work, sports, or travel requires long exposure, they (and you) should always wear a hat and long sleeves. Experts generally recommend sunblock, but Dr. Maas and others think this may not be the best way to protect your skin from the sun. Higher doses of essential fatty acids, orally and topically, along with other antioxidant nutrients, may be an overall safer approach to skin protection. This does not inhibit the development of helpful skin pigments, nor does it expose you to petroleum products and other chemicals that are absorbed from tanning lotions and sunblocks. Your babies and grandbabies, too, need to be protected. Skin cancer is no laughing matter and the pits and scars that come from surgery to remove those growths that may begin to show up in middle age (although they took years to develop) aren't too nice to look at either.

Other practices that hurt your skin are exposure to excess wind and temperature extremes. Protect your skin with clothing and salves if you know you'll be roughing it. Avoid also overdoing the caffeine and alcohol, both of which dry out your skin. Remember, smoking tends to worsen wrinkles, particularly around the mouth; give it up if you care about your looks *and* your health. Stress and emotional upheaval take their toll on your face, so pay attention to diet, relaxation, stress management, and the amount and quality of sleep you're getting.

Regular strenuous exercise helps you cope with stress, and increases the blood circulating to all parts of your body, imparting a healthful, more youthful glow.

When bathing, consider adding a tablespoon or two of sesame or other oil. Or rub a thin film of oil onto your skin while it's still moist after bathing or showering—this helps seal in the moisture. Consider sponge baths or washcloths for those body parts that especially need it: genitals, armpits, and feet. When showering, use mild soap on those areas, too—the rest of you really doesn't need to be covered in lather in order to be sufficiently clean, and most soaps strip your skin of their natural oils. Use a loofa or brush to remove old, dead skin layers and the dirt they hold. One of the best things you can do for your skin is to buy a hand shower that attaches to your regular shower fixture to use as a bidet after sex or other activities that require a washing off. If you're bleeding a lot and passing big clots during your period, you may also want to rinse off—but there's no sense in washing everything just because a couple of places need it!

Your clitoris, urethra, and vulva can be very sensitive to chemicals. Perfumed soaps can cause variable amounts of burning, immediately or days later. Irritation can set off yeast or bacterial infections owing to the change in the acid balance, flora balance (bacteria and other microorganisms), or your own defenses owing to the inflammation.

Women have found the following specific natural approaches to be particularly helpful for keeping skin healthy-looking.

Nutritional Supplements

A good multivitamin-mineral formula containing the doses recommended in Chapter 3, pages 61–64, generally supplies the nutrients you need to protect your skin from environmental damage. Be especially diligent in taking your antioxidant supplements, such as vitamins C and E and beta-carotene. Beta-carotene seems to be especially protective against sun damage. You may also take:

• *Essential fatty acids,* 45 g of gammalinoleic acid (GLA), which calms skin irritations. GLA is found in evening primrose oil, black currant seed oil, or borage oil supplements; or take 1 tablespoon of fresh flax seeds or flax oil. Other essential fatty acids are found in hemp and safflower oil.

Massage and Aromatherapy

Your skin looks healthier if it has a good supply of blood carrying oxygen and nutrients. Massage can help, but some cosmeticians recommend that you leave massaging the delicate skin on your face to a professional. However, you can give yourself an invigorating scalp massage to increase the blood supply to your face. Simply rub your scalp with your fingertips as if you were giving yourself a shampoo. For dry skin, add *geranium, jasmine,* or *rose oil* to a rich carrier oil such as jojoba, avocado, or peach kernel, which will help restore the natural oils that diminish as we age. Skin that is dull and crepy benefits from *sandalwood, patchouli,* or *frankincense* added to a carrier oil and applied to your skin. The Egyptians used frankincense for embalming, and it seems to help preserve living skin as well! Oil of *chamomile* and *rose,* added to a bland carrier oil, help improve the fine network of broken capillaries that sometimes appears with age, but they must be applied daily and take quite some time to show their effects. (*See* Chapter 3, page 84, for more information about aromatherapy.)

Natural Hormone Therapy

If the above approaches are not effective enough, before considering taking conventional hormone replacement therapy, you may want to try *natural progesterone cream.* Women who use it report it not only eases menopausal symptoms, but is a wonderful moisturizing cream and makes their skin look smoother. However, Dr. Brown feels it is inappropriate for women to use any kind of hormonal therapy for cosmetic purposes. She feels that all hormones—even natural ones— are powerful substances that should be used only in true cases of hormone deficiency, and for problems directly linked to such deficiencies. Dr. Maas points out that, on the other hand, the skin may be one of the only clues a woman has of a hormone imbalance. Because of the safety of the natural progesterone, Dr. Maas feels it is not unwise for a woman to give it a clinical "trial" and see how she feels.

You may also want to eat more foods high in plant estrogens; these include flax seeds, soybeans (and foods made from them, such as tofu); fruits such as figs and dates; plants and vegetables such as alfalfa, garlic, sprouted green peas, fennel, and anise seeds; nuts and legumes such as cashews, peanuts, almonds, and whole grains.

Urinary Tract and Bladder Infections

When the level of estrogen decreases, the tissues in your urinary tract (urethra and bladder) become thinner and drier and lose their tone. This means that after menopause, tissues become more delicate, leaving them more vulnerable to irritation and infection, sometimes with symptoms of burning and itching. (Your vaginal tissues also undergo similar changes, and these are discussed in the sections "Vaginitis" and "Vaginal Dryness.")

When the tissues in and around the urethra thin out and become dry, the urethra becomes easily inflamed. Your urethra swells and turns red, causing burning when urine passes through it. The swelling may also cause a partial obstruction. In other words, your bladder doesn't empty completely, and instead becomes a breeding ground for bacteria. You may feel this constriction as a change in your urine stream, or you may feel nothing unless the bacteria grow out of hand and cause a bladder infection. This infection may extend to other parts of your urinary tract—including the kidneys—if it's not attended to.

Urinary tract and bladder infections are common in middle-aged and older women. About 15 percent of postmenopausal women experience more frequent bladder infections than premenopausal women. Bladder infections or "cystitis" usually cause very painful urination and a feeling that one has to urinate all the time. Urinary infections are often treated with antibiotics, but there are natural treatments you may try instead. If you start your home treatment as soon as you feel symptoms, and follow a complete program for urinary health, you may eliminate the troublesome overgrowth of bacteria. However, this self-treatment is not for everyone, so please refer to the section on "Precautions" as well.

See also "Incontinence."

General Nutrition

As you follow the Balanced Life Plan in Chapter 2, make a special effort to eat foods high in immune-supporting nutrients such as vitamins C and E, beta-carotene, zinc, and garlic. Drink at least two quarts of fluids every day, most of it in the form of plain water. This increases the amount of urine produced and flushes out bacteria. Avoid coffee, tea, alcohol, and sweet drinks. Avoid sugary foods, which impede your immune system.

Cranberry and blueberry juice have been found to contain a substance that prevents most types of bacteria from growing on the bladder lining. In a 1994 study of 153 elderly women, the women who drank 10 ounces of cranberry juice a day had half the number of bacterial infections, after 1 month. Interestingly, many of the women drinking the cranberry juice had tested positive for bacteria before the study began. Since unsweetened cranberry juice is so unpalatable, and sugar encourages bacterial growth, the cranberry juice was sweetened with saccharine in the study. We believe it's wise to avoid artificial sweeteners as well as sugar, so we recommend taking cranberry tablets or cranberry extract diluted and sweetened with a small amount of stevia honey, instead, both of which are available at health food stores.

Some women may suffer from recurrent bladder problems because of food allergies or sensitivities (for information about food allergies, *see* Chapter 2, page 38). Another possibility is that calcium supplements may be causing recurrent infections in sensitive women, by causing the bacteria to adhere to the bladder wall. The solution is to drink 10 ounces of cranberry juice from unsweetened extract or its equivalent in tablets.

General Considerations

Many of the recommendations in the "Vaginitis" section will also help prevent urinary tract problems because the urethra is so close to the vagina. Avoid holding in urine if you feel the urge to urinate; there's evidence that women who have frequent infections tend to ignore nature's call and hold in urine for an hour or longer after feeling the urge to go. In addition, drinking water and emptying your bladder before and after sexual intercourse prevents irritation and flushes out bacteria.

Women have found the following specific approaches to be particularly helpful for treating urinary infections.

Nutritional Supplements

A good multivitamin-mineral formula containing the doses recommended in Chapter 3, pages 61–64, generally supplies the nutrients you need to keep your urinary tract healthy and able to withstand infection. You may also increase your daily intake of:

• *Vitamin C,* up to 500 to 1,000 mg every 1–2 hours during an active urinary infection (you have reached the upper limit of your personal dosage for vitamin C when your bowels become loose). Not only does this support your immune system, but vitamin C accumulates in the urinary tract, where it causes the urine to become more acidic, which discourages the growth of most bacteria.

You may also take:

• *Essential fatty acids,* up to 9–30 g of gammalinoleic acid (GLA), found in evening primrose oil, black currant seed oil, or borage oil supplements; or 1–1½ teaspoons a day of fresh flax seeds or flax oil. This omega-6 fatty acid helps reverse tissue thinning, dryness, itching, and burning.

Herbal Remedies
Several herbs offer help with urinary atrophy and infections. For instructions on herbal remedies, *see* Chapter 3, pages 70–75. Use an all-purpose menopausal herbal remedy to balance hormones. Or choose among these herbs, which are particularly effective in treating this condition. Use them singly or in combination, or look for a commercially prepared herbal formula that contains them.

• *Uva-ursi* is known for its antiseptic properties. The crude plant extracts seem to be more effective than the powdered products that contain only one isolated substance from this herb called arbutin. Take as tea, 1 teaspoon of tincture, or 1 cup of infusion up to three times a day during an active infection.

• *Goldenseal* is known to be a highly effective infection fighter; it is often combined with *echinacea,* another infection fighter. Take ½–1 teaspoon of tincture three times a day, or up to 2 cups daily of infusion during an active infection. If you have frequent bouts of cystitis, after sex you may prevent future infection by brewing a strong solution of goldenseal tea (2 teaspoons in 1 cup of water). Use this to wash your labia and urethral area before and after intercourse.

• *Motherwort* (½ teaspoon tincture up to twice daily, up to 2 cups of infusion daily, or 10–15 drops of extract in warm water up to three times a day) and *agnus castus* in similar amounts taken several times a day aid in restoring lubrication and tone to your urogenital tissues.

Homeopathic Remedies

Homeopathy offers several remedies for urinary problems. Following the instructions in Chapter 3, pages 75–81, you may want to use a combination remedy formulated to restore hormone balance, or choose a formula designed specifically to combat cystitis that contains one or more of the remedies listed below. You may also choose from among one of the many single remedies that are useful for the constant or frequent burning sensation of cystitis, according to your symptoms. Follow the instructions on the package; if your symptoms are severe, it is usually recommended that you take a dose as often as every 5 minutes; for milder symptoms, take every 3 hours. One dose usually equals 2–3 pills or 5–10 drops.

• *Apis* soothes cystitis if you feel better in the fresh air and worse in the heat, and are irritable generally.
• *Cantharis* soothes cystitis if the pain is violent and spasmodic, and if you feel worse after having a cold drink.
• *Sulfur* is best if your symptoms are worse when you get up in the morning, or at night, or when you urinate; if you are generally restless and irritable.

Aromatherapy

Some women have found relief for urinary tract infection from *bergamot, eucalyptus, lavender,* and *sandalwood.* You may add them to your bath at least once a day; but be aware that any essential oil can be irritating if it comes into contact with swollen or inflamed urethral tissues. Use diluted amount for a short time to test oils, or simply inhale them as directed in Chapter 3, page 84. Or add *bergamot* or *chamomile* to a carrier oil and gently massage over your abdomen.

Spinal Manipulation

If you have frequent urinary tract infections, you should have your alignment checked by an osteopath or a chiropractor because manipulation of the pelvis may be needed.

Natural Hormone Therapy

Hormones are a useful treatment for urinary tract infections only if you clearly have atrophy of the urogenital tissues. Most physicians prescribe estrogen in vaginal suppositories or creams, patches, or oral medication. They all bring the hormone to the tissues where it is needed, although vaginal preparations provide the bulk of the effect directly to these tissues. Dr. Maas prescribes estriol, sometimes in combination with estradiol and estrone, and sometimes with other hormones, especially progesterone. According to health professionals and women who use it, natural progesterone cream on its own helps reverse tissue atrophy and dryness with no or minimal side effects. *See* Chapter 4 for more information about hormone therapy. You may also want to eat more foods high in plant estrogens; these include soybeans (and foods made from them, such as tofu); flax seeds; fruits such as figs and dates; plants and vegetables such as alfalfa, garlic, sprouted green peas, fennel and anise seeds; nuts and legumes such as cashews, peanuts, almonds, and whole grains.

Precautions

Natural therapies can help some women restore hormone balance and fight off minor infections. However, if natural therapies don't relieve your symptoms or if your symptoms get worse, especially fever, back pain, nausea, or decreased appetite, or if you feel ill, be sure to see a doctor. Symptoms such as pelvic pressure similar to menstrual cramps and frequent urination have other causes that require a doctor's evaluation. If untreated, these infections, like others, can cause a lot of trauma to the system. So even if you get these infections often and take them casually, remember that all untreated infections can play havoc with your body. One of the ways women don't take themselves seriously may be in neglecting these common infections until they can't be ignored.

Vaginal Dryness

As we noted in Chapter 2, estrogen production diminishes—sometimes dramatically—as you reach menopause and continues to dwindle as you pass into the postmenopausal years. Deprived of their customary supply of estrogen, vaginal walls tend to become thin and dry. The cervix secretes less mucus and the entrance to the vagina can actually become smaller. The blood supply to your entire genital area decreases. All these changes explain why intercourse can become uncomfortable and sometimes painful, even if you are able to have sexual feelings and achieve a climax. Some women are simply uncomfortable with dry, delicate tissues, which become easily irritated with or without intercourse; in some women dry vaginal tissues tend to become infected more easily with yeast and bacteria.

Some believe that, in addition, estrogen contributes significantly to sexual desire and that low estrogen would therefore also affect our sensations during intercourse in another way. That's because being sexually aroused is a prerequisite to producing the lubrication that bathes the vagina with the fluids that make intercourse smooth. When these juices don't flow copiously, intercourse can become painful and achieving an orgasm is more difficult because dry stimulation of the clitoris just hurts and is less likely to produce a sexual "excitation." The clitoris is more likely to respond to a well-lubricated penis or finger stimulating it.

The conventional treatment for a dry vagina is estrogen cream. The cream, which you apply to the vagina and vulva, is very effective in many women; you should notice a difference in 1 or 2 weeks. Estrogen cream will help thicken your vaginal walls, and it usually solves your lubrication problem, but some women find they still need to use one of the lubricating creams or gels mentioned below. Although many women are satisfied with the results, there are a few problems with using the cream. If you have a dry vagina, it usually indicates that you have low levels of estrogen throughout your body—including your brain and heart—not just your vagina. Since your sexual hormones affect all of your tissues, this suggests that the health of all your tissues may be suffering as well. Some women may feel that they don't "need" vaginal health or that estrogen cream is all they need if vaginal thinning or dryness is their main or only problem. Because the estrogen in the cream is applied directly to the vagina, most of the hormone stays right there; however, some of the estrogen (about 25–50 percent) will still enter your bloodstream (*see* Chapter 4). Estrogen cream is not to be used as lubrication before intercourse, since it was not designed for this and the estrogen may be absorbed into your partner's bloodstream too. Although estrogen cream does help and seems relatively safe, for those who cannot or prefer not to use hormones, there are other alternatives to explore.

See also "Urinary Tract and Bladder Infections" and "Vaginitis."

General Nutrition and Lifestyle Considerations

The most pleasurable and natural way to deal with vaginal dryness that makes intercourse painful is to set aside time for the extended foreplay that you may need to stimulate your own natural lubrication. If that's still insufficient, you may also use one of the lubricating products especially made for sexual activity, such as K-Y Jelly or Astroglide. They are water-soluble, and unlike non–water-soluble creams and lotions or petroleum jelly, they will not increase suscepti- bility to infection or interfere with birth control or condoms. A prod- uct called Replens, available in drugstores without a prescription, is specially formulated to plump up your vaginal cells with water, which aids in lubrication and keeps your tissues healthy whether you have sex or not. It also helps restore alkalinity to your vagina, which helps prevent some vaginal infections. Adult ''sex shops'' may have a greater selection of lubricants.

Women have found the following specific natural therapies to be particularly helpful for minimizing vaginal thinning and dryness.

General Lifestyle Considerations

Vaginal atrophy can be made worse if you're out of shape and have sluggish circulation. Regular exercise pumps up and improves circula- tion all over your body, including your pelvic area. Some women report that doing pelvic exercises improves their vaginal tone; Kegel exercises strengthen the muscles surrounding your vagina and may help make intercourse more comfortable at this time of your life. (*See* ''Incontinence'' for information on how to perform Kegel exercises.) And remember, this is a case of ''use it or lose it.'' Research suggests that regular sexual activity—either with a partner or by self-pleasur- ing—helps keep the vagina toned and lubricated. This may be due to estrogen produced by the adrenal glands as well as the increased blood flow and toning effect of muscle contractions before and after arousal and orgasm. Avoid medications such as antihistamines, which dry out the delicate mucous tissue all over your body, not just in your nose and sinuses.

Nutritional Supplements

A good multivitamin and mineral formula containing the doses rec- ommended in Chapter 3, pages 61–64, usually supplies the nutrients you need to help balance hormones and maintain healthy vaginal tis- sue. You may increase the total daily dosage of certain nutrients up to the following amounts:

• *Vitamin E,* up to 600 IU for 4–6 weeks, to help treat atrophy of the vagina and increase lubrication. You may take this vitamin orally, or apply it directly to your vaginal tissues.

• *Essential fatty acids,* 9–45 g of gammalinoleic fatty acid (GLA), three times a day. GLA, found in evening primrose oil, black currant oil, or borage oil supplements, may help improve vaginal tissues and lubrication. Essential fatty acids are also found flax seeds and flax seed oil; 1–3 teaspoons per day minimizes symptoms within 1 month.

Herbal Remedies

Herbs may help with vaginal thinning and dryness because they help balance hormones. For instructions on using herbal remedies, *see* Chapter 3, pages 70–75. You may decide to use the all-purpose menopausal herbal formula that helps menopausal symptoms generally, or use a commercially prepared menopause formula. *Black cohosh, licorice,* and *motherwort* are particularly effective in relieving this symptom; you may use them either singly or in combination. The usual dose is 1 capsule or 1 teaspoon of tincture up to three times a day.

Homeopathic Remedies

Following the instructions in Chapter 3, pages 75–81, use a combination remedy for general menopausal symptoms, or try *bryonia,* which is appropriate for women who suffer from dryness everywhere, including the mouth, eyes, and vagina and who are generally very thirsty. Follow instructions on the package; if your symptoms are severe, it is usually recommended that you take a dose as often as every 5 minutes; for milder symptoms, you might get results with a single dose 3 times a day. One dose usually equals 2–3 pills or 5–10 drops.

Natural Hormone Therapy

If after following the Balanced Life Plan and using natural therapies, you still suffer from vaginal dryness and atrophy, you may want to try *natural hormone therapy* such as progesterone cream under a doctor's supervision (*see* Chapter 4). According to health professionals who recommend it and some women who use it, natural progesterone cream sometimes restores tone and lubrication to these tissues. You may apply progesterone cream directly to the affected tissues, but it is usually applied twice a day to areas of your body where your skin is soft and thin and covers a layer of fat, particularly the breasts, abdomen, inner arms, and inner thighs. Most often the dose is $1/2$ teaspoon per day, but be sure to check with your physician about how much progesterone cream you should use, if any. You may also want to eat more foods high in plant estrogens; these include flax seeds, soybeans (and foods made from them, such as tofu); fruits such as figs and dates; plants and vegetables such as alfalfa, garlic, sprouted green peas, fennel, and anise seeds; nuts and legumes such as cashews, peanuts, almonds, and whole grains. In one study, women who ate a diet including soy foods high in plant estrogens were able to increase the cells lining their vaginas.

Precautions

Dryness and thinning out of the vaginal walls can cause small tears in the tissue during intercourse. This makes more possible the entry of viruses and bacteria. Remember to practice safe sex with anyone other than your longtime trusted lover. (*See* ''Safer Sex'' in Chapter 7.)

Vaginitis

Your vagina and cervix are anatomically designed to secrete fluids. These fluids vary according to the phase of your menstrual cycle, sexual excitement, and whether or not you are pregnant. A vaginal discharge is not necessarily a sign of illness, but you should be aware of any changes in your normal vaginal secretions: the amount, the consistency, color, and odor, as well as any other symptoms such as inflammation and itching. Such changes are indications that you have vaginitis, which is an overgrowth of microorganisms.

Certain conditions can change the balance of normally present microorganisms in the vagina and encourage the overgrowth of one type over another. Menopause is one of them; so is a weakened immune system (for example, from stress or overwork), medications that cause a hormone imbalance, use of products such as spermicidal creams and jellies that contain irritating chemicals, certain foods, and others. There are several types of vaginitis, caused by different organisms, and characterized by a variety of symptoms.

Yeast infections are probably the most common. They are due to the overgrowth of a yeast or organism (usually *Candida albicans*) which normally exists in smaller quantities on our skin and in our intestinal tracts and vaginas. They are often triggered by an excess of sugar in the diet; in some women even fruit or white bread can cause yeast overgrowth. A yeast infection of the vagina is characterized by a thick whitish discharge that may look like cottage cheese; sometimes it smells like baking bread and sometimes it smells acrid. Yeast infections also can be maddeningly itchy and the external genital tissues become red and irritated. Yeast may grow out of control after a woman has been treated with a course of antibiotics for a bacterial infection because the drugs also wipe out beneficial vaginal bacteria that kept the normally present yeast in check.

Bacterial infections may be due to an overgrowth of a variety of different bacteria. This type of vaginitis is often referred to as nonspecific vaginitis and results in a white or yellow discharge; you may have burning with urination, itching, and an odor. Chlamydia and gonorrhea are sexually transmitted bacterial infections that you should have identified through a professional examination; they can have serious consequences if not diagnosed and treated.

Trichomonas infections involve a tiny parasitic organism and are characterized by a thin, foamy yellowish or greenish discharge that smells offensive. Trichomonas is sometimes sexually transmitted and requires a professional examination to identify; however, it is not serious.

Noninfectious vaginitis may be due to irritation from chemicals (such as douches or spermicide), sexual activity, or a tampon particularly if it has been inadvertently left in. Your vagina becomes red and swollen and may produce a discharge to rid your body of the irritation.

General Nutrition and Lifestyle Considerations

As you follow the Balanced Life Plan provided in Chapter 2, make a special effort to emphasize whole foods and to cut out sweets (even fruit) from your diet during an infection; this is especially important if you are getting one vaginal infection after another. Adding acidophilus supplements, which restore normal bacteria, often helps.

Try soaking in a ''sitz bath''—a bathtub containing 6 inches of warm water and $1/2$ cup of vinegar. Or douche twice a day with a cleansing douche using 1–2 tablespoons of white vinegar diluted in a pint of warm water. Vinegar helps change the acid balance of the genital area and helps restore the normal population of organisms. If the acidic vinegar wash doesn't bring relief, try the opposite: an alkaline wash of 4 tablespoons of baking soda in a pint of water. Wash your genital area gently and frequently, using mild soap or no soap at all; pat dry.

If it contains active yogurt cultures (check the label), plain yogurt may help soothe irritated tissues and restore balance. Apply it directly to the outer tissues, or insert a tampon dipped in yogurt and remove in an hour, or dissolve 2 tablespoons of yogurt in a pint of warm water and use as a douche. Or introduce yogurt's beneficial organisms into your system by eating it; a daily half-cup of plain yogurt has been shown to significantly reduce the number of yeast infections that women have.

Avoid wearing tight or synthetic clothing that encourages overgrowth of organisms by reducing air circulation. Exercise helps keep your immune system in good working order, but spend as little time as possible in wet or damp clothing such as bathing suits or workout clothing. If you suspect your vaginitis may be caused by irritation rather than an infection, avoid the suspected irritant for a time, or switch brands. Especially avoid bubble baths and vaginal deodorants, which can irritate delicate genital tissue.

Women have found the following specific natural approaches to be particularly helpful for preventing vaginitis and speeding up recovery from mild vaginal infections, if your immune system is not very depleted.

Herbal Remedies

Many women find that herbs help with vaginitis. For instructions on herbal remedies, *see* Chapter 3, pages 70–75. Use an all-purpose menopausal herbal remedy to tone and strengthen vaginal tissues. Or choose one or more of these herbs, which are particularly effective in treating this condition. Use them singly or in combination, or look for a commercially prepared herbal formula that contains them.

• *Citrus seed extract, caprylic acid, undecylenic acid,* and *garlic* are key oral herbal treatments used at the MEND Clinic.

• *Beth root, false unicorn root, white poplar,* and *cranesbill* are useful when you have a discharge that is thin and watery. Take 1 teaspoon of tincture of these herbs up to three times daily for 3 months.

• *Goldenseal* and *cranesbill* help reduce mucuslike discharge and many bacterial infections. The usual dose is ½–1 teaspoon of tincture up to three times a day, or up to 2 cups of infusion daily. Your symptoms should gradually disappear; continue to take the herbs for a month after symptoms have gone.

• *Goldenseal* and *echinacea* together, or *blue cohosh, comfrey, raspberry leaf,* or *oatstraw* are generally useful for vaginitis. If your problem is chronic, try *St. Johnswort* as an infusion (1 cup), or an extract (1 teaspoon) up to three times a day.

In addition to taking herbs internally, you may also douche with herbs. A general formula for vaginitis is 2 teaspoons each of powdered *goldenseal* and *myrrh* plus ½ teaspoon of *ginger* per pint of water. Boil the herbs, let cool, and strain the formula, then use once a day until you are better. Add *calendula* for tissues that are very irritated.

Homeopathic Remedies

Homeopathy offers several remedies for vaginitis. Following the instructions in Chapter 3, pages 75–81, you may want to use a combination remedy formulated for menopause or vaginitis that contains one or more of the substances listed below. Or choose the single remedy that most closely matches your symptoms. Follow the instructions on the package; if your symptoms are severe, it is usually recommended that you take a dose as often as every 5 minutes; for milder symptoms, take 3 times a day. One dose usually equals 2–3 pills or 5–10 drops.

• *Sepia.* For a discharge that is yellow-green and smells offensive, and that is worse in the morning, from walking, and before a menstrual period. Accompanying symptoms are a feeling of pressure or heaviness in the pelvis, cramping, and burning pain and irritation of the vulva.

• *Graphites.* For a thin, nonodorous, white, burning discharge that gushes out. Accompanying symptoms are weakness or abdominal tension. Symptoms are worse from walking and in the morning.

• *Mercurius vivus.* For a greenish, irritating discharge accompanied by rawness of the vulva; symptoms are often worse in the evening or at night; the vulva feels better after washing with cold water.

• *Pulsatilla.* For creamy yellow discharge; when the discharge is either bland or irritating. This remedy is especially useful for vaginitis that changes in character from day to day, and that occurs during pregnancy or in young girls.

• *Calcarea carbonica.* For thick white or yellow discharge that causes severe itching, may flow in gushes, and doesn't have much odor.

The following homeopathic remedies are also helpful for vaginal problems:

• *Belladonna* is useful when your vagina is hot, tender, and red and you are generally an oversensitive person.

• *Cantharis* is useful for a raw, burning vagina that feels better from applications of cold or gentle massage.

• *Sulfur* may help when vaginal itching is intense or burning.

Spinal Manipulation

Recurrent infections in the pelvic area may occur when a woman holds tension in the area. However, manipulation by an osteopath or a chiropractor, acupuncture, and appropriate exercise can often dramatically helps these problems, be they acute or chronic.

Precautions

Seek medical care if you have significant pelvic or lower abdominal pain; nausea; fever; pain during sex; trouble with your bowels or bladder; if you feel ill; you have had a recent new sexual partner; or you have a heavy discharge that does not improve with natural therapies. Vaginal discharge can have several noninfectious causes which may be serious.

Weight Gain

It's no secret that women tend to gain weight around the time of menopause. But is this inevitable? And is it unhealthy? When it comes to middle-aged spread, the evidence so far shows us that while it is possible to be too thin, being lean—even leaner than average—is healthier overall than being pleasantly plump.

The most recent figures show that 52% of all American women

aged fifty to fifty-nine are overweight. This is higher than other age groups. Recent surveys show that the average weight of the typical American adult has gone up by 8 pounds since 1985; and that 32% of Americans are considered to be obese, compared with 25% in 1980 and 24% in 1962. It may be small consolation, but teenagers are getting fatter, too.

So we're all getting heavier—clearly it's not just our fluctuating hormones. The real culprit is too little activity in relation to too much fat and refined carbohydrates in our diets. As a nation, we *all* need to eat less and exercise more; as we age, our metabolism gradually slows down, meaning that unless we make some lifestyle changes, we'll gain even more.

But how unhealthy is it to be heavy? High blood pressure, hardening of the arteries, diabetes, gallbladder disease, heart disease, and increased risk of many types of cancer including cancer of the breast, colon, and uterus are all associated with obesity. Although there is an accepted definition of ''obesity'' as being 20% over your ''desirable'' weight, the definition of ''desirable'' is not carved in stone. And even women who are not ''obese'' are at higher risk of premature death from all causes.

A recent study involving 115,000 middle-aged women shows that the lowest death rates occurred among the leanest women, including those 15–20% below average weight. It also showed that even middle-aged women of average weight have a 30% greater risk than those 20 pounds lighter. The lead researcher of the study, Dr. Jo-Ann Manson, co-director of Women's Health at Brigham and Women's Hospital, said, ''Being overweight is second only to cigarette smoking as a cause of premature death.'' The study corrected for participants who were smokers and who had existing heart disease, diabetes, or cancer.

On the other hand, it is possible to be too thin, especially if you're an older woman. For one thing, eating a low-calorie diet makes it virtually impossible to consume the nutrients you need to maintain strong healthy bones (*see* ''Osteoporosis'' in Chapter 6 for more information). And it's definitely unhealthy to go on a crash diet to lose 20 or 30 pounds to reach a more desirable weight. For another, women who carry around a bit more fat tend to have fewer menopausal difficulties, probably because fat cells take over the production of estrogen when the ovaries stop. In addition, the added weight puts good stress on the bones, which strengthens them. However, as we have seen in previous chapters, there are dietary and lifestyle changes we can make to help balance hormones and maintain bone strength without relying on extra body fat.

How Much Is Too Much?

Do you weigh more than is good for you? It depends on your body-mass index. A study published in the September 1995 *New England Journal of Medicine* concludes that thinner is usually better. But figuring out a healthy weight requires calculating a single number so that those with different heights can be compared. This number, called the body-mass index, is your weight in kilograms divided by the square of your height in meters.

Figuring body-mass index
1. Multiply your weight in pounds by 0.45 to get kilograms.
2. Convert your height to inches.
3. Multiply this number by 0.0254 to get meters.
4. Multiply that number by itself.
5. Divide this into your weight in kilograms. Your answer will probably be a number in the 20s or low 30s. It is your body-mass index.

Interpreting results
How body-mass indexes relate to risk of death in middle-aged women

Below 19	Lowest risk
19 to 24.9	20% higher
25 to 26.9	30% higher
27 to 28.9	60% higher
Over 29	100% higher

Source: Associated Press

Besides the health impacts mentioned above, there are other reasons to stay lean. Too much flesh on our bones is going to make it even harder to move around and get the exercise we need as we age, and exercise has many psychological benefits in addition to physical ones. Furthermore, it's almost impossible in our "think-thin" culture to feel really good about ourselves if we don't measure up to the ideal. It's also tiresome and humiliating to hear health care professionals admonish us to "just" lose weight. All these dire health warnings must be balanced, of course, by the advantages of having a positive self-image. Feeling good about your body the way you are is a key component of a holistic approach to good health. It may be that the superthin woman who regards every gram of fat as evil incarnate is no healthier than the plumper woman who occasionally indulges in rich food, but thoroughly enjoys every minute of it. Even if you can't whittle your weight down to the most desirable category, it would be a mistake to throw in the towel and sink into a spiral of self-loathing. Any movement in the right direction still lowers your risk of disease—and offers you an emotional lift that goes beyond its physical benefits.

Recent research indicates that even a small weight loss—of 10 or 15 pounds—can lower health risks, no matter how heavy you are. The natural approaches suggested below have helped many women get on the right track. We are not suggesting that modifying your weight is easy. We urge you to consider your weight problem, if you have one, as a potentially serious illness, but one that is quite treatable. With the help of a caring health professional and a balanced weight loss program, even hundreds of pounds can be dropped in time.

General Nutrition and Lifestyle Considerations

The best way to lose weight is to combine sensible eating with appropriate exercise. See Chapter 2 for our Balanced Life Plan, which provides eating and exercising guidelines. As most everyone who's tried knows, it's much easier to get weight off initially than it is to keep it off. The key is to make habitual your healthy eating and activity pattern. Once you start, it's just as easy—and more rewarding—than just counting calories to commit to a fun, nourishing, and social physical activity to keep you young and energetic. Food addictions, like any addiction, can be seen as a self-treatment for a spiritual longing. This can sometimes be overcome with love, meditation, and deep spiritual commitment.

Addictions may also be related to food sensitivities and allergies, and these in themselves cause some women to gain weight. In Dr. Brown's experience as a nutritional counselor, she rarely sees a weight problem that is not associated with a food sensitivity or allergy. By incorporating an allergy screening and elimination diet in her clinical program for weight loss, 80 percent of her clients are successful at eliminating cravings, reducing appetite, raising energy, and losing weight.

For some reason, it's also easier in the short run for us to cut way down on calories than it is to step up our physical activity. All recent evidence shows that this is the completely wrong way to go about it. According to Dr. Walter C. Willet, a prominent researcher at the Harvard School of Public Health, "the crucial factor in controlling weight gain is exercise, not dieting. People who exercise regularly can maintain their weight," he states.

The reality is that there are lots of reasons why we're less active as we age. One is that we don't feel as good getting out there and moving around. Our joints and muscles may ache; we can't go as fast as our younger companions; and many of us have full-time jobs now, so we honestly feel too tired to exercise or just plain don't have time.

So what's a larger woman to do? The answer is to join a group—or if need be, one group for weight loss and one for exercise. (A group can be just you and one other person, by the way.) While research indicates that a lot of people who lose weight gain it back, the chances that you'll keep it off are greater if you're in a group such as Weight Watchers that lets you stay on a "maintenance" program and keep coming to meetings for as long as you want. Weight Watcher meetings are held almost everywhere in the world and at most hours of the day and evening. They're a lot of fun: the leaders are former fatties who've kept it off and have wonderful stories to tell and snapshots of their former selves to pass around for the thousandth time; the participants are helpful, full of low-cal recipe ideas, and home-grown psychological advice, otherwise known as common sense. You're sure to find some buddies there who'll walk, hike, dance, or play tennis or swim with you and give you a hand when you drop a couple of pounds.

Nutritional Supplements

A good multivitamin-mineral formula containing the doses recommended in Chapter 3, pages 61–64, generally supplies the nutrients most women need to keep their metabolism humming and their weight under control. To lose weight, some women also have found increasing the total daily dose of the following to be helpful:

• *Chromium,* 100 mcg three times a day after meals. It's a key ingredient in many of the latest over-the-counter weight-loss products, and is also available as individual supplements. Chromium plays a role in stabilizing glucose levels in the blood, which in turn may help diminish mood swings and sugar cravings. According to some researchers, this nutrient helps you eat less by decreasing appetite. Because it is involved in metabolizing fat and carbohydrates, it may also decrease fat and increase lean muscle and thus improve your fitness. Chromium is contained in many foods (liver, broccoli, mushrooms, cheese, apples) but 90 percent of all Americans don't get enough from their food.

• *CitriMax* is a formula that supports natural weight loss without stimulating the central nervous system, unlike popular over-the-counter diet pills. In addition to chromium, it contains HCA, hydroxycitric acid, a substance extracted from a South Asian fruit, which redirects calories from fat production and helps reduce appetite. (Available from Pure Encapsulations, Inc., 490 Boston Post Road, Sudbury, MA 01776, 1-800-753-2277.)

Herbal Remedies

Many women find that herbs help with weight loss and control. For instructions on herbal remedies, *see* Chapter 3, pages 70–75. Use an all-purpose menopausal herbal remedy to balance hormones and metabolism. You may also find these herbs helpful. Use them singly or in combination, or look for a commercially prepared herbal formula that contains them.

• *Chickweed, cleavers,* and *pokeroot* are herbs that stimulate weight loss by helping to burn fat.
• *White ash bark* also helps weight loss, and *yerba maté* and *fennel* decrease appetite and aid digestion.

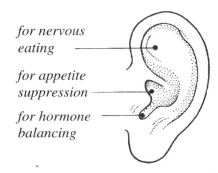

Acupressure Points
For Weight Control

for nervous eating

for appetite suppression

for hormone balancing

Acupressure and Massage

Acupressure massage (*see* Chapter 3, page 81) may help control appetite and food cravings, regulate your endocrine system, and reduce water retention. Press or massage the points shown in the diagram above once or twice a day. Massage of any type decreases stress and may decrease the "itch" to eat; some women find this occurs because it helps them literally to get in touch with and learn to accept their body as it is.

In addition, video and audiotapes may help you relax and dampen nervous eating. Dr. Maas has produced a series of tapes designed to ease tension that have proved an invaluable component in many of her patients' weight control programs. (*See* Resources section.)

Natural Hormone Therapy

A hormone imbalance may cause you to gain weight and make it more difficult to take it off. Although we don't recommend any type of hormone therapy for the sole purpose of weight control, if you do decide to take hormones, thyroid hormone is the most important. If you have trouble losing weight, feel cold, sluggish, constipated, are losing hair, your skin is dry and your head hair is coarse, you may have low thyroid. When thyroid is replaced, even to normal levels, metabolism and weight loss step up. Other hormones, for complicated reasons, can affect weight. Check with your health care provider for testing and treatment. Dr. John Lee, the foremost expert on natural progesterone, says natural progesterone helps you lose or maintain weight in a number of ways. Unlike synthetic progestins, progesterone is a natural diuretic, helps use fat for energy, helps thyroid function, and normalizes blood sugar levels. Estrogens,

DHEA, and testosterone also affect mood and metabolism and can help balance weight when prescribed to restore normal hormone ratios.

Precautions

Rapid weight loss accomplished through low-calorie beverage meals, even with a medically supervised program that includes nutritional supplements, can have serious consequences. Some of these programs can fail to nourish heart, muscles, brain, and other nerves and destroy the immune system as well—all of which can be difficult to repair.

CHAPTER 6

The Risks of Getting Older:
Beyond Hot Flashes

This chapter covers four of the most common and serious health problems that women face as they get older. Cardiovascular disease, osteoporosis, breast cancer, and diabetes—your risk for these conditions begins to rise at the time of menopause, and continues to increase as you age. Interestingly, breast cancer is the disease that strikes the most fear in the hearts of women, and as epidemic as it is, breast cancer is a far less common cause of death than the other three we discuss here.

While science hasn't yet unraveled all the possible causes of such diseases, they all appear to be diseases of modern civilization, and the seeds for most of them are sown in our youth and young adulthood. It's unfortunate that these health problems have been associated with menopause, when they actually result from a high-stress life in an increasingly toxic environment, compromised nutrition, and diminished physical strength and endurance. These hazards increase the risk of these four diseases as well as the symptoms of menopause.

Following the Balanced Life Plan in Chapter 2 can help you reduce your risk. Research also suggests that switching to certain drugless therapies can also contribute to managing and treating these diseases once they have occurred. For example, natural therapies can provide support and comfort for women with breast cancer before, during, and after conventional treatment. Certain nutritional supplements may protect the body from the harmful effects of radiation and chemotherapy, without lessening the therapy's beneficial effects. Visualization/ guided imagery can reduce certain side effects, and homeopathy and herbs are used to lessen the detrimental effects of anesthesia and speed recovery from surgery. The results of one study conducted at Stanford University suggest that support groups improve not only the quality of life of breast cancer patients, but their length of life as well.

Cardiovascular Disease

Until recently, the medical community and women themselves thought heart disease to be mostly a problem for men. Nothing could be farther from the truth. You may be surprised to learn that more American women die of heart attack than do men—500,000 each year, according to the American Dietetic Association. In fact, cardiovascular disease is the major cause of death in women. It kills six times as many women as does breast cancer; there is twice as much cardiovascular disease as osteoporosis in American postmenopausal women, and the death rate is over ten times as much.

Unfortunately, most of what we know about preventing and treating heart disease is based on studies done on men. Also, for unknown reasons, some of the indicators of heart disease, such as the stress test (treadmill with EKG) are not as predictive for women as they are for men. Women also respond to medication differently—and do *even better* with lifestyle changes than do men. Heart disease is less likely to be diagnosed early or correctly in women than in men, and women who have heart attacks are twice as likely to die shortly following the attack. Women's health issues are receiving more funding now; however, these new studies will take years to complete. In the meantime, women are encouraged to follow screening and treatment guidelines similar to those developed for men, and to wholeheartedly embrace the lifestyle advocated in Chapter 2. Yet a recent Gallup survey showed that only a small percentage of women are concerned about heart disease, and presumably aren't aware that they can reduce their risk by adopting the natural approaches covered in this book.

What Is Cardiovascular Disease?
The cardiovascular system includes the heart and the blood vessels. Coronary arteries are the blood vessels of the heart, which supply the

heart muscle with oxygen- and nutrient-rich blood. Coronary heart disease is the end result of a long, multistep process that threatens the flow of blood to the heart.

We now believe that free radicals begin the process by damaging the blood vessel wall. (*See* Chapter 3 for a discussion of free radicals— molecules with an electron charge—and how antioxidants reduce their damage.) Blood vessels that are in poor health are more susceptible to damage, and poor diet increases the free radical load and reduces antioxidants as well. Once damaged, the wall becomes inflamed, and *plaque*—made of cells, protein, cholesterol, and other fats—accumulates on their walls in a process called *atherosclerosis.* The plaque calcifies and hardens in time.

Angina, or chest pain, is a danger signal that the arteries are partially blocked and the heart isn't receiving enough oxygen. It's important that you do not ignore chest pain—your heart is in danger of suffocation, and the longer you are in pain, the higher the risk of irreversible death to your heart tissue. What's commonly called a *heart attack* occurs when the coronary artery is blocked by a threshold amount of plaque, or when the vessel, even without much plaque cramps—a reaction to an as yet unknown factor—completely blocking the blood flow. Deprived of blood for a long enough time, heart cells die and the heart becomes permanently damaged. Sometimes chunks of plaque get pulled off the wall and lodge elsewhere as a clot—this can cause damage to the brain, a lung, or a leg. *Stroke* occurs when the blood flow to the brain is disrupted because a blood vessel is blocked by atherosclerosis or has ruptured. Without oxygen, brain cells die, causing the loss of the ability to sense and/or control certain functions related to the affected part of the brain.

Hypertension—high blood pressure—increases the risk of cardiovascular disease as well as of stroke, kidney failure, and other serious diseases. About half of all women over fifty have high blood pressure; it is called a silent killer because usually there are no symptoms and few early signs, other than a high blood pressure reading. Diet and lifestyle are the main risk factors for atherosclerosis and heart attack, and they play a huge role in high blood pressure in some people.

There are cholesterol-lowering drugs that reduce cholesterol by an average of 35 percent, and blood-pressure-lowering drugs as well; both have side effects and we're only now beginning to see studies showing how lowering these measurements translates into preventing heart attacks or strokes. As we discuss later, hormone replacement therapy is another preventive offering for women.

Risk Factors for Cardiovascular Disease

After menopause (heart attack is uncommon in women under fifty), the major risk factors for cardiovascular disease are thought to be similar to men: high blood pressure and elevated cholesterol and other fats in the blood—both of which are influenced by diet and lifestyle. For example, in men, for each 1% increase in cholesterol, the risk of heart attack increases by 2% (some researchers believe it is closer to 3%).

In the United States we have come to expect cholesterol levels and the risk of heart disease to increase along with the candles on our birthday cakes. Yet in many countries, these measurements do not change much with age. For example, cholesterol levels are rarely above 150 in Africa, the Solomon Islands, Tasmania, the New Guinea Highlands, or among the Congo Pygmies, Masai, Navajo, bushmen, and Australian aborigines. As the chart below shows, however, the picture is changing as countries adopt a modern Western lifestyle and diet. The United States ranks ninth highest in women with heart disease, higher than Japan, France, Switzerland, Italy, Poland, the former Yugoslavia, Belgium, the Netherlands, Austria, Norway, Sweden, Romania, Bulgaria, Denmark, Canada, Finland, and Israel.

Percentage Increases in Mortality in Women Between 1960 and Most Recent Year (1989 if not otherwise marked)

Country	Year to, if not 1989	Heart diseases, %	Stroke, %
Canada		48	5.3
Costa Rica	1961–1988	184	168.4
United States	1988	55.4	10.4
Colombia	1984	195	181
Ecuador	1988	263	270
Hong Kong		178	148
Singapore		275	167
Thailand		156	350
France		8.4	−25
Germany, West		135	3

Source: U.N. Demographic Yearbook, 1993.

Cholesterol and Other Factors

Because cholesterol is one of the substances that causes plaque in artery walls, high cholesterol is a factor in cardiovascular disease. However, the relationship seems to be more complicated than we thought and is becoming controversial. Cholesterol is found throughout our bodies and is needed for many functions; for example, it is a precursor for progesterone and all the sex hormones. As you may know, there are two main types of cholesterol which are carried in the bloodstream. *Low-density lipoprotein (LDL)* transports cholesterol to the tissues; it is thought to be the bad cholesterol—too much increases the risk of cardiovascular disease. *High-density lipoprotein (HDL)* transports cholesterol to the liver, where it is metabolized and then excreted; it is thought to be the good stuff—high levels of it seem to protect us from coronary mishap. *Triglycerides* are another type of blood fat that raises the risk of cardiovascular disease; it appears that even when women have normal cholesterol, high triglycerides increase heart disease. Generally, triglycerides should be between 50 and 150 mg per dl (deciliter), but in women anything over 100 may be too high.

What may be more important is what happens to cholesterol and your arteries when they become damaged from oxidation by free radicals. Free radicals damage the vessels and oxidized cholesterol creates more free radicals, and your body lays down plaque over the damaged area as a protective mechanism. That's why there's been so much interest in antioxidant nutrients, such as vitamins C and E and beta-carotene for cardiovascular protection.

Other fatty and protein substances have been implicated in atherosclerosis. A blood fat called *lipoprotein(a)* may be the first to adhere to the wall, and LDL then adheres to this sticky substance. Vitamin C seems key in preventing this process. Elevated amounts of *homocysteine,* an amino acid, have recently been associated with clogged arteries and an increased risk of heart attack and stroke. Folate and vitamins B-6 and B-12 help get rid of excess homocysteine.

Platelets, the blood cells responsible for blot clotting, also play a role. When platelets form blood clots, they release inflammatory substances that damage the lining of the arteries; the clots also contribute to closing off the blood supply in arteries narrowed by atherosclerosis. This is why aspirin, which decreases the blood's tendency to clot, is recommended as a preventive.

The Hormone Connection: Estrogen and Your Heart

Since the incidence of heart disease rises in women after menopause, it is generally thought that estrogen exerts a protective effect. The latest large study to evaluate estrogen replacement therapy found that estrogen does lower LDL and raise HDL; however, some studies also show that at the same time it raises triglycerides. Another theory is that part of estrogen's protective effect relates to its ability to act as an antioxidant—if true, it may be more prudent to get more antioxidant protection through nutritious food or supplements. Definitive studies are under way to show whether there is any long-term benefit of taking HRT to prevent cardiovascular disease. It will take decades of controlled studies, however, to prove definitively if estrogen therapy reduces the death rate from heart disease.

Assessing Your Risk for Cardiovascular Disease

The more of these risk factors you have, the higher your risk and the more enthusiastically you'll want to embrace a heart disease prevention program. Fortunately, most of these risk factors are within our control—we can change them with our diet and lifestyle. And even if a close relative has died of heart disease, you can still overcome all but the most extreme type of family history—you have the power to lower your risk.

1. Are you age fifty or older?
2. Do you have high blood pressure?
3. Do you have diabetes?
4. Do you have a family history of premature heart disease (before age fifty-five in male relatives, age sixty-five in female relatives)?
5. Do you smoke?
6. Is your HDL cholesterol low (under 35 mg/dl)?
7. Is your total cholesterol high (200–239 mg/dl is borderline; 240 and over is high risk)?
8. Is your LDL cholesterol high (130–159 mg/dl is borderline; 160 and over is high risk)?
9. Are you overweight?
10. Did you have a total hysterectomy (surgical menopause) before age forty-five?

11. Do you take birth control pills *and* smoke?
12. Do you get very little exercise or have a sedentary occupation?

Reducing the Risk of Cardiovascular Disease

When we look at other cultures, we see that heart disease is rare in less technologically advanced societies; it's also less common among people who live low-stress, vegetarian, and physically active lives. It seems the measures you can take to reduce your risk for heart attack, stroke, and high blood pressure are exactly the same. The bonus is they also reduce your risk of the other major conditions discussed in this chapter—breast cancer, osteoporosis, and diabetes. The Balanced Life Plan provided in Chapter 2 makes it easy.

Changing Your Diet

You may be surprised to learn how effectively simple changes in diet can lower cholesterol, which may be due to their vitamin and mineral content, to their fiber content, or direct chemical activity, as is the case for garlic. For example, in one study, eating just two carrots a day reduced cholesterol levels by 11%. A daily bowl of oatmeal can decrease cholesterol by 8–23%. Including two fruits rich in pectin (such as apples), a type of soluble fiber, in your daily menu can produce a 15% drop in cholesterol. Foods containing water-soluble fiber bind cholesterol in the intestines and increase excretion—so eat your beans, fruits, vegetables, and whole grains.

Dr. Dean Ornish conducted the famous Lifestyle Heart Trial, consisting of a vegetarian, low-fat (10%) diet of mostly whole grains, legumes, and vegetables—plus exercise and stress reduction techniques. This program actually *reversed* the atherosclerosis in their coronary arteries—while the control group, managed with the best prescription medical care and a 30% of calories fat diet, showed that the atherosclerosis actually got worse.

The cholesterol in your food doesn't raise cholesterol as much as saturated fat does. Fish may be the preferable source of animal protein, especially cold-water fish such as salmon, mackerel, and herring. Some say that shellfish are heart-healthy because although they contain cholesterol, they contain little saturated fat and are rich in EPA. This essential fatty acid protects your heart by lowering triglycerides, raising HDL cholesterol, and reducing blood clots. (Essential fatty acids also appear to protect against heart disease, but very little is found in commonly eaten foods—*see* "Nutritional Supplements," pages 256–257.) A vegetarian diet may be healthiest of all—several studies show that replacing meat protein with plant protein (for example, found in wheat and soybeans), is more effective in lowering cholesterol levels than simply switching to a lower-fat diet. (*See* Chapter 4.)

Flax seed oil and sesame oil contain some essential fatty acids and other nutrients. Olive oil while low in EFAs is particularly interesting because heart disease and cancer are much less common in the Mediterranean countries, where olive oil is used in traditional cooking. Avoiding processed foods containing hydrogenated polyunsaturated and tropical oils (such as margarine and cookies—read labels carefully) can also help because they, too, damage blood vessels.

Emphasize green leafy vegetables, fruit, and other foods rich in the antioxidant vitamins C and E and beta-carotene, which several studies associate with a lower risk of heart disease. Vitamin C also helps form collagen, a kind of "glue" that holds cells together, strengthening them and enabling artery walls to withstand damage from free radicals, further preventing atherosclerosis.

Eating plenty of garlic and onions is another tasty way to lower blood pressure and cholesterol—a recent review of studies found that one clove of garlic a day lowered cholesterol by an average of 9 points, which translates into about a 20 percent drop in the risk of heart disease. Ginger may also lower cholesterol and reduce blood clotting, and cayenne pepper is a confirmed blood pressure reducer. A primary risk factor for hypertension is eating too much salt (sodium) in relation to potassium, so replace sodium with potassium in your salt shaker and cut back on processed foods, which are often high in sodium. Low calcium and magnesium also contribute to high blood pressure, so be sure to eat foods high in these minerals such as leafy green vegetables and whole grains.

Changing Your Lifestyle

Other risk factors are excess caffeine and alcohol, so make the effort to cut down. If you still smoke, do everything in your power to quit. Nearly three times more smokers die of heart disease than of lung cancer. Women who smoke have twice the risk of stroke as do nonsmokers, and heavy smokers have six times the risk. Smoking combined with oral contraceptives or other estrogens is especially risky for stroke and other clotting problems.

A sedentary lifestyle is a risk factor for atherosclerosis, heart attack, hypertension, and stroke. Regular aerobic exercise brings down blood pressure, and it appears to raise HDL cholesterol and lower your risk of heart attack. Women who don't exercise have three times the risk of heart disease as those who lead active lives. Recent evidence suggests that you don't have to make a big deal out of exercise, or even work up a big sweat—even moderate exercise will lower your risk.

Being overweight is a factor in all forms of cardiovascular disease. A recent study of 116,000 female nurses found that gaining only 11–18 pounds after age eighteen increased the risk of heart attack by 25%; a gain of 18–25 pounds bumped the risk by 60%; and a more than 25-pound gain doubled or even tripled the risk.

Stress is another universal risk factor for cardiovascular disease, so try to lower your stress level or learn to manage what you can't change, and remember that exercise is a superb stress-buster. In a recent Swedish study, a work stress reduction program raised HDL cholesterol (the good kind) by 6 percent. Anger, whether you admit to feeling it or not, is a significant factor which increases blood pressure and adrenaline levels and brings a higher incidence of death from heart attacks. Harvard University conducted a series of studies in which 1,600 people were asked to recall the events occurring in the 26 hours before a heart attack. According to the study, if you've already suffered a heart attack, getting angry makes you 2.3 times more likely to suffer an attack within 2 hours of the angry outburst.

Another possible risk factor is depression, which is more common in women than in men; yet cholesterol-lowering drugs have recently been tied to an increase in depression and suicide. *See* "Depression" in Chapter 5 for natural approaches to treating this condition.

The following natural therapies appear to be particularly helpful in preventing cardiovascular disease.

Nutritional Supplements

A good multivitamin-mineral formula containing the doses recommended in Chapter 3, pages 61–64, supplies the nutrients you need to keep your cardiovascular system in tip-top form. You may also take the following, in divided doses:

- *Vitamin C,* up to a total of 5,000–10,000 mg per day.
- *Vitamin E,* up to 800–1200 IU per day. A recent study of over

80,000 middle-aged women suggests that vitamin E supplements had reduced their risk of coronary heart disease to the levels of women on estrogen therapy.

• *Beta-carotene,* up to 50,000 IU per day.

• *Chromium,* up to 200 mcg twice a day.

• *Niacin,* 50–500 mg (up to 2,000 mg under professional supervision). We recommend the inositol hexaniacinate form of this vitamin.

• *Essential fatty acids,* up to 15,000 mg of EPA and up to 240 mg of GLA. EPA is available in fish oil capsules, or take flax seed oil, hemp, or safflower oil (1 tablespoon) which the body converts to EPA.

• *Garlic,* up to 1,200 mg per day (best as fresh or lightly cooked cloves).

• *Co-enzyme Q-10,* 25–100 mg per day. Studies have shown that this natural substance benefits people with high blood pressure and other cardiovascular disease.

• Supplements of water-soluble fiber such as *psyllium seeds, guar gum,* and *pectin.*

• *Lecithin* helps remove cholesterol from artery walls and reduces its ability to cling to arteries; it also reduced blood clotting.

• *Gamma-oryzanol,* 300 mg a day. In several studies, this naturally occurring component of rice bran oil significantly lowered cholesterol and triglycerides and increased HDL.

• *Carnitine,* 50 mg per day. This amino acid has been shown to increase HDLs while lowering LDL and triglycerides.

• *Magnesium,* 500–1500 mg per day in chelated glyconate form.

Herbal Remedies

For instructions on herbal remedies, *see* Chapter 3, pages 70–75. You may want to try a combination herbal formula designed to balance hormones during menopause, or choose one or more of the following herbs, which are particularly effective in reducing risk factors:

• *Bromelian,* which is an enzyme from pineapples, lessens blood clotting, lowers blood pressure, and breaks down atherosclerotic plaque.

• *Hawthorn berry and flower extracts* have been shown to lower blood pressure, reduce angina attacks, prevent cholesterol deposits, prevent heart rhythm problems and reduce cholesterol; they are very popular in Europe. Take up to 2 cups of infusion per day, or $1/2$–1 teaspoon of tincture three times a day.

Precautions

Be familiar with the signs of heart attack, hypertension, and stroke; have regular checkups to monitor your blood lipids and blood pressure. Symptoms of heart attack are not always the typical squeezing pain in the center of the chest. There may be uncomfortable pressure, fullness, aching, or heaviness in your shoulders, neck, jaw, arms, or upper back; and sweating, dizziness, fainting, shortness of breath, nausea, or sudden weakness. There may be only fatigue or indigestion.

Symptoms of stroke are numbness, weakness or loss of strength in your arm, leg, or side of your face; difficulty walking; blindness in one or both eyes; trouble speaking; there may or may not be headache. High blood pressure usually has no symptoms; however, in severe cases, there may be headache, dizziness, ringing in the ears, and nosebleeds. Some people just feel different in ''some way'' when their blood pressure is up.

If you have any of these symptoms, it's paramount to get medical help immediately—people with heart attacks who are treated within one hour suffer half the heart damage and have a death rate of 1 in 100, compared with 1 in 12 for those whose treatment is delayed. Aspirin not only seems to cut the risk of heart attack, but can be valuable first aid once a heart attack occurs. So if you experience any symptoms of heart attack, chew an aspirin immediately—it helps reduce the damage to the heart and improves your chances of surviving the attack. Take deep breaths and call 911.

Osteoporosis

Osteoporosis is more common and more serious than most people believe. About 7 to 8 million Americans—80 percent of them women—have this bone-weakening condition and another 17 million are at risk for the disease due to low bone density. And the sad truth is, osteoporosis may have no obvious symptoms until fractures of the spine, hip, or wrist occur—about 1.5 million of them each year. Fractures due to this condition cost at least $18 billion a year in health care, and immeasurable pain and suffering.

Spinal fractures, responsible for 30 percent of all osteoporosis-related fractures, involve collapse of the vertebrae that form your backbone, usually in the midback region. Full-blown spinal fractures begin as a series of poorly healed microfractures and eventually the vertebra collapses. Over the years, the effects of multiple vertebral fractures accumulate and result in curvature of the spine, a stooped posture ("dowager's hump"), and loss of height. Some—but by no means all—women experience great pain, especially when the nerves exiting the spine are compressed. Hip fractures account for 25 percent of the total fractures. They frequently require hospitalization and major surgery, which can cost up to $35,000. Despite treatment, half of all hip fractures lead to an inability to live independently; 20 percent of those women suffering such fractures die from conditions related to the fracture or the surgery. One out of every six white women in the United States—and one in twelve men—are expected to suffer a hip fracture in her or his lifetime. It's figures like these that should convince you to do everything you can to prevent osteoporosis and to reverse it if you already have it.

What Causes Osteoporosis?

Simply stated, with osteoporosis bones become more porous—abnormally thin, with loss of the calcified architecture *(osteo* means "bone"). You have two types of bone: *compact or cortical bone,* which seems solid and hard, and *trabecular bone,* which is spongy and lighter. The compact bone is found mainly in the shafts of your long bones such as your legs and arms; trabecular bone is found in the ends of your long bones, in your spinal vertebrae, and in your heel bones, ribs, and jaw.

You may be surprised to learn that bone is not a permanent, static substance. It is a dynamic, ever-changing, living tissue. Our bone tissue is alternatively being broken down and built back up in a process called remodeling. Specialized cells called *osteoclasts* break down small segments of old, worn-out bone (a process called *resorption).* The specialized *osteoblast* cells build this segment back with fresh new bone *(formation).* It has been estimated that by this process we replace one-fifth of our entire skeleton each year!

Bones are continually remodeling and repairing themselves in response to wear and tear, mechanical stress, and to the metabolic demands placed upon them. As we shall see, metabolically our bodies need to have access to the calcium and other minerals stored in bone. During our growing years, the osteoblasts stay way ahead of the osteo- clasts, creating more bone than is destroyed. In early adulthood, with the proper nutrition and exercise, and good health in general, our bones not only grow *larger,* they grow *denser.* It's believed that our bones reach their peak density between our mid-twenties and late thirties.

As mature adults, both men and women continue to grow bone, but more slowly. Eventually, the balance shifts as the osteoclasts catch up to and surpass the osteoblasts. Bone breakdown exceeds formation, and bone becomes less dense and can become more brittle. Generally around our early forties, we begin to lose bone mass. This gradual bone loss (1% or less a year) seems to be a normal part of aging, but not a disaster—if we grow properly dense bones during our early years, the bones stay strong enough to support us for the rest of our lives. However, instead of losing 1 percent or less each year some people lose more bone. For example, rapid bone loss occurs with bed rest, anorexia, malabsorption, from several diseases and medications. It is also common for the transition into menopause to be a period of rapid bone loss. With prolonged and accelerated rapid loss, compact bone becomes thinner, the trabecular bone becomes spongier, with larger holes, and the bones become weak and vulnerable to breakage.

Most physicians in the country now prescribe hormone replacement therapy (HRT), calcium supplementation, and vitamin D for osteo- porosis. Occasionally the hormone calcitonin is prescribed. Etidronate showed promise for a few years, but has not been approved by the Food and Drug Administration (FDA) for osteoporosis. The new nonhormonal bisphosphonate drug Fosamax was approved for osteo- porosis treatment by the FDA late in 1995. To date it has been studied for only three years. It appears to halt spinal bone loss but it is not clear if it will be effective for the hip. Also Fosamax works by inter- fering with the bone remodeling process and it is not clear if it leads to "worn-out" or unrepaired bone over the long haul.

There is much research ongoing but we don't yet know all the long- term effects of HRT, yet many doctors prescribe estrogen and proges- togins for the duration of your life. Studies show that women who take estrogen for at least seven years cut their risk of hip fractures in half during the time they use the drug. However, once you stop the ther- apy, bone loss resumes at the usual accelerated rate found in early stages of menopause. HRT has risks and undesirable side effects, as described in Chapter 4.

Who Is at Risk?

Who is at risk for osteoporosis? As a whole in the U.S., women are at much more risk than men, Caucasian women much more than African Americans or Latinos and the risk increases with age. It is interesting to note, however, that while one half of all Caucasian American women aged 50 will suffer one or another osteoporotic fracture during her lifetime, this high incidence of osteoporosis is not universal. The United States has one of the highest rates of osteoporosis in the world, and other highly industrialized/Western societies such as Finland, Norway, Sweden, and England are not far behind. On the other hand, people in less industrialized/Westernized countries living more traditional lifestyles like the native populations of Africa and New Zealand, the Japanese and Chinese, have much lower rates of osteoporotic fracture. In fact, around-the-world hip fracture rates for women vary thirty-fold for women and sixteen-fold for men. Unfortunately, the osteoporotic fracture rate is gradually rising in developing countries as they "modernize," changing their lifestyle, eating, and exercise patterns.

Risk Factors

All in all osteoporosis occurs when the forces encouraging bone breakdown well exceed those stimulating bone renewal. Unfortunately, in our culture the factors encouraging bone breakdown are many and include: low nutrient intake; high intake of nutrient robbers like sugar, coffee, alcohol, excess sodas, phosphorus, protein, and fat; an overall acid-forming diet; drugs and medications; inactivity and a profound lack of exercise; food allergies; malabsorption; and endocrine factors like ovary removal, low hormone levels, adrenal or thyroid weakness.

Before we show you how to change your diet and lifestyle to protect your bones, let's take a look at two of the most highly publicized factors that play important roles in maintaining bones through life—calcium and hormones.

Osteoporosis Rates Around the World

	Females	*Males*
USA (Rochester, MN)	319.7	177.0
USA (District of Columbia)		
whites	231.8	82.0
blacks	118.8	109.7
Finland	212.8	136.1
Norway (Oslo)	421.0	230.5
Sweden (Malmo)	237.2	101.4
Holland	187.2	107.9
United Kingdom (Oxford-Dundee)	142.2	69.2
Yugoslavia	74.4	69.2
Israel (Jerusalem)		
American/European born	201.8	113.9
Native-born	168.0	107.5
Asian/African-born	141.7	109.2
Hong Kong	87.1	73.0
Singapore (total)	42.1	73.1
Indian	312.9	131.4
Chinese	59.0	106.1
Malay	24.2	35.4
New Zealand		
whites	220.4	98.6
Maori	104.4	84.0
South Africa (Johannesburg)		
whites	256.5	98.8
Bantu	14.0	14.3

Yearly Hip Fracture Per 100,000 People Age 35 and Older
Melton, J. and Riggs, L. ''Epidemiology of Age-related Fractures.'' In *The Osteoporotic Syndrome,* Editor Avioli, L. New York: Grune and Stratton, 1983.

Calcium and Your Bones

Let's begin by taking a look at the roles bone plays in your body. Bone is made primarily of the support structures (protein and collagen) studded with calcium and several other minerals. Calcium is what gives bone its strength, but it also serves many other functions. It is needed for our muscles to grow, contract, and relax—most importantly our heart muscle needs calcium to function. It also allows the smooth muscles of our blood vessels to relax and therefore plays a role in lowering blood pressure. Calcium is required for a healthy nervous system. About 99 percent of the calcium in our bodies resides in our bones; in order to be available to perform these crucial functions, there is a give-and-take of calcium between our bones and our other tissues via the bloodstream.

So, our skeleton not only holds us up so we can go shopping or dance the tango, but also functions as a calcium bank, and when too much calcium is withdrawn from the bank and not replaced, osteoporosis is the result.

Bone is largely composed of calcium, and calcium intake clearly plays a role in building and maintaining strong bones. However, ingesting lots of calcium—either from food or supplements—isn't the only answer to preventing this condition. In spite of all the hype about milk and calcium supplements, the scientific evidence that humans need huge amounts is weak. Women in less-developed countries consume much less calcium and milk than we do, yet they have much less osteoporosis. Studies among populations as diverse as those of Peru, Ceylon, Central America, and Africa show that women maintain healthy bones on calcium intakes of 200–475 mg—amounts easily gotten from their diets. However, American women even on 800–1,000 mg per day still lose calcium from their bones. What causes us to withdraw too much calcium from our bones and redeposit too little, resulting in an epidemic of osteoporosis in this country? As we'll see later, it's a combination of diet and lifestyle factors.

The Hormone Connection

Hormones from the ovaries, adrenals, thyroid, parathyroid, and pituitary, hypothalamus, and kidney all play important roles in bone health. To date, however, most attention has been given to ovarian estrogen and an association drawn between the estrogen drop at menopause and the rapid spurt of bone loss many women experience the 4 or 5 years around menopause. More recent studies suggest, however, that menopausal changes in progesterone as well as estrogen play a role in this accelerated bone loss.

As we explain in Chapter 1, estrogen production dips around menopause; estrogen limits or depresses the osteoclasts, so lowered levels would allow these bone-dissolving cells to get the upper hand. Fortunately, nature has given our bodies a second system of producing sex hormones, which kicks in after menopause. Our ovaries continue to produce some estrogen, as well as androgens; androgens are also produced by our adrenal glands. Androgens are the "male" hormones that are related to sex drive, muscle strength, and vaginal health; they are also converted to estrogen by our fat cells. So, after menopause, our body should still be producing enough estrogen to maintain bone strength, provided our adrenals are in good working order. However, emotional and physical stress can burn out the adrenals, providing less androgens to be converted to estrogen. Stress can also cause the adrenals to produce cortisol, a hormone that mobilizes calcium from the bone to the blood where it is filtered and excreted by the kidneys in urine.

Progesterone also appears to be a factor in bone health, and unfortunately we also produce less of this hormone after menopause. Progesterone stimulates the bone-building cells, the osteoblasts, so a lack would slow the bone-rebuilding process—a disastrous scenario when combined with the bone-dissolving cells becoming more active in the absence of estrogen. Androgens and progesterone, in addition to DHEA and thyroid have a potent effect on our bones. Both Dr. Maas and Dr. Brown recommend getting your salivary or blood levels checked before replacing these hormones to be sure of what you need.

Studies have shown that taking estrogen, particularly soon after menopause, and continued life long can decrease the risk of hip fracture by 30–40 percent and spinal fractures by up to 50–75 percent. Progesterone also appears to protect against osteoporosis, but we have only Dr. John Lee's small clinical study to demonstrate this; other studies are ongoing. However, there is evidence that postmenopausal hormone deficiency is not the only culprit. Researchers at the Mayo Clinic have shown that sex hormone levels do not correlate with osteoporosis in postmenopausal women; they also found that an American woman has already lost a full half of all the bone she will lose during her lifetime between the ages of thirty-five and fifty.

Assessing Your Risk for Osteoporosis

Bone mineral density testing by the dual energy X-ray absorptiometry (DEXA) method is the best way to determine if you already have osteoporosis and if so, how severely. New urine tests which indicate if you are currently breaking down bone at a normal or accelerated rate are also now available. While these urine tests cannot determine if you have osteoporosis, they can help monitor the results of your treatment or indicate that it might be important to have a bone density measurement because you were breaking down bone at a rapid rate. These urine tests are inexpensive, noninvasive, and require no irradiation. The following factors increase your risk of developing osteoporosis. Ask yourself the following questions—the more "yes" answers, the higher your risk and the greater measures you should take to prevent or reverse bone loss.

1. Are you 65 or older?
2. Have you had a "total" hysterectomy, that is, uterus and ovaries removed?
3. Do your older relatives have osteoporosis—have any of them fractured a hip or do they have curvature of the spine?
4. Are you thin or petite, or do you have a small frame?
5. Have you used cortisone, antiulcer medication, antibiotics, Depo-Provera or antacids containing aluminum for a long period of time?
6. Do you drink alcohol heavily (more than two drinks a day)—or have you in the past?
7. Do you get very little exercise or have a sedentary occupation?
8. Do you smoke, or have you in the past?
9. Do you have problems digesting food or have you had gastrointestinal surgery?
10. Do you drink two or more servings daily of soft drinks, coffee, or other caffeine-containing beverages?
11. Do you eat a diet low in green leafy vegetables, fruits, and whole grains, and high in fat and sugars, or did you in the past?
12. Do you eat a diet high in protein, especially animal protein, or did you in the past?
13. Do you have food allergies?
14. Have you been on many crash diets or undereaten for a long period of time?
15. Did your menstrual periods ever become irregular or stop when you were younger? Or did you have an early menopause (before age forty)?
16. Are you Caucasian? (African-Americans and Hispanics have a lower incidence of osteoporosis.)

17. Did you have salt-and-pepper hair in your twenties or a lot of gray hair before the age of forty? (In one study, those who did had four times the risk of developing osteoporosis.)
18. Did you have no full-term pregnancies?
19. Do you have any chronic disease including diabetes, thyroid disease, rheumatoid arthritis, kidney disease, or gum disease?
20. Did you dislike milk as a child? Do you not drink it now, or avoid it possibly because you have trouble digesting it?

Reducing Your Risk: Preventing, Halting, and Reversing Osteoporosis

It's never too late to build more bone mass instead of losing it. Even women who have already suffered a fracture can reduce their risk of another fracture. Remember that for every 1 percent increase in bone mass, the risk of fracture from osteoporosis decreases by 6 percent.

Although hormones and calcium play key roles in maintaining strong healthy bones throughout our lives, bone metabolism is far more complex than taking aim with either of those two magic bullets. The more we learn about this condition, the clearer it becomes that osteoporosis is the result of a lifetime of unbalanced nutrition, too little exercise, and other bad habits. Lowering our risk of getting osteoporosis—as well as slowing or reversing it—involves maintaining a healthy lifestyle, and that may mean changing a number of things about the way we live. For example, in addition to taking in enough calcium, we also need to be able to absorb calcium, keep it from being excreted, and keep it in balance with other nutrients. Our comprehensive bone-building strategy works on four fronts. They are:

1. Maximize bone-building nutrient intake.
2. Exercise.
3. Minimize antinutrient intake.
4. Promote endocrine balance.

Why a Comprehensive Plan

A few studies suggest that calcium supplementation alone is able to reduce, halt, and even begin to reverse bone loss in some cases. Others show stronger results combining calcium supplements with other nutrients in balanced amounts. For example, while calcium is important to bone, so are nearly two dozen other nutrients. The minerals magnesium, zinc, manganese, copper, phosphorus, silica, boron, and fluorine are all essential for bone health as are the vitamins D, C, A, B-6, K, and B-12, and folic acid, essential fatty acids, and protein. Unfortunately, our intake of most of these nutrients is below the minimal RDA, and considerably less than the more ideal optimum intake level, which is summarized in the Nutrient Table of Vitamins and Minerals on page 61. Some studies show that exercise alone can stop and begin to reverse bone loss; but still other studies show that optimum bone growth requires exercise and good nutrition. What's important is that ground-breaking results have been achieved with only partial measures. How much bone regeneration could have been achieved with a truly comprehensive program? Remember: Estrogen replacement therapy alone does not reverse bone loss; studies show it only stops more bone loss from occurring, and in only 75–80 percent of the women using it. On the other hand, fascinating research from the University of California, San Diego, showed that postmenopausal bone loss can be halted and even minimally reversed simply by taking daily supplements of calcium (1,000 calcium citrate malate), zinc (15 mg), manganese (5 mg), and copper (2.5 mg). Interestingly, a study published in the *Journal of Nutritional Medicine* showed that while bone loss was only halted in postmenopausal women who were taking estrogen replacement, those who also made dietary and life-style changes and took a broad-spectrum nutritional supplement *gained 11 percent trabecular bone mass* in just one year, and 50 percent of them moved out of the fracture risk zone. The nutritional supplement contained all the essential vitamins and minerals including 600 mg magnesium and 500 mg of calcium per day; the women lowered their intake of meat, sugar, caffeine, alcohol, and fat while increasing their complex carbohydrates, beans, and whole grains. When Dr. Lee added natural progesterone to a good diet, exercise, and nutritional supplement program (with or without estrogen therapy), he got even better bone-building results. On the average the osteoporotic women in his studies gained 15 percent bone mass in three years.

Studies with younger women show that those with adequate nutrition and exercise have a higher bone mass, which is obviously an advantage to a woman by the time she reaches menopause. It's never too early to be concerned about building healthy bone, so encourage your daughters to follow this plan: A 5 percent increase in peak bone mass in young adolescents can translate into a 50 percent reduction in risk of fractures in their later years.

What about the woman who is perimenopausal? This is the time around the menopause during which bone loss is accelerated. During this 5- to 10-year period, you can lose one-quarter of all the hip bone density you will lose during your lifetime, and an even greater percentage of your spinal bone. This is likely due to the rates of change of hormones during this time, and that's why many researchers suggest that perimenopausal bone loss cannot be halted without the use of estrogen replacement. There has not yet been a study including a systematic, holistic approach applied to the prevention of this phase of accelerated bone loss. Without waiting for scientific trials, it seems wise to include all the major elements that have been shown to individually affect bone health. If you are perimenopausal, you will more likely avoid considerable bone loss, and if you already have osteoporosis, these measures will help you restore bone health.

General Dietary Changes

Following the Balanced Life Plan in Chapter 2 is your foundation for reducing your risk of osteoporosis as well as improving and maintaining overall health. Increase your intake of green leafy vegetables such as broccoli, kale, bok choy, and collards, which are rich in *calcium;* so are canned salmon and sardines (including the bones), shellfish, and tofu. Foods that are high in calcium are also rich in many other nutrients needed by healthy bones, and may be one reason why vegetarians have less osteoporosis than meat eaters. Dairy products are rich in calcium but may not be the best source for many women (*see* Box, page 269).

Remember, we need other *minerals* besides calcium to keep bones strong. Phosphorus, magnesium, manganese, boron, strontium, silica, zinc, fluorine, and copper, all need to be present in the right amounts in order for calcium to do its job. Several other studies have shown the minerals manganese, zinc, and copper to be key elements in bone development and maintenance. Several other studies suggest that magnesium may as important, if not more important, than calcium in building bone. Make sure you are eating foods high in magnesium as well, such as whole grains, leafy greens, beans, and almonds.

The Problem with Dairy

In our culture, increasing calcium intake generally helps to build stronger bones, but calcium is just one of the twenty-odd nutrients essential for bone health. Also, when we think of calcium we think of dairy products and suppose a diet high in dairy will solve the osteoporosis problem. Unfortunately, it is not so simple.

Milk and other dairy products such as cheese are usually touted as good sources of calcium—but are they really? First, milk is high in animal fat and protein; animal fat is linked with many serious diseases including heart disease and cancer, and excess animal protein causes calcium to be excreted in the urine. Even skim or low-fat milk isn't the answer—by getting rid of the fat, you increase the proportion of acid-forming protein! In addition, milk contains too little magnesium in relation to the calcium, which could lead to an imbalance in these minerals; this could interfere with the absorption of magnesium, which is also needed for strong bones. Finally, many adults cannot digest milk because they have sensitivities, allergies or lack the enzyme, lactase, to digest milk sugar, lactose. This causes bloating, gas, cramps, and sometimes diarrhea; it also decreases absorption of bone-building nutrients.

All *vitamins* play their individual roles in maintaining healthy bones. Vitamin D (in fish liver oils, fortified milk, and synthesized in our skin from sunlight) is needed to absorb calcium. Vitamin C, found in citrus fruits and other fruits, tomatoes, and leafy vegetables, is needed to form collagen, the connective tissue that is a major component of bone. Vitamin B-6 (in many foods, particularly eggs, fish, spinach, walnuts, wheat germ) is also needed in collagen formation. Vitamin K (in many foods, especially vegetables) is essential for bone building and repair, since it is needed to produce a specific protein in which calcium crystalizes. Vitamin A (found in meat, fish, eggs; its precursor, beta-carotene, is found in green and yellow-orange fruits and vegetables) helps in the development of osteoblasts and aids calcium metabolism; these bone-building cells also require vitamin B-12 (meat, fish, chicken eggs, and dairy). There is also evidence that vitamins and minerals work synergistically to prevent osteoporosis. Dr. Brown recommends two ways of judging the adequacy of your diet. One is through a computerized three-day diet analysis and the second concerns use of a self-help workbook entitled *The Nutrition Detective.* (*See* Appendix B.)

Another factor is *poor digestion*—even those who take supplements regularly may not be absorbing as much as they think. Calcium—whether in food or supplements—is usually in the form of salts. In order for these salts to be bioavailable, they need to be broken down by hydrochloric acid in our stomachs. But as we grow older, we frequently produce less digestive juices and so absorb less of the calcium we take in. Adults may absorb as little as 15–30 percent of the calcium they ingest, depending on bowel health, digestion, hormone balance, and other factors. Many components of our contemporary lifestyles such as stress, eating too rapidly, inadequate chewing, overeating, and using certain drugs weaken digestion. Food intolerances and allergies may also be a factor in some people. (*See* Chapter 2, page 38.)

Other Lifestyle Considerations

Getting enough exercise is the most important lifestyle change you can make for bone strength. An inactive lifestyle causes you to lose bone strength and increase your risk of fractures. We know this partly because of studies that evaluate the benefits of exercise (see below), and also because of studies of people who have required long bed rest due to illness or injury. For example, adults who stay in bed because of back pain lose almost 1 percent of their lumbar spine mass per week.

Exercise protects against fractures in several ways. The jarring or pressure stresses the bones, creating a mild electrical charge which stimulates growth and calcification. During exercise, muscles pull on the bones, which respond to the stress by buttressing their strength with new cells, collagen, and minerals. Gravity—which often makes life difficult—is your ally in this instance. *Weight-bearing exercise* has long been considered to be the most effective osteoporosis fighter. This includes anything that forces your body to work hard against gravity, such as jogging, walking, aerobic and other types of dancing, and team or racket sports such as volleyball and tennis. Weight training is a great weight-bearing exercise and also seems to be beneficial because it stresses the bones by pulling on them. According to a Mayo Clinic study, women with stronger back muscles have stronger vertebrae. A recent small study of women aged fifty to seventy showed that a high-intensity strength training program increased both bone mass and muscle mass—without changes in diet or estrogen therapy. The program lasted a year and consisted of about an hour twice a week of using an exercise cycle, a stretching device, and weight-resistance machines. The researchers pointed out that the women also improved their strength and balance—an important additional factor in reducing falls and fractures—and were more motivated to participate in spontaneous physical activity.

Although other forms of exercise such as swimming, bike riding, and yoga may be good for burning calories, cardiovascular fitness, relaxation, and keeping you limber, they have been thought to be less effective for preventing or reversing osteoporosis because they don't put much of a demand on your bones. Even so, several recent studies show these also help maintain bone.

(*Note:* if you already have osteoporosis, be sure to consult with a knowledgeable health professional about the types of exercise you may safely do. You need to take care not to put excessive stress on weakened bones.)

An exercise program that Dr. Brown endorses was developed by Gail Dalsky. It consists of 50–60 minutes of weight-bearing and non–weight-bearing aerobic exercise three times a week. In a study of this program with a minimal nutritional plan of 1,500 mg calcium (from both supplements and diet) and 50 IU of vitamin D every day, at the end of 9 months, exercisers showed a 5.2% increase in bone density; after 22 months, they gained 6.1% bone density. These gains were maintained as long as the women followed the exercise program—the gains made were lost when they stopped.

On the other hand, *being too thin*—either through excessive exercise or drastic dieting—can starve your bones too. Very low-calorie diets without adequate nutrients pull calcium and other minerals out of your calcium bank, depleting your bones of critical minerals and pushing them into bankruptcy. Chronic dieters have less bone mass going into menopause. In addition, having too little fat means less conversion of other hormones to estrogen, which lowers bone mass at any age.

Avoid Nutrient Robbers

Certain foods contain substances that deplete your body of calcium and other nutrients that work hand in hand with calcium to build bones. For example, too much *protein* in the diet—especially animal protein—pulls calcium out of the bones. When protein is metabolized, it creates acid by-products that are excreted in the urine; the more acid by-products, the more calcium is needed to reduce or buffer them. Countries with lower protein consumptions have lower rates of osteoporosis than do Western countries, where women eat a lot of protein. Eating a lot of *sugar* will also deplete calcium, by increasing excretion of calcium and other nutrients in the urine, by interfering with their absorption, by adding to the acid load, and because it usually is eaten in foods that contain little calcium and other nutrients to begin with. And while we are usually low in most minerals, we often get too much *phosphorus*—large amounts are found in soft drinks, which are this country's favorite beverage, as well in meat and other high-protein foods and artificially preserved foods. The problem is largely with high phosphorus intake in the face of low calcium intake. This causes the parathyroid gland to become overactive, which pulls calcium from the bones in order to increase blood calcium levels to match the blood phosphorus levels. In addition, excess phosphorus binds to magnesium and prevents its absorption.

Caffeine acts as a diuretic, which increases calcium excretion in the urine; in addition the 29 acids in coffee cause calcium to be taken from bone in order to neutralize them. Three cups of coffee can leach 45 mg of calcium from your bones; in one study, women who drank more than two cups of coffee or four cups of tea had a 59 percent increased risk of fracture; another study found that women who drank four cups of coffee per day had triple the risk of hip fracture compared with women who almost never drank coffee.

Smoking accelerates bone loss and doubles your risk of osteoporosis, so now's the time to quit. Researchers have found that smoking is so anti-estrogenic that it can cancel out the beneficial effects of estrogen therapy. Limit your use of alcohol because excessive drinking of alcohol also increases the risk of osteoporosis. Certain medications including diuretics, corticosteroids, and other medication including antibiotics depletes bones of calcium as well; check with your physician to see if you can keep these to a minimum or substitute other treatments. Whether thyroid hormone itself decreases bone mass is debatable, although most doctors believe that this is the case.

Practice meditation and other stress reduction techniques, since stress affects your endocrine system and this can cause calcium to leach out of your bones. Exercise is another superb stress-reliever, in addition to building bone.

The following natural therapies, described in Chapter 3, may also be specifically helpful in preventing or reversing osteoporosis.

Nutritional Supplements

A good multivitamin-mineral formula containing the doses recommended in Chapter 3, pages 61–64, supplies most of the nutrients you need to keep your bones healthy. Be especially vigilant about obtaining the following nutrients:

• *Calcium,* up to 1,200 mg a day for children and young people up to 24 years, with up to 1,500 mg during adolescence; 1,000 mg a day for women up to menopause; 1,500 mg for postmenopausal women not on estrogen; 1,000 mg for postmenopausal women on estrogen. Some studies show that calcium citrate is the most absorbable form for women over forty, who tend to have low stomach acid. Other research suggests that calcium in the form of microcrystalline hydroxyapatate concentrate (MCHC) is particularly useful for helping to rebuild lost bone. Calcium carbonate is one of the most popularly recommended forms of calcium, found in antacids such as TUMS. While OTC antacids are readily available, pleasant tasting, and calcium carbonate has been well studied, there are disadvantages. The calcium is not well absorbed by the body; antacids are not a complete supplement for bone (most particularly it is unwise to take calcium, as in antacids, without magnesium); antacids reduce the hydrochloric acid necessary for proper digestion of many nutrients.

• *Magnesium,* equal amount as calcium.
• *Vitamin C,* 1,000–3,000 mg per day.
• *Vitamin D,* not to exceed a total of 800 IU per day without profes-

sional supervision. Amounts higher than found in a good multivita-min-mineral are generally only needed by older people who get very little sunlight.

- *Boron,* a total of up to 2–4 mg per day.
- *Copper,* 2–4 mg per day.
- *Fluorine,* 1.5–4 mg per day.
- *Silica,* 100–1,000 mg per day.
- *Vitamin B-6,* 50–100 mg per day.
- *Manganese,* 10–15 mg per day.
- *Zinc,* 20–25 mg per day.

Herbal Remedies

For instructions on herbal remedies, *see* Chapter 3, pages 70–75. Herbs can be useful as part of your bone health program, but not as useful as nutrition and exercise. You may use a hormone-balancing menopausal herbal formula, or choose one or more of the following herbs which are particularly high in calcium:

- *Horsetail, comfrey, oat straw, nettle, dandelion greens, water-cress, mustard greens, chickweed.*
- There is also a combination remedy called Dr. Christopher's *Bone, Flesh, and Cartilage,* which we recommend for some of our patients. It contains horsetail, chaparral, plantain, parsley, burdock, marshmallow, and slippery elm. This supplement is available at many health food stores, and by calling 1-800-634-1308.

Natural Hormone Therapy

There's some evidence that *natural progesterone* can help prevent and reverse osteoporosis. Dr. John E. Lee, a physician in Sebastopol, California, followed 100 postmenopausal women with osteoporosis who were using progesterone cream in addition to watching their diet, using supplements, and exercising. All but three of the women were able to reverse osteoporosis; the average improvement was 15 percent in 3 years, and virtually no fractures. Many women with the lowest bone mineral density (as measured by bone density tests) improved 40 percent over 3 years. A few of the women also took low doses of estrogen because of hot flashes and vaginal dryness. Under Dr. Lee's regimen, women on estrogen used the cream daily during the last two weeks of estrogen use or three weeks per month if estrogen was not used. Dr. Lee's results are impressive, but we caution that his small study has never been duplicated. If you consider using hormone therapy of any type, be sure to check your blood levels or saliva levels to make sure you don't overdo it. Dr. Maas has seen women with progesterone levels thirty times normal for premenopausal women; she finds progesterone cream particularly concerning because even when a woman rotates application areas, the hormone accumulates in time. See Chapter 4 for a fuller discussion of hormone therapy.

Precautions

Osteoporosis is a "silent disease"—you usually don't know you have it until you have suffered a fracture or your spine becomes deformed. Pay attention to warning signs—receding gums that indicate you have lost bone from your jaw; chronic back or hip pain; loss of height; and a curving spine known as "dowager's hump." Today, we have screening tools that are relatively sensitive and report how dense your bones are compared with women of your height, weight, age, and race. These are somewhat useful for monitoring the effectiveness of treatment as well. Bone density tests such as dual-energy X-ray absorptiometry (DEXA) are the easiest way to definitively diagnose osteoporosis and they are also most commonly used to monitor it. If your assessment puts you at high risk for osteoporosis and you are concerned, discuss with your physician the advisability of getting a baseline bone density test. They cost $145 to $250 depending on your geographic location, but not all medical insurance plans cover them. We recommend bone density tests as a screening only if you are willing to change your life based on the result, or if a good-news result will help you rest easier.

A low-tech test for osteoporosis is for your health professional to measure your height compared with your arm span over time; if you're shrinking, it may indicate vertebral compression due to microfractures. Biomarkers—substances in the blood and urine that reflect bone loss—are being used to monitor the progression or reversal of bone breakdown. Such measurements might be able to detect changes within two months and therefore are more useful tools in monitoring treatment. The new urine tests for bone breakdown are coming into general use and they represent a good way to check the efficacy of your treatment regimen. Women seeking more detailed information on understanding, preventing, and reversing osteoporosis can refer to Dr. Susan Brown's book *Better Bones, Better Body: A Comprehensive Self-Help Program for Preventing, Halting and Overcoming Osteoporosis* (Keats, 1996).

Breast Cancer

Breast cancer is the most common cancer among women and is probably the disease that women fear the most. Breast cancer can be fatal—in 1995 approximately 182,000 American women were diagnosed with it and 46,000 died of it. (The cancer that kills more women than any other, however, is lung cancer, most of which is attributable to cigarette smoking.)

Even when the prognosis is good, women diagnosed with breast cancer suffer both physical and emotional scars that can take a long time to heal. Worldwide, breasts are symbolic of nurturing and femininity; many cultures—particularly the United States—equate breasts with desirability and beauty as well. They are all too frequently the framework of our self-esteem. For some women the thought of losing a breast to cancer is as distressing a thought as losing their life.

The incidence of breast cancer has been rising steadily in American women and is now double the rate of 1940. According to the American Cancer Society, the current risk for specific ages is:

By age 50:	1 in 50
By age 60:	1 in 23
By age 70:	1 in 13
By age 80:	1 in 10
By age 85:	1 in 9

In spite of the war on cancer, and some small advances regarding early detection and treatment, the death rate for women diagnosed with breast cancer has remained essentially unchanged for the past 70 years. One-fourth of the women diagnosed with breast cancer are dead in 5 years; one-half are dead in 10 years—breast cancer is the leading cause of death among women aged 40–45.

Thank goodness we no longer routinely remove the entire breast when the cancer is small and localized—the preferred treatment is now *lumpectomy* to remove just the lump, possibly followed by radiation treatment. Still, a *mastectomy* (removal of the entire breast) is sometimes performed when the disease is advanced or for other reasons. Chemotherapy is often prescribed in addition to the above treatments, in order to kill any remaining cancer cells. These powerful drugs cause unwanted effects such as hair loss, nausea, and vomiting, debilitating fatigue, a suppressed immune system, and many other problems. High-dose chemo, combined with bone marrow transplant, is becoming more common. Tamoxifen and similar antiestrogen drugs are now commonly prescribed and are being studied. They are less toxic than chemotherapy, which kills cancer cells outright, but still can bring on loss of libido, inability to concentrate, depression, vision changes, hot flashes, weight gain, and other more life-threatening side effects as well such as an increased risk of uterine cancer.

There is evidence that such aggressive drug therapy lengthens the lives of some women, regardless of the stage of breast cancer. However, once the cancer is advanced, and cells from the original tumor in the breast have spread to vital organs such as the liver, lungs, bone, or brain, the goal of chemotherapy for breast cancer is to slow the progress and relieve pain—but a cure is considered unlikely. There is increasing interest in the role of alternative therapy in breast cancer. We recommend that women research their alternatives and find a caring and well-informed health practitioner when diagnosed with a serious disease such as breast cancer.

Early Detection

Catching a breast cancer early when the lump is small and confined to the breast greatly increases the chance of a cure. It also increases the likelihood that a lumpectomy rather than a mastectomy will be appropriate. The most important step you can take for early detection is to do breast self-exams because, unlike your doctor, you can examine yourself monthly. Eighty percent of all lumps are found by women themselves, and most lumps are not cancer.

Yet women don't examine breasts regularly because they are afraid of "finding something." Christiane Northrup, a holistic physician, notes that our breasts deserve as much or more loving attention than our hair or complexion. She recommends that you transform the breast exam—don't do it necessarily to find suspicious lumps, but to "send energies of caring and respect to this area of [your] body." While in the shower or bath, explore your contours with soapy hands. Imagine you have healing power in your fingertips and feel your breasts in the spirit of curiosity and love for this area of your body, rather than a spirit of fear. As you get to know your breasts, you will become much more comfortable and trusting of yourself. For a free brochure about how to perform a self-exam, call the National Cancer Institute (1-800-4-CANCER), or contact your local American Cancer Society chapter. The MEND Clinic also publishes a brochure on breast self-exam.

In addition, you should get a thorough professional breast exam once a year, which may include a mammogram. Although they are imperfect, most health professionals feel that mammograms are our best method for detecting breast cancer early enough to hope for a cure. However, mammograms miss 10–15 percent of all cancers (false negative); and 6–10 percent of the suspicious lumps they detect turn out to be benign (false positives) upon biopsy.

While mammography is controversial for the dense breasts of women who are under thirty years old, it is less controversial for women over fifty. If you are fifty or older, you are advised to get a mammogram (breast X-ray) every year; however, if your breasts appear healthy, you may skip 1 or 2 years if you are not at high risk. These recommendations vary from one organization to another, and also are periodically revised; if you have no or few high risk factors, discuss with your doctor about whether and how often you should have a mammogram.

Based on a pooling of the six studies on the efficacy of mammograms, it appears that routine screening would reduce death from breast cancer in women age fifty and over by 30 percent. However, two scientists recently published a critical evaluation of the studies (in *The Lancet,* July 1, 1995). They discovered that when you look at the studies separately, only the two earliest studies show a reduction in the death rate that is statistically significant. Presumably, mammography has improved since the early studies were done, in 1982 and 1985. Why, then, have results not improved, but worsened?

Even if the 30 percent death reduction held up under further scrutiny, clearly screening isn't enough—there are many other things you can do to reduce your risk of getting breast cancer in the first place.

Risk Factors for Breast Cancer
Prevention is clearly the best course of action, but in spite of the increase in media attention that breast cancer advocates have

achieved, we still don't know much about the causes of breast cancer. Only about 25 percent of all women with breast cancer have one or more of the "known" risk factors. There must be other factors at play which have yet to be discovered. We know that breast cancer is "genetic" in the sense that damage to DNA, the genetic material of the cell, leads to the uncontrolled growth that characterizes cancer. Some women may inherit faulty genes and need only a few more "hits" to turn the cell cancerous. Imbalanced hormones, an unhealthy diet, and environmental pollution are prime suspects. Again, as we see in the chart showing the range of death rates from country to country, the risk is greatest in industrialized countries, and lowest in countries where women live a traditional lifestyle.

Breast Cancer Death Rates Around the World, 1986–1988

Country	Breast Cancer Deaths (per 100,000 Women)
England/Wales	29.3
Denmark	28.3
Scotland	27.5
Ireland	27.0
United States	22.4
Japan	6.0
Ecuador	5.7
China	4.7
Korea	2.6
Thailand	1.0

Known Risk Factors

• *Genetics/family history:* The risk is greater if your mother, sister, or aunt has had breast cancer. According to a study involving over 2,000 nurses with breast cancer, the risk is doubled if your mother had breast cancer before the age of forty. The risk is only 1.5% greater if your mother developed breast cancer after age seventy, however. In this study, only 2.5% of the women with breast cancer had a close relative with the disease. Researchers have pinpointed certain gene mutations that run in families; one of them, BRCA1, confers an 85% chance of developing breast cancer and is responsible for 5% of all breast cancer cases. We now have a diagnostic test, not widely available, to ferret out women who carry these high-risk breast cancer genes, but the test is controversial, since it is not clear what we should do with the results.

• *Age:* The older you get, the higher the risk, probably because there are more chances for genetic damage to occur. As shown on page 276, the rate doubles from age fifty to age sixty, and doubles again to age seventy.

• *Overweight:* Obese women have two to four times the risk of breast cancer. Obesity is also associated with ovarian and uterine cancer.

• *Age at menarche:* Women who begin menstruating at a young age (under twelve) have a higher risk.

• *Age at menopause:* Women who stop menstruating later (after age fifty-five) have a higher risk.

• *Childbearing history:* Women who have no children or children after age thirty are at higher risk.

• *Other risk factors* are living in a North American or Western European country, living in an industrial society, a history of exposure to radiation, abnormal menstrual cycles (irregular, short, or long, which indicate a hormone imbalance), and one rare type of fibrocystic breast disease.

The Hormone Connection

The evidence is overwhelming that hormone imbalance is somehow related to breast cancer. Breast tissue has estrogen and progesterone receptors in it and breast cells are sensitive to hormones. Interestingly, many of the known and suspected risk factors are associated with hormonal imbalance: menstruating early and stopping late exposes a woman's body to more estrogen over the course of her lifetime; so does never being pregnant. There's some evidence that irregular periods, a sign of hormone imbalance, also increase the risk. A diet high in animal fats stimulates production of estrogen, and the more body fat you have, the more hormone precursors are converted to estrogen by fat cells. Also, in our country, animal fats are generally laced with estrogenlike drugs unless labeled ''organic.'' Furthermore, alcohol can disturb the menstrual cycle and may alter hormones in a way that encourages breast cancer to grow.

Prescription hormones (such as in hormone replacement therapy or birth control pills) may also effect breast cancer risk as well as the progression of the disease. We have reviewed selected studies, which point to a 50%–70% increase in breast cancer risk with the use of estrogen replacement therapy. Interestingly, European studies show an even greater increased risk (of up to 200%). Dr. Alan Gaby, a nutritional medicine expert, conducted a "meta-analysis" in 1992. He looked at many studies and estimated that, compared with women who had never used estrogen, women who had ever used estrogen showed a slight increase in risk. As for the long-term users of estrogen, the pooled studies revealed a 30% increase for women who had used estrogen for at least 15 years, and a 25% increase in those who had used estrogen for 8 years. Some of these studies showed increases of up to 50% or more in long-term users. Recent findings of the Harvard Nurses' Health Study, which monitored 121,700 women since 1976, concur. A significant increase in breast cancer was found among women who have ever used estrogen, and women on long-term hormone replacement therapy had nearly a 50% higher risk of breast cancer as compared with women who had never used the drug. As Christiane Northrup writes in her book, *Women's Bodies, Women's Wisdom,* "It makes sense that in a woman potentially at risk for breast cancer, ERT could start a tumor growing that might otherwise have been dormant." Also worrisome is the fact that estrogen makes breast tissue denser so it resembles that of a younger woman—and this makes mammograms more difficult to interpret.

Some data suggest that adding progestins to hormone replacement therapy could theoretically raise the risk of breast cancer; a recent study found that women who started using a progestin-based contraceptive within the past five years had a doubled risk of breast cancer. This may not be true for natural progesterone, which is being studied.

Environmental Factors

Breast cancer is increasing in virtually all the industrialized countries. There's compelling evidence that chemical compounds called organochlorines may be partly to blame. According to a report by Greenpeace, there are thousands of organochlorines in the environment from pesticides such as DDT, dioxin, solvents, and plastics and vinyls such as PVC and PCBs. They mimic or interfere with sex hormones including estrogen, and thus may promote breast cancer. The evidence against exogenous estrogens or xenoestrogens is compelling: When Israel banned DDT and other toxic pesticides, breast cancer rates dropped dramatically; women with breast cancer have high levels of DDE, a DDT metabolite, in their blood; and women with breast cancer have twice as many PCBs and DDEs in their breast tissue than cancer-free women. Some experts believe that it's not the fat in our diets per se that increases breast cancer, but the chemical contaminants such as organochlorines that accumulate in the fat. Other possible factors being studied are electromagnetic energy such as that emitted from electric power lines, chlorinated water, and patterns of exposure to certain types of light.

Assessing Your Risk of Breast Cancer

In addition to the above ''known'' risk factors, there are several ''suspected'' risk factors that need further study. The more of these known and unknown risk factors you have, the higher your risk and the more enthusiastically you'll want to embrace a cancer prevention program. Unfortunately, many of the known risk factors are beyond our control, especially by the time we reach menopause. However, many of the suspected risk factors are under our control—we can change them with our diet and lifestyle. And even if breast cancer runs in your family, you still have the power to lower your risk.

KNOWN RISK FACTORS

1. Does breast cancer run in your family—has your mother, sister, or aunt had breast cancer before the age of forty?
2. Are you age fifty or over?
3. Are you overweight?
4. Did you have an early menarche (before age twelve) and/or late menopause (after age fifty-five)?
5. Did you never have children or have them late in life (after age thirty)?
6. Did you have irregular periods before reaching menopause?
7. Do you live in the United States, Canada, a Western European country, or another industrialized country?
8. Do you smoke?
9. Do you drink alcohol?

SUSPECTED RISK FACTORS

10. Do you eat more than three servings a week of meat, cheese, or other animal fat?
11. Do you eat fewer than five servings of fresh vegetables and fruits every day?
12. Have you been exposed to excessive radiation?
13. Have you been exposed to excessive organochlorines such as pesticides or chlorinated water?
14. Did you or do you now take estrogen (oral contraceptives or estrogen replacement therapy) for 8 or more years, within the last 10 years?

Reducing the Risk of Breast Cancer

Conventional medicine has little to offer in preventing breast cancer. For high-risk women, the two main strategies are prophylactic mastectomy (removal of healthy breasts before cancer develops) and taking the antiestrogen drug tamoxifen. These are both drastic measures that remain unproven. Some suggest that natural hormones such as progesterone and estriol might accomplish the same thing as tamoxifen, but this is also unproven. Even the American Cancer Society recommends that we eat more fruits and vegetables, and reduce fat.

Although we can't change factors such as our personal or family history that account for 25 percent of breast cancer risk, we can change the lifestyle factors thought to increase the risk. Because of the long latency period for breast cancer—it can take up to fourteen years for a single damaged cell to grow into a detectable lump—much breast cancer begins way before menopause. So it is probably wise to decrease risks as much as possible even in our youth. Lifestyle changes affect our immune system and metabolism dramatically, so we can probably influence cancer cell growth even once it has begun. Measures aimed at prevention may also influence the prognosis once breast cancer is diagnosed. For example, a 10-year Canadian study of women with breast cancer found that for each 5 percent increase in saturated fat (mainly animal fats), the risk of dying from breast cancer increased by 50 percent, but there was no significant increase in risk with total fat intake.

Preventive steps revolve around three goals: (1) reducing exposure to carcinogens and cancer-promoting substances such as alcohol, cigarettes and exogenous estrogens; (2) maintaining a healthy estrogen-progesterone balance; and (3) boosting the immune system to support its ability to detect and destroy cancer cells before they cause trouble.

Changing Your Diet

The two most important changes to make go hand in hand: reducing fat intake and increasing fruits, vegetables and beans. Although much has been written about the link between high fat intake and increased risk of breast cancer, there are so many nutritional, environmental, and social influences, we believe you can't blame breast cancer on high fat intake alone. For example, women who eat a high-fat diet are usually not eating fruits and vegetables and so are getting paltry amounts of cancer-protecting vitamins, minerals, fiber, and other plant chemicals. The type of fat you eat is critically important. Hydrogenated fats such as margarine and damaged fats such as overheated polyunsaturates are harmful to cells and our immune systems. Essential fatty acids (*see* Chapter 3, page 66) are generally healthy, even necessary, for the immune cells that fight cancer. That's why it's not enough to switch to no-fat cakes and cookies. And that's why following the Balanced Life Plan is something that every women should do to reduce risk of breast cancer.

According to Maureen Henderson, M.D., head of the Cancer Prevention Research Program at the Fred Hutchinson Cancer Research Center in Seattle, cutting our fat intake (which averages 37% of calories) in half would cut the breast cancer rate by 60%. Evidence suggests that if you do eat fat, most of it should be unsaturated. A 1995 Harvard study of over 2,000 Greek women found that women who consumed olive oil (a monosaturated fat) twice a day had 25% less cancer than those who consumed it once a day. A Spanish study found similar results. Animal fats from animals given estrogen hormones or nonorganic feed should be avoided. Interestingly, many European countries will not import our beef because it is so laced with estrogen. Organic, range-fed beef is more lean, and small amounts may be important for some women to include in their diets.

Many studies show that the more fruits and vegetables you eat, the less cancer you will generally develop. The same Harvard study mentioned above found that women who ate the most vegetables had a 48% lower risk of developing breast cancer than those who ate the least; women who ate the most fruits had a 32% lower risk than women who ate the least.

Fruits and vegetables contain hundreds of substances—many of which are still being discovered—that work together and may protect us in several ways. They are high in fiber, which encourages excretion of estrogen from the body. Soybeans and soy foods contain plant estrogen-like compounds (*see* Chapter 4) which help normalize estrogen in the body and are thought to be one of the major reasons that Japanese and Chinese women have low rates of breast cancer. Vegetables containing substances called indoles also affect estrogen metabolism and may protect against cancer; these foods include cabbage, kale, broccoli, brussels sprouts, and collard greens. Foods containing antioxidant vitamins and minerals such as vitamins C and E, beta-carotene, and selenium blunt the effects of free radicals, which are linked with cancer. Research conducted at the University of Washington in Seattle found that the tissue of women with breast cancer has more free-radical damage than women without breast cancer.

Because of the likely pesticide connection to breast cancer, we emphasize the importance of buying organic fruits and vegetables. Although DDT has been banned in the United States, it is still used freely in many of the countries who export food to America. Residues of past use persist in our own soil and in our fat cells almost indefinitely. One theory is that the increase in breast cancer in women over fifty is due to their exposure to DDT, which appeared in 1945. In all, more than 220 million pounds of chemicals thought to alter our hormones are currently used on sixty-eight different crops each year, according to the Environmental Working Group. These accumulate in the meat and dairy products of animals who are fed nonorganic feed.

Changing Your Lifestyle

Limiting alcohol to less than three drinks a week and stopping smoking will also lower your risk of getting breast cancer or dying of it. Studies have consistently found that drinking three or more alcohol beverages a week increases breast cancer risk by 20–70%. Smokers generally have a 25% higher death rate from breast cancer than do nonsmokers; smoking two packs a day bumps the rate up to 75%.

Regular exercise during the reproductive years can substantially lower a woman's breast cancer risk. One study found a lower than average rate of breast cancer among young women who had been college athletes. Strenuous exercise may exert this effect by reducing the production of estrogen. In another study, women who jogged, swam, or worked out strenuously for 4 hours a week had a 60% lower risk of breast cancer than sedentary women. The protective effect of exercise persisted through the age of forty, but we don't know whether this benefit holds true for women in their menopausal years. Interestingly, the highest incidence of breast cancer (and colorectal cancer) is in areas where people get the least amount of sunlight. Since sunlight forms vitamin D in the skin, some researchers believe insufficient vitamin D is the connection. So, try to spend about a half-hour each day in natural sunlight.

If you are at higher than average risk for breast cancer, consider trying the natural therapies described in Chapter 3 to help balance hormones, reduce the detrimental effects of too much stress, and help your body's immune system handle unavoidable toxins. The following therapies are particularly promising in cancer prevention.

Nutritional Supplements

Many studies suggest that nutritional deficiencies increase the risk of all cancers, including breast cancer. A good multivitamin-and-mineral formula containing the doses recommended in Chapter 3, pages 61–64, supplies what we now consider to be the optimum amounts of nutrients that are associated with reducing cancer risk or have cancer-fighting properties. If you are at high risk you may also increase the dose of:

• *Beta-carotene,* up to 100,000 IU per day. Beta-carotene is a precursor for vitamin A, which slows the progression of breast cancer in animals.
• *Vitamin C,* up to 10,000 mg per day. Vitamin C is a potent antioxidant and enhances the immune system. Bioflavonoids work together with vitamin C and some of them modify the effects of estrogen in the body. (*See* "Natural Hormone Therapy," pages 287–288.)
• *Vitamin D,* up to 800 IU per day. Improves immunity.
• *Vitamin E,* 400–800 IU per day. Vitamin E is a powerful antioxidant and immune booster.
• *Selenium,* 200 mcg per day. Selenium is an antioxidant that appears to be particularly effective in preventing breast cancer; most women with breast cancer have below normal levels of selenium in

their blood. Methio-selenium contains methionine, which helps the liver detoxify harmful substances such as carcinogens.

• *Essential fatty acids,* 250 to 6,000 mg per day to boost immunity. Foods and supplements containing a combination of EFAs are best; these include flax, hemp, and safflower oil. Coldwater fish oils are high in EPA, which also boosts immunity; Eskimos consume diets high in EPA from fish oil and have a low incidence of breast cancer despite their fatty diet. In an animal study of advanced breast cancer, EPA prolonged survival and slowed tumor growth.

You may also wish to add:

• *Lactobacillus acidophilus,* a friendly bacteria that is thought to help the body metabolize estrogen. It is available in capsules and liquid form at health food stores.

• *Aloe vera drink,* 1 ounce three times a day. This plant has been used since antiquity and appears to boost immunity and aid in general detoxification.

• *Garlic* supplements, 200–1,200 mg per day, or 1–4 ounces of fresh garlic. Garlic has many remarkable properties, including the ability to boost the immune system; it may also directly affect the growth of cancer cells, and prevent cells from turning cancerous in the first place.

• *Chinese* or *Korean ginseng,* which appears to reduce the risk of cancer.

• *Shiitake mushrooms,* which are available in powdered form. They are a mainstay in the Japanese diet and contain substances that are associated with improved immunity and anticancer effects.

• Maitake mushrooms have even greater anticancer effects, and are part of a successful breast cancer treatment regimen in Japan. The "D fraction" is the most important anticancer element.

Natural Hormone Therapy
There is evidence that commonly prescribed hormone regimens increase the risk of breast cancer. As of this writing, the standard of care is not to prescribe estrogens for women with or at high risk of breast cancer. That having been said, the question is: Are plant estrogen-like compounds safe for high-risk women? There is some evidence that consumption of natural plant hormones actually reduces the risk of

breast cancer. For example, high intake of plant phyto-estrogens contained in foods such as soybeans appear to lower breast cancer incidence as among the Japanese.

The same question arises when we look at pharmacological-grade natural progesterone made from plant compounds. According to Dr. Lee, a proponent of natural progesterone, it is high levels of unopposed estrogen (that is, accompanied by low levels of progesterone) that increase breast cancer risk. He believes that natural progesterone is protective against breast cancer—and endometrial cancer as well. This remains to be proven and appears to depend on the individual cancer's hormone receptors. A significant opposing view suggests that both synthetic and natural progesterone may increase breast cancer risk.

The two types of estrogen, estradiol and estrone, which are used in commonly prescribed ERT, have been associated with an increased risk of breast cancer. However, a third type called estriol has been suggested by some to actually protect against breast cancer. In a small unpublished study by Dr. Henry Lemon in 1975, women with breast cancer had lower estriol than healthy women. When Dr. Lemon gave estriol to women with advanced breast cancer, 37 percent had a remission or their cancer stopped growing. More recent epidemiological studies show that women who live in countries with low breast cancer rates have more estriol than women in countries where the breast cancer rates are high. Limited as the research is, estriol appears to be a more user-friendly form of estrogen drug and comprehensive studies on its efficacy and safety are clearly overdue. Estriol is available by prescription from compounding pharmacies and it is the major estrogen in Dr. Jonathan Wright's "Tri-Est" postmenopausal estrogen replacement formula. (*See* Chapter 4 for more information about hormone replacement therapy.)

Precautions

Be sure to perform a breast self-exam every month, and get regular mammograms; consult a physician immediately if you feel anything suspicious. Early detection greatly improves your prognosis if you are diagnosed with breast cancer.

Diabetes

It is estimated that nearly 14 million Americans have sugar diabetes, or diabetes mellitus. (Although there are other types of diabetes, in this chapter we refer to the most common type, also known as non–insulin-dependent diabetes mellitus, Type II or "adult-onset" diabetes, which usually starts after age forty.) Of the 14 million, 85 percent have non–insulin-dependent diabetes. Adult-onset diabetes is the third leading cause of death in some ethnic/gender groups in the United States, particularly African-American women. Diabetes leads to infection, worsens heart disease, and is associated with many other causes of illness and death.

When you have diabetes, your body has too much sugar (glucose) in the blood. In excess, glucose and its products wreak havoc on blood vessels, nerves, and other tissues. Glucose, which our body gets from food, is the fuel used by cells to create energy. Insulin is a hormone produced by the pancreas that regulates the amount of glucose in the blood. Insulin "escorts" glucose into our cells, where it is taken in through an insulin receptor on the cell membrane. Glucose is then used immediately or stored and used later on; this prevents our blood sugar from going too high, as occurs in diabetes. Insulin fits into cell wall receptors like a key fits into a lock; they open the cell wall to let the sugar in.

Some people are genetically susceptible to developing diabetes. After a lifetime of eating too much simple sugar, the cell may sprout more and more receptors to handle the load. It is suspected that in time these receptors become chemically numb to the onslaught, although the mechanism of this is unknown and there are other factors involved. In any event, more and more insulin is needed to get lower blood sugar.

Although very common, diabetes is a serious disease and can be ugly in its later stages: with blindness, lingering sores, amputation of toes or feet, heart disease, and nerve pains which are very difficult to relieve. All this suffering is usually unnecessary because diabetes is, to a very large extent, preventable. In our experience, only a minority of diabetics cannot control their disease with diet and exercise. Nonetheless this disease can render someone so "brittle" that a single piece of chocolate or a banana can send them into a ketoacidic coma, and a missed meal after a full dose of insulin causes hypoglycemic coma. The vast majority of diabetics have tremendous difficulty letting go of their freedom to indulge in sweets. They forget that processed breads may have sugar; that dates, raisins, honey, powdered milk, and fruit concentrates are powerfully sweet, and they brag about their "sugar-free" desserts, which are actually chock-full of these little devils. Sugar is an addiction and often the only way to quit it is to quit it.

Detection and Treatment

Diagnosing diabetes mellitus requires a fasting blood sugar test, which should be repeated if the diagnosis is in doubt. Normal fasting blood sugar levels are about 70–120.

In addition to watching their diet, people with diabetes can often control their blood sugar levels by controlling their weight and getting regular exercise. The latter is very important, since the metabolism needs to be speeded up to get the insulin moving into the cells and to use the calories. Many people with diabetes also take oral medications that help their own pancreas produce more insulin and/or get it into the cells more easily. There are also newer agents which decrease absorption of glucose from the gut. It should be noted that there is *no* oral insulin. The stomach cannot process insulin. Therefore, anyone who takes insulin must take it by injection. It is not uncommon for adult diabetics who have been taking oral medication successfully for a number of years to become unresponsive to it. In those cases, insulin taken by injection will be recommended by their health care professional.

Diabetes self-care includes regular blood testing, either spot checks or a specific number of times per day, including a fasting glucose test early in the morning after no food for 9–12 hours. People who inject insulin learn from their health care providers how to adjust their insulin requirements to the blood glucose readings. Most home readings are obtained by pricking the finger with an automatic needle-prick device and then putting the drop of blood onto a test strip inserted into a small machine that gives a digital reading of the glucose present in that drop of blood.

Risk Factors

Major risk factors for diabetes in those over forty are excess weight and a lack of regular exercise. In the United States, over 80 percent of all people with adult-onset diabetes are obese. A Scandinavian study found that moderate obesity increases the risk of diabetes tenfold; and people who are extremely obese (45 percent above normal weight) have thirty times the risk. In the United States, the rate of diabetes is increasing much faster than the rate of population growth, so we can't blame it on the fact that we're just getting older. During the past several decades we have, however, gradually switched to a sweeter, more refined diet, with less fiber and nutrients, and we have been steadily been gaining weight. Sugar intake in particular is linked to increasing rates of diabetes.

In industrialized societies, the estimated rate of diabetes for men and women is 3–10 percent; in most traditional societies, the average rate is just over 1 percent. However, these figures are changing because diabetes is increasing all over the world, as more countries give up their traditional diets and lifestyles and adopt a more industrialized way of life. As the chart below shows, the greatest increase in death from diabetes for women between 1960 and 1989 has occurred in traditional countries.

Percentage of Increase in Diabetes in Women Around the World, 1960–1989

Country	Percentage Increase
Canada	75
Costa Rica (to 1988)	237
US (to 1988)	31
Colombia (to 1984)	194
Ecuador (to 1988)	767
Hong Kong	681
Thailand	498
France	79
Germany	52
Singapore	585

Source: U.N. Demographic Yearbook, 1993.

Genetic predisposition is thought by many to be a risk factor; if it is, it seems to work in conjunction with diet and lifestyle. For example, diabetes was rare among indigenous Native Americans, but with colonization, diabetes is common among these people and one tribe in particular (the Pima) has been studied for its highest rates in the world. With modernization and an increased intake of sugar and refined foods, diabetes has increased among other traditional peoples such as the Bushmen, Eskimo, and some Pacific Islanders, who now have an incidence of up to 35 percent.

Assessing Your Risk of Diabetes

The more risk factors you have, the higher your risk and the more enthusiastically you'll want to embrace a diabetes prevention program. Fortunately, only one risk factor—heredity—is beyond your control. The others are under your control—you can change them with our diet and lifestyle.

1. Does diabetes run in your family?
2. Are you overweight?
3. Do you live a sedentary lifestyle?
4. Do you eat a lot of sugar, fruit, and refined foods?

Preventing and Controlling Diabetes: General Nutrition and Lifestyle Considerations

The major factors in preventing and controlling diabetes are diet, weight loss, and exercise. The recommended diet to reduce the risk of developing diabetes and reduce complications is similar to the eating plan outlined in our Balanced Life Plan in Chapter 2. According to the American Diabetes Association, research shows that a vegetarian diet (vegetarians generally follow the guidelines provided in our recommended basic eating plan) reduces the incidence of diabetes. You may initially have feelings of deprivation as you leave behind familiar foods. Focus on all the good foods you *can* eat until they become your habit, and remind yourself that choosing healthy foods is a choice of self-care and nurturance.

An antidiabetes way of eating concentrates most of all on a diet high in complex carbohydrates and minimizes simple sugars including fruit and limits fat. Look for the hidden sugar in foods, and avoid artificial sweeteners, which take you a step backward from changing your taste sensibilities. Many studies show that eating a high-fiber diet helps prevent diabetes and normalize blood glucose levels in people who already have diabetes. So favor high-fiber foods; vegetables, beans, and oats, which are particularly high in soluble fiber, the type that slows down glucose absorption by your intestines. This in turn reduces the surge in glucose (and thus, insulin) and increases the sensitivity of tissues to insulin. Stevia is an excellent natural sweetener with no calories and may actually help control blood sugar.

If you enjoy them, eat more garlic and onions (at least 2 ounces a day, cooked or raw) because substances in these foods normalize glucose levels, either by increasing liver metabolism of glucose, by increasing insulin secretion, or by increasing the lifespan of insulin in the body. The mineral chromium is needed for insulin to work, so be sure to include foods rich in this trace mineral, such as brewer's yeast, and whole grain cereals and breads. Foods containing zinc are essential as well; this mineral is a component of insulin, and is required for immunity and wound healing—important because people with diabetes have trouble healing and warding off infections.

Exercise plays a crucial role in diabetes control and prevention. Aerobic exercise lowers blood sugar, helps in weight reduction, oxygenates tissues, and stimulates the metabolism.

Stress triggers the production of adrenaline, which in turn raises blood sugar, so yoga, tai chi, walking and other relaxing movements, as well as meditation, massage, and visualization are recommended.

All the natural therapies in Chapter 3 are generally helpful in reducing the risk of diabetes; many also help control diabetes once it's been established and reduce the risk of complications, but should be used under professional care. The following specific approaches may also be particularly helpful in preventing and controlling diabetes.

Nutritional Supplements

People with diabetes seem to have a deficiency in and/or an increased need for certain nutrients. These nutrients tend to be related to the complications of diabetes, and some studies suggest that supplementation can prevent or reverse these conditions. Certain nutrients are required for the production of glucose tolerance factor (GTF), a substance that augments the action of insulin. For example, chromium is the major mineral involved in GTF production. In experiments, chromium piccolinate supplements improved glucose tolerance in diabetics. Vitamin B-3 (niacin) is also a component of GTF, may reduce insulin requirements, and may prevent diabetic kidney disease. Vitamins B-6 and B-1 (thiamin) may prevent or reverse nerve damage from diabetes. Vitamin C supplements may improve glucose tolerance, and protect diabetics in several ways from atherosclerosis. Vitamin E may reduce insulin requirements, and prevent heart disease and eye disease. Manganese is needed to activate enzymes the body produces to use sugar for energy. Magnesium improves regulation of blood sugar levels and may prevent diabetic heart disease.

A good multivitamin-mineral formula containing the doses recommended in Chapter 3, pages 61–64, usually supplies these nutrients and all the others you need to help keep your blood sugar normal and reduce the complications of diabetes. Under professional supervision, you may increase the daily total dose of the following:

• *Chromium,* up to 200 to 600 mcg daily in divided doses. If you are on insulin, begin with 200 mcg and increase slowly, as chromium supplements can lower the need for insulin.

• *Vitamin E,* up to 1,000 IU daily. If you have diabetes, start with no more than 100 IU daily and slowly increase the dosage—vitamin E may reduce your insulin requirements and affect your heart and so dosage should be monitored carefully.

• *Vitamin B-complex,* up to 100 mg daily.

• *Vitamin C,* 3,000 mg daily in divided doses. Be sure to ask your pharmacist (or the manufacturer of the blood sugar strips you are using) if the strips are susceptible to false vitamin C readings.

You may also take:

• *Vitamin A,* 25,000 IU per day.

• *Vitamin D,* 400 IU per day. (The D-3 form is best if you have kidney problems.)

• *Garlic supplements,* up to 5,000 mg per day (about 4 capsules per meal).

• *Guar gum, apple pectin, or psyllium,* 5 to 10 g, up to three times a day. These are concentrated sources of soluble fiber that have been shown to be helpful in stabilizing blood sugar. Be sure to drink extra water to avoid constipation when using these fiber sources.

• *Essential fatty acids,* up to 4,000 mg total, instead of other fats.

Take as oil of flax seed, soy, sesame, canola, safflower, or as supplements of evening primrose oil, black currant oil, and borage oil, or fish oil.

• *Brewer's yeast,* up to 9 g daily. An excellent source of GTF, brewer's yeast has many benefits for diabetics: it improves glucose tolerance, increases insulin sensitivity, and lowers blood fats. However, it is not well tolerated by women with yeast sensitivities and is difficult to digest.

Herbal Remedies

Many herbs are used in folk medicine to support the medical treatment of diabetes, either because they reduce blood sugar, increase the production or effectiveness of insulin, or reduce the harmful effects of diabetes on tissues. They can have a rapid effect on blood sugar, which varies from person to person, so herbal therapy should be tailored to your individual needs and closely monitored by a health professional. For instructions on herbal remedies, *see* Chapter 3, pages 70–75. The following herbs are most often used and best documented to be effective.

• *American ginseng* is used in folk medicine to treat diabetes and is believed to lower the blood sugar level. There are fifty-five substances in ginseng that may affect blood sugar, but these are found only in standardized crude extracts, not purified ginsenoside extracts. The usual dosage is 1 capsule or ½–1 teaspoon of tincture up to three times a day, or 1 cup of decoction twice a day.

• *Fenugreek* (25–100 mg per day) and *aloe vera* (2 teaspoons per day) have also been shown to lower blood sugar.

• *Antioxidants* and *flavonoids* protect diabetics in many ways. *Gingko biloba* is a free radical scavenger circulation enhancer which has been shown to prevent diabetic retinopathy in rats and may also protect humans. *Pycnogenol* is a product containing a variety of flavonoids; 150–300 mg per day has been shown to increase circulation of tiny capillaries. *Bilberry* (500 mg per day) has flavonoids, which increase circulation in capillaries.

• *Maitake mushrooms* bring down blood sugar.

• *Prickly pear juice,* 1 tablespoon has been shown to decrease blood sugar.

Precautions

The above recommendations can have a powerful effect on your blood sugar. Be sure to enter your regimen thoughtfully, with careful home and professional blood sugar monitoring. Be aware of the signs and symptoms of blood sugar out of balance. These include fatigue, abdominal or chest pain, trouble concentrating, shortness of breath, blurring of vision or the sensation that your eyes are out of focus, increased thirst or hunger, numbness or tingling in feet or hands, trouble healing, frequent yeast infections, and bladder problems.

CHAPTER 7

Enjoying Sex During Menopause and Beyond

To be sure, hormones and other physical factors are significant players in the lifelong sexual dance. But the way we express our sexual selves is also influenced by our emotions, the society we live in, and our culture's values. In this chapter we discuss all of these as they affect the sex lives of menopausal and postmenopausal women living in the United States in the 1990s. Here, too, you'll read about practicing safe sex and birth control, finding a partner, and maintaining a sexual relationship—these issues may change as you age, but they continue to be topics of concern through menopause and beyond.

Perhaps our most important message is that it's a myth that once a woman hits menopause, sex is over. (Unless, of course, the woman, herself, believes it or wants it to be over!) Menopause may mean the end of your periods, but it doesn't mean the end of sex. In fact, many women experience greater desire and pleasure now that pregnancy worries are past. Some even report a surge in sexual energy along with a deeper, more sophisticated appreciation, open attitude, and technical expertise.

Although having a satisfactory sex life can be difficult for you if you are a middle-aged or older woman—you may lack a partner, be experiencing vaginal changes that make sex uncomfortable, be in a marriage gone stale or sour, or be going through emotional difficulties—in these cases we hope that you find this chapter reassuring. A happy love life, including wonderful sex, is every woman's right, if she wants it. It has many health benefits, too. Gratifying sex releases endorphins in the brain that promote the immune system, sex also helps lower blood pressure, relax us, and deepen our bond with our partners. As Picasso said at the age of ninety-three, "Love is a great refreshment!"

Getting Help if You Need It

Fortunately there are many places to turn to if you and your partner want to improve your love life, assuming you've already tried listening and looking into each other's eyes, expressing sincere caring and acceptance of each other—even your faults and neediness. Counseling services for couples are widely available and there are many types, depending on your specific needs. A general counselor can help place you if you need a specialist in marriage, self-esteem, or sex. A consultation with an experienced and reputable therapist can help you better define the issues that need work. Referrals to a therapist can be provided by your church, any social service agency such as Catholic Family Services or Jewish Family Services, your physician, your health plan, or the state licensing board for that specialty. It's best to take a referral from someone you know and trust, if possible.

There's help, too, if you are experiencing specific physical problems that are hampering your sexual enjoyment. Please refer to Chapter 5 for natural remedies for a variety of common concerns including vaginal dryness, painful intercourse, breast tenderness, fatigue, and insomnia.

Self-esteem and Changing Body Image

Women who are menopausal and older today grew up at a time when girls rated themselves on the success of their flirtations. Remember, women are only as attractive as they feel. Thanks to powerful, self-assured role models, it's becoming less of a social/sexual crime to have an unusual nose or physique. Look at Cher, Whoopie Goldberg, Barbra Streisand—these women would never be confused with Barbie, and yet they get top billing.

And don't forget that how we look and what we project depends a great deal on how well rested we are, what we've been eating, our exercise habits, sexual activity, work accomplishments, what we are wearing, and—perhaps most importantly—our attitude and frame of mind. Do we carry ourselves proudly and speak our minds? It's the hunched shoulders, knitted brow, and timid voice which turn people off—and the genuine smile and attentiveness which wins the hearts and minds of those who are worthy.

We don't have to buy into anyone's devaluation of older women. It may not have been considered "proper" for grandmothers of yester-year to enhance their sexuality and vitality with attractive clothes; they didn't run out to the gym or take fitness walks, as we are now free to do. That may be because they never thought of themselves as having a sexuality that would appeal to anyone, and because of past societal puritanism and a Victorian Age sense of propriety that accompanied getting older. Now women are running marathons in their menopausal years and enjoying their peak years of love and adventure.

In spite of the conscious change in older women's thoughts about themselves as sexually desirable and desirous, there remains in many an underlying anxiety about their appeal. This anxiety may find expression in low sexual desire, rejection of masturbation as an alternative to having a partner, or even turning off the idea of looking for a new sex partner when a former one is no longer available.

Many women find that such anxiety evaporates when exposed to the light of day—that is, when you can openly talk about it with other women. You could turn to friends, relatives, or special groups. If you feel deflated and discouraged about your impact on the world, you might seek out a group like OWL (Older Women's League) or the Grey Panthers. Make sure you get together regularly with others in the same boat, not to gripe but to apply your energies to upholding and building strong self-images. That will bring joy not only to yourself, but to everyone, and especially to younger people and people who set policies in the workplace and in government.

Either in a group or on your own, you can practice building self-esteem in your heart and mind. Clear the corners of your mind of any thoughts which do not bring you images of fulfillment and emotions of joy, energy, and self-esteem.

The only way to gain power is to
    act powerful.
The only way to gain respect is to
    give respect.

300 / Natural Medicine for Menopause and Beyond

The only way to gain love is to
    give love.

Self-pleasuring and Sensuality

As noted above, some older women may feel unappealing sexually, or embarrassed, or "too old for that" and so they put sexual feelings and activities out of their lives, including self-pleasuring. Masturbation is but one way to give the self erotic pleasure. Before moving on to the others, please note that if you do masturbate and find this physically uncomfortable, use the same palliatives that you would with a partner: soothing lubricating creams and jellies and frequent, gradual penetration with a dildo or other suitably shaped object will keep your vagina toned and in shape, whether you have planned for penetration with a partner or not. (*See* "Vaginal Dryness," pages 232–33.)

Erotic pleasures are extremely personal and can add some spice to your life. We're never too old for sexual stimulation, whether that be listening to luscious, soulfully sexy music, writing and reading erotic poetry and literature, looking at sexy pictures or videos. Fantasies of your own devising can be immensely enriching, as long as they are not hurtful of yourself, your partner, or your own sense of propriety and respect.

And not all sexuality is specifically erotic. For example, when we extend our concept of sexuality to include sensuality, we see that there are a great many activities that can pleasure us. Water and warm sun are great sources of sensuality (though watch those ultraviolet rays and read our section on skin problems in Chapter 5). Massages by a lover, a friend, or a sensitive massage professional can help us feel very luxuriant and calmed. Probably the best nonhuman providers of sensuality are the pets who love us. Research shows that those with pets live longer than those without them and that blood pressure goes down while people stroke or groom their pets. So keep in touch with your sexuality and sensuality—you'll feel the better for it psychologically and those raging endorphins released when we feel sexy and loving are good for the immune system, too! For a refreshing take on health and sensuality, read *Healthy Pleasures* by Robert Ornstein and David Sobel—a liberating compendium of the science, theory, and how-to of enjoying life to its fullest.

Safer Sex

While finding a new partner can be achingly difficult for a woman of any age, the next step can be just as difficult—and awkward, especially if you've been out of circulation for some time. A new sexual partner brings excitement and regeneration, but it also can bring a new concern: sexually transmitted diseases. Unfortunately, age is not protective against these diseases. The list is daunting: gonorrhea, syphilis, herpes, genital warts, chlamydia, hepatitis, and AIDS. AIDS may especially be overlooked as a risk to older people (and therefore, to their health care providers, who may assume an older person is not infected and neglect to take the proper precautions).

It's very difficult to ask a new man to wear a condom. It's embarrassing, or we've been brought up to defer to men. Maybe you feel you're just lucky to have a lover again; better not to hassle him too much. Maybe your former partner never used a condom. Maybe you've never even seen one before; maybe you have but don't like them. If you feel awkward and are at a loss for what to say and how to say it, consider saying something like the explanation below. It helps to actually say the words out loud—a kind of rehearsal—beforehand, so you feel more comfortable when the time actually comes. For example, you might say:

"It's been a long time since I've felt so comfortable and attracted to a man. I think it's time to break the ice about an intimate subject. When you kissed me last night, I felt we might go further—did you feel that way too? I trust my intuition and I feel you are a man of your word, who is cautious and honorable. I need you to tell me honestly now of any possible risks to my health if we are to become intimate. Could you be at any risk at all for any sexually transmitted disease?"

Give him time to answer—be very patient and look at him supportively so that he can tell you about having herpes, or a one-night stand, or a prostitute. You have to be patient with yourself, too, to let the opportunity pass if you don't feel 100 percent comfortable with his answer.

These conversations are best done sitting at a table fully clothed—not in the heat of passion. Give yourself time to think about his answers before diving in. Search for a look in the eye, or a tone of voice, which opens up a window to sincerity—or not. He may be trying to be honest, and fear of rejection may edit his speech. Until you know each other very well, it's really hard to know whether a partner is being truthful.

Remind him that by wearing a condom he's protecting himself, too, which he might consider reasonable. Please remember that there are many ways the most respectable-looking man may have contracted an STD. Think about it for a minute. If he's a widower, did he have sex with anyone else—maybe a prostitute in search of comfort? Does he know the medical histories of any of the men with whom any lovers of his had sex? Could he be a closet bisexual? Could one of his lovers have had a transfusion with tainted blood? A partner doesn't have to have AIDS but only be HIV-positive to transmit the virus. The best thing is to learn how to use a condom until the two of you have been monogamous for at least 6 months after you've both tested negative for HIV.

This is a good time to discuss your feelings about monogamy, frequency and/or types of sex you enjoy, and future goals. Recognize that relationships are living creatures which change us, their constituents. Feel free to cast aside the way you used to be if you feel you could be different with this potential mate—especially if doing so is healthy and supportive of your individual growth and fulfillment.

Birth Control

Although it's true that we produce fewer and tireder eggs and ovulate less frequently as we approach menopause, it's also true that there are many midlife babies toddling around out there. Unless you wouldn't mind getting pregnant late in life (or mistakenly thinking you're pregnant because of irregular periods), you still need to use birth control if you are sexually active with a potent man. Until when? Until a year has gone by without your having any periods.

You still have the same less-than-satisfactory contraceptive methods available as younger women, but the pros and cons shift as we age so be sure to discuss them with a trusted practitioner. For example, many experts advise against using birth control pills once you hit forty, but among many other practitioners, the pill is "in" for perimenopausal women. Older women have a risk of heart attack or stroke from the pill that is sixteen times higher than for women in their thirties. Intrauterine devices (IUDs) may make more sense to you now than when you were younger because one of their most disturbing risks—infertility—would not be as catastrophic if your childbearing years are over. On the other hand, if you are bleeding heavily because of menopausal changes, an IUD could make it worse.

An increasingly attractive option is the "barrier" methods such as condoms, diaphragms, cervical caps and contraceptive jellies, foams, and creams. Because of your declining fertility, the chance of some sperm getting through is less significant, especially as you are more sensible and realistic than the average teenager who leaves the diaphragm at home and forgets to pick up more spermicidal cream. Some older women may have medical conditions, such as a prolapsed uterus or uterine fibroids, which may make it difficult to get a diaphragm or cervical cap to fit and function properly. And diaphragms increase the risk of urinary tract infection, which women are susceptible to as they age. Many women and men are sensitive to spermicides, latex, or both. Seek a practitioner who is familiar with all of your options and potential problems.

Remember, with irregular menses, you must use birth control every time to prevent pregnancy. Another important caution is that only condoms can prevent sexually transmitted diseases. So if you're using another type of birth control and you're not 100 percent sure of your partner's health status—either because he's new on the scene or a regular lover but not monogamous—we recommend that you ensure your safety and insist that he wear a condom.

Does Sex Change for Men and Women?

Some researchers have concluded that as testosterone levels decrease in the aging man, he becomes more "feminized" in a way that's good for women; that he is more sensuous over his whole body rather than being "penis driven"; that he is more nurturing; and usually he takes longer to have an orgasm! Younger men may turn some older women on but older men may actually make the best lovers for them.

Some other physical changes are worth knowing about. For example, men's nipples tend to become more sensitive as they age. A man may discover pleasure from stroking, licking, and gentle biting of his nipples more so now than in his youth. More penile stimulation may be required to help him to erection, so again all kinds of touching from gentle to vigorous stroking to sucking and licking may do the trick. Why not ask your lover if you might try something new; ask him if he would like you to explore his body like a new lover to see if there are hidden ecstasies you might discover together. An older man may want his partner to stimulate his penis orally, or with hands, or by rubbing with other parts and using other means to orgasm if he's having trouble achieving and maintaining an erection.

Women undergo changes as well. Like men, testosterone levels in women decrease as we age. Progesterone and estrogen diminish, as well as other hormones of youth and vigor. Lack of sexual hormones also leads to vaginal dryness, a major complaint that can hinder sexual play unless treated (see "Vaginal Dryness" on pages 232–33 in Chapter 5 for natural remedies). We recommend having your hormones checked; a new, affordable, and highly sensitive way to check tissue levels of steroids and other hormones is by saliva testing. Correcting deficiencies to resemble normal premenopausal levels can make a wonderful difference in your physical and emotional sexual well-being.

The shape of your vagina may change after menopause—shorter, narrower, but still able to accommodate sexual activity. Your clitoris may become more sensitive and require extra lubrication to enjoy being stroked. Usually, women experience less blood flow to the genitals as they age, and this may noticeably blunt the sharp edge of arousal. Breast size no longer increases with arousal, but this shouldn't dampen their sensitivity.

These naturally occurring changes needn't hurt your sex life if you and your partner are open with each other about the way your body is feeling and both of you are willing to experiment until you are mutually satisfied. If you feel inhibited about doing these things because you were raised in a sexually conservative atmosphere, but you would like to persist, some sessions for the two of you with a licensed sex therapist may be helpful.

Long-Lasting Sexual Pleasure

In closing, we'd like to reassure you that in most respects women (and men) can enjoy a long and satisfying sex life as long as good health prevails. You deserve this if you want it, but may need to help your health care professionals recognize that you intend to be a sexy and sexually active aging woman and find out what they can provide that will help you achieve that. You may also need to retrain your longtime partner and that calls for sensitivity, too. Your sexual responsiveness and needs have changed, as have your partner's. And finally, if you are single now and desirous of a mate you will have to go out there and let your love light shine. Other potential partners are out there if you no longer have the former one available. Don't be pessimistic because of the statistics—they are numbers, not people. You are a unique and lovable "catch," and the more you enjoy life, practice love and laughter, stay healthy, and prioritize your own development, the more attractive you are to everyone, including potential new lovers.

Appendixes

Appendix A
Glossary of Terms

Adaptogenic: any chemical agent that helps the body adapt to stress, and return to a balanced state.

Adrenal glands: two small glands located on the top of each kidney;

they secrete adrenaline and cortisol, the stress hormones, DHEA and other rejuvenating and mineral-balancing hormones; as well as some sex hormones.

Androstenedione: an androgen secreted by the ovaries and adrenal glands; it is the major precursor of estrogen after menopause.

Antioxidant: a molecule made by our bodies or eaten as a food or supplement which chemically prevents oxidation of cells by replacing electrons which are "stolen" by free radicals. Free radical damage has been implicated in many diseases and conditions, including cancer, heart disease, and arthritis.

Bioflavonoids: a group of chemicals found in fruits and plants that are essential for health and are helpful in many processes of cell structure and function, including the absorption of vitamin C.

Endocrine system: the body's system of glands that secrete hormones.

Endometrium: the lining of the uterus which grows during each menstrual cycle and then is shed.

ERT: estrogen replacement therapy.

Estrogen: a group of "female" sex hormones needed for the development of female sexual characteristics and reproduction; produced by the ovaries, adrenal glands, placenta, and fat cells. Estradiol, estrone, and estriol are the three major forms found in women.

Fibrocystic disease: a misnomer for any benign lumpy changes in the breast.

Free radicals: molecules lacking an electron; they easily react with molecules in the body, which can harm the cells.

Hormone: a chemical produced by the endocrine glands that the blood carries to other parts of the body where they cause specific effects.

HRT: hormone replacement therapy; usually consists of estrogen and synthetic progesterones called progestins.

Hypothalamus: the part of the brain that is responsible for regulating visceral and chemical activities including temperature, water balance, sleep, and hormone production by the pituitary gland.

Hysterectomy: surgical removal of the uterus; a total hysterectomy includes removal of the uterus, cervix, ovaries, and fallopian tubes.

Incontinence: inability to control urine release from the bladder, or bowel incontinence resulting in inadvertent soiling.

Libido: sex drive.

Menarche: the beginning of menstruation.

Perimenopausal: the period of time around menopause; may be 5–10 years.

Progesterone: a hormone produced by ovaries during the second half of the menstrual cycle; it promotes the growth of the uterine lining prior to menstruation.

Progestins: synthetic progesterones which have similar, but not identical, effects on the body as the naturally occurring hormone.

Phytoestrogens: also called plant estrogens, these substances are chemicals found in plants that have an estrogen-enhancing or estrogen-like effect on the body.

Phytosterols: hormones found in plants.

Testosterone: a ''male'' sex hormone thought to be responsible for sex drive; also is produced by women.

Uterus: the female sex organ also known as the womb, which carries the fetus during a pregnancy.

Vagina: the canal in a woman's body that extends from the vulva to the cervix.

Vulva: the female sex organ consisting of the labia majora and labia minora (major and minor lips), the clitoris, and the vaginal opening.

Appendix B
Diagnose Your Own Food Allergies and Sensitivities

One of the best ways to test for food allergies and sensitivities is the simple elimination and challenge procedure.

Step 1. List the foods you suspect might be causing you a problem. The foods that you like and crave the most are likely the ones to which you have special sensitivities. So, if you cannot imagine living without pasta or bread, cheese or milk, then you should include these foods on your list of foods to test. The most common food allergens are corn, wheat, dairy products, chocolate, peanuts, eggs, soy, yeast, and any of the more than 3,000 additives and preservatives found in processed food.

Step 2. Eliminate from your diet—for at least four days—the most common allergens listed above plus any additional foods which you suspect might be causing you a problem.

Step 3. On the fifth day, begin to reintroduce the eliminated foods back into your diet. Add one at a time, beginning in the morning for breakfast, on an empty stomach. Eat the food in its simplest form— for wheat, test plain spaghetti, or plain wheat cereal such as Wheatena. Do any symptoms appear? If not, have another form of wheat for lunch and then dinner, and see how you fare.

Step 4. Use the pulse test. Many people are "pulse responders" and notice that their pulse rises or lowers significantly after eating a food to which they are sensitive. Measure your pulse before eating the food and then 15 minutes and a half hour afterward. If your pulse changes by ten beats in either direction, this is a significant reaction.

Step 5. If no symptoms occur after testing a food for a full day, then go on to test the next food on your list the next day. If you noticed symptoms, go off the offending food and wait for the reaction to clear before testing the next food.

Delayed reactions: Food allergies and sensitivities can cause immediate, obvious symptoms in as little as 5 minutes or 5 hours. They may also cause delayed reactions in as much as 5 hours to 5 days after eating the food—these are often called hidden allergies. For uncovering hidden allergies, we recommend the Elias/Act™ Lymphocyte Response Test from Serramune Physicians Laboratory, 800-553-5472.

Precautions: Do not test any food if you know or even suspect it may cause a serious problem. Some people cannot breathe after eating shellfish or nuts—this do-it-yourself test is not for them! Nor is it for folks who have severe asthma that gets worse when they eat certain foods. If you fall into either of these categories, allergy testing should be handled under professional care.

Those seeking more information on food allergies are referred to Dr. Susan Brown's workbook: *Is the Right Food Wrong for You?: A Self-Help Program to Detect and Overcome Food Allergies.* (*See* Appendix C.)

Appendix C
Resources

Organizations

Menopause and Women's Health
North American Menopause Society
Department of Ob/Gyn, University Hospitals of Cleveland
2074 Abingdon Road
Cleveland, OH 44106
216-844-3348
  Referral to menopause specialists; publishes a quarterly journal and sponsors annual meetings.

Midlife Wellness Center for Climacteric Studies
University of Florida
901 NW 8th Avenue, Suite B
Gainsville, FL 32601
  Publishes a quarterly journal on menopause and aging.

Women's Health Connection
P.O. Box 6338
Madison, WI 53716-0338
800-366-6632
  This educational division of Women's International Pharmacy publishes a bimonthly newsletter on menopause, PMS, and other hormone-related disorders.

A Friend Indeed Publications, Inc.
P.O. Box 1710
Champlain, NY 12919
  Publishes a monthly newsletter on recent menopause research.

Menopause News
2074 Union Street
San Francisco, CA 94123
800-241-6366

Publishes a bimonthly newsletter on recent information about medical and psychological aspects of menopause.

National Women's Health Network
514 10th Street, NW, Suite 400
Washington, DC 20004
202-347-1140
A membership education and advocacy organization that publishes a newsletter and packets of information on ERT/HRT and alternative treatments.

Older Women's League (OWL)
666 11th Street, NW, Suite 700
Washington, DC 20001-4512
202-783-6686
A membership and advocacy organization that publishes a newsletter.

Dr. Christiane Northrup's
Health Wisdom for Women
7811 Montrose Road
Potomac, MD 20854
800-804-0935
(a monthly newsletter)

Specific Conditions and Diseases
The Osteoporosis Education Project
East Genesee Medical Building
1200 East Genesee Street
Syracuse, NY 13210
315-471-0264
(Send SASE for information)

National Osteoporosis Foundation
2100 M Street, NW
Washington, DC 20037
202-223-2226
Publishes the free information kit called *Bonewise.*

American Diabetes Association, Inc.
1660 Duke Street
Alexandria, VA 22314
800-232-3472

National Alliance of Breast Cancer Organizations
9 East 37th Street, 10th floor
New York, NY 10016
212-889-0606
Publishes a newsletter.

Alternative Therapies

For more information about the these therapies and listings of knowledgeable practitioners in your geographical area, contact these organizations.

American Association of Naturopathic Physicians
P.O. Box 20386
Seattle, WA 98112

American Chiropractic Association
1701 Clarendon Boulevard
Arlington, VA 22209

National Center for Homeopathy (NCH)
801 N. Fairfax Street, Suite 306
Alexandria, VA 22314
703-548-7790

American Institute of Homeopathy (AIH)
1585 Glencoe Street, #44
Denver, CO 80220
303-370-9164

International Foundation for Homeopathy (IFH)
2366 Eastlake Avenue E, #301
Seattle, WA 98102
206-324-8230

American Academy of Osteopathy
3500 DePaulo Blvd, Ste. 1080
Indianapolis, IN 46268-1136
317-879-1881
  osteopaths who specialize in manipulation.

American Academy of Environmental Medicine
P.O. Box 16106
Denver, CO 80216
303-622-9755
  doctors who specialize in environmental medicine.

American Holistic Medical Association
4101 Lake Boone Trail, Ste. 201
Raleigh, NC 27607
  doctors who specialize in holistic medicine.

International and American Associations of Clinical Nutritionists
5200 Keller Springs Road, #410
Dallas, TX 75248
214-392-2355

American Aromatherapy Association
P.O. Box 1222
Fair Oaks, CA 95628

American Society of Acupuncture and Oriental Medicine
1424 16th Street, NW, #501
Washington, DC 20036
202-265-2287

American Academy of Medical Acupuncture
5820 Wilshire Boulevard, Suite 500
Los Angeles, CA 90036
880-521-2262

The Garlic Information Center
The New York Hospital–Cornell University Medical Center
515 East 71st Street, S 904
New York, NY 10021

Free brochure on the possible benefits of garlic suggested in the scientific literature.

Products

In addition to homeopaths, herbalists, nutritionists, health food stores and pharmacies, you can get homeopathic, herbal and nutritional remedies (either single remedies or combination formulas designed for menopause, headache, PMS, insomnia, and other complaints) through the mail from the following reputable companies. Ask for a specific remedy, or request a catalog (usually free) before ordering:

Homeopathic Remedies
Boericke and Tafel, Inc.: 800-876-9505
Boiron, USA: 800-BLU-TUBE
Dolisos America, Inc.: 800-365-4767
Hahnemann Medical Clinic: 510-524-3117
Medicine from Nature: 800-293-1133; 801-489-1500
Standard Homeopathic Company: 800-624-9659

Homeopathic Educational Services
22124 Kittridge Street
Berkeley, CA 94704
415-547-2492; 800-359-9051
This is the premier mail-order resource for books, remedies (individual, combination, and kits), tapes, software, home study courses, and general information. Their catalog is a course in itself.

Herbal and Nutritional Remedies and Supplements
Products from BHI, Heel Pharmaceuticals, and Vitality Works Herbals are available through:
Shanah Azee Distributors
800-945-0409
Homeopathic remedies: BHI Feminine, BHI Mulimen, Hormeel, Klimaktheel, Nervoheel, Ovarium Compositum. Herbal remedies: Fem Complex, Energy.

Rainbow Light
207 McPherson Street, Dept. P
Santa Cruz, CA 95060
800-635-1233
Herbal remedies.

Frontier Copperative Herbs
800-669-3275
Herbal remedies.

Biotanica
P.O. Box 1285
Sherwood, OR 97140
800-572-4712
503-625-4824
This company sells Dr. Tori Hudson's herbal formulas for menopause and PMS.

Phyto-Pharmica
P.O. Box 1745
Green Bay, WI 54305
800-553-2370
They manufacture and distribute the formulas of Dr. Murray. These
include the "Fem-Tone," "Remifemin," and other formulas for
menopause.

Maharishi Ayur-Ved Products International, Inc.
P.O. Box 541, 417 Bolton Road
Lancaster, MA 01523
800-255-8332
They produce two Ayurvedic herbal formulas for menopause called
"Golden Transition."

Pioneer Nutritional Formulas, Inc.
P.O. Box 259
Shelburne Falls, MA 01370
413-625-8212
800-458-8483

They produce a high-potency herbal support product for menopause.

NEEDS
527 Charles Ave. 12A
Syracuse, NY 13209
800-634-1380
A mail order supplement company offering a wide range of nutrition products.

Allergy Resources
P.O. Box 444
Guffey, CO 80820
800-USE-FLAX
A mail order company that offers a wide range of nutrition and health products.

Cardiovascular Research Ltd.
1061-B Shary Circle
Concord, CA 94518
415-827-2636

Hormone Replacement Therapies

These companies manufacture and/or distribute natural progesterone, the three forms of estrogen, and DHEA; most of these products require a doctor's prescription. This is a rapidly growing area, so call or write for their most recent catalog.

Women's International Pharmacy
5708 Monona Drive
Madison, WI 53719-3152
800-279-5708

Professional and Technical Services
333 Northeast Sandy Boulevard
Portland, OR 97232
800-648-8211

College Pharmacy
833 North Tejon Street
Colorado Springs, Colorado 80903
800-888-9358

Delk Pharmacy
1602 Hatcher Lane
Columbia, TN 38401
615-388-3952

Testing Laboratories

Laboratories Offering Saliva Tests for Hormone Levels
Diagnos-Techs, Inc.
6620 South 192nd Place, #J-104
Kent, Washington 98032
1-800-87-tests
206-251-0596
   This laboratory works only with physicians, but the interested public can receive information on these tests from Dr. Rebecca Wynsome.
Send a SASE for information.

National BioTech Laboratory
3212 NE 125th Street
Seattle, WA 98125
800-846-6285
206-363-6606

Aeron Biotechnology
1933 Davis St. Ste. 310
San Leandro, CA 94577
800-367-3296

Urinary Tests for Bone Resorption
Great Smokies Diagnostic Laboratory
18A Regent Park Blvd.
Ashville, NC 28806

800-522-4762
704-253-0621

Meredian Valley Clinical Lab
515 Harrison St., Suite 9
Kent, WA 98042
800-234-6825
206-859-8700

MetaMatrix Medical Laboratory
5000 Peachtree Ind. Blvd.
Suite 110
Norcross, GA 30071
404-446-5483
800-221-4640

Ostex International
2203 Airport Way South
Suite 301
Seattle, WA 98134
206-292-8082
800-99-OSTEX

Audio and Videotapes

Dr. Maas has created a series of audio and videotapes for breathing, relaxation, and relief of lower back pain; and movements to relieve pain and release stress.

The MEND Clinic
9121 E. Tanque Verde #105
Tucson, AZ 85749
520-749-0800

Appendix D
Bibliography and Recommended Reading

Although we may not agree with everything the authors of the following books conclude or recommend, each has valuable information to offer.

Books

Barbach, Lonnie. *The Pause: Positive Approaches to Menopause.* New York: Dutton/Penguin, 1993.

————. *Shared Intimacies: Women's Sexual Experiences.* Garden City, NY: Anchor Press/Doubleday, 1980.

Bailey, Covert, and Bishop, Lea. *The Fit or Fat Woman.* Boston: Houghton Mifflin, 1989.

Baron-Faust, Rita, with the Physicians of NYU Medical Center. *Breast Cancer: What Every Woman Should Know.* New York: Morrow, 1995.

Brown, Susan. *Better Bones, Better Body: A Comprehensive Self-Help Guide to Preventing, Halting, and Overcoming Osteoporosis.* New Canaan, CT: Keats, 1996.

Bruning, Nancy. *The Natural Health Guide to Antioxidants.* New York: Bantam Books, 1994.

————, and Corey Weinstein. *Healing Homeopathic Remedies.* New York: Dell, 1995.

The Burton Goldberg Group. *Alternative Medicine: The Definitive Guide.* Puyallup, WA: Future Medicine Publishing, 1993.

Castleman, Michael. *The Healing Herbs.* Emmaus, PA: Rodale Press, 1991.

Castro, Miranda. *The Complete Homeopathy Handbook.* New York: St. Martin's Press, 1990.

Chopra, Deepak. *Ageless Body, Timeless Mind.* New York: Harmony Books, 1993.

————. *Perfect Health: The Complete Mind/Body Guide.* New York: Harmony Books, 1990.

Cobb, Janine O'Leary. *Understanding Menopause.* New York: Penguin, 1994.

Cone, Faye Kitchner. *Making Sense of Menopause.* New York: Simon & Schuster, 1994.

Coney, Sandra. *The Menopause Industry: A Guide to Medicine's "Discovery" of the Mid-Life Woman.* New York: Penguin Books, 1991.

Cummings, Stephen, and Ullman, Dana. *Everybody's Guide to Homeopathic Medicines.* New York: Putnam/Tarcher/Perigee, 1991.

Cutler, Winnifred. *Hysterectomy: Before & After: A Comprehensive Guide to Preventing, Preparing For, and Maximizing Health After Hysterectomy.* New York: Harper & Row, 1988.

Davis, Patricia. *Aromatherapy: An A–Z.* Essex, England: C. W. Daniel Company, 1988.

Doress-Worters, Paula B., and Siegal, Diana Laskin. *The New Our Bodies, Ourselves, Growing Older.* Boston: Boston Women's Health Book Collective, 1994.

Elias, Jason and Masline, Shelagh Ryan. *Healing Herbal Remedies.* New York: Dell Publishing, 1995.

Erasmus, Udo. *Fats That Heal, Fats That Kill.* Burnaby, BC Canada: Alive Books, 1993.

Faelton, Sharon. *The Allergy Self-Help Book.* Emmaus, PA: Rodale Press, 1983.

Gaby, Alan. *Preventing and Reversing Osteoporosis: Every Woman's Essential Guide.* Rocklin, CA: Prima Publishing, 1994.

Gach, Michael. *Acu-Yoga.* Tokyo: Japan Publications, Inc., 1981.

———. *Arthritis Relief at Your Fingertips: Your Guide to Easing Aches and Pains Without Drugs.* New York: Warner Books, 1989.

Gittleman, Ann Louise. *Supernutrition for Menopause.* New York: Pocket Books, 1993.

Golan, Ralph. *Optimal Wellness.* New York: Ballantine Books, 1995.

Greenwood, Sadja. *Menopause Naturally,* second edition. Volcano, CA: Volcano Press, 1992.

Hendler, Saul. *The Doctors' Vitamin and Mineral Encyclopedia.* New York: Simon & Schuster, 1990.

Ito, Dee. *Without Estrogen: Natural Remedies for Menopause and Beyond.* New York: Carol Southern Books/Random House, 1994.

Kamen, Betty. *Hormone Replacement Therapy: Yes or No—How to Make an Informed Decision.* Novato, CA: Nutrition Encounter, Inc., 1993.

Kano, Susan. *Making Peace with Food.* New York: Harper & Row, 1989.

Krohn, Jacqueline. *The Whole Way to Allergy Relief and Prevention.* Point Roberts, WA: Hartley & Marks, 1991.

Lamb, Lawrence E. *The Weighting Game.* New York: Lyle Stuart, 1989.

Lark, Susan. *The Menopause Self-Help Book.* Berkeley, CA: Celestial Arts, 1992.

Lee, John R. *Natural Progesterone: The Multiple Roles of a Remarkable Hormone,* 1993. Available from: BLL Publishing, P.O. Box 2068, Sebastopol, CA 95473.

Lerner, Michael. *Choices in Healing: Integrating the Best of Conventional and Complementary Approaches to Cancer.* Cambridge: MIT Press, 1994.

Lieberman, Shari, and Bruning, Nancy. *The Real Vitamin & Mineral Book.* Garden City: NY: Avery Publishing Group, Inc., 1990.

Love, Susan. *Dr. Susan Love's Breast Book,* Reading, MA: Addison-Wesley, 1991.

Maas, Paula, and Mitchell, Deborah. *The Natural Health Guide to Headache Relief.* New York: Pocket Books (forthcoming).

Mandell, Marshall. *Dr. Mandell's 5-Day Allergy Relief System.* New York: Pocket Books, 1980.

Messina, Mark, and Messina, Virginia. *The Simple Soybean and Your Health.* Garden City, NY: Avery Publishing Group, 1994.

Murray, Michael T. *Menopause: How You Can Benefit from Diet, Vitamins, Minerals, Herbs, Exercise,* Rocklin, CA: Prima Publishing, 1994.

————. *The Healing Power of Herbs.* Rocklin, CA: Prima Publishing, 1992.

————, and Pizzorno, Joseph. *Encyclopedia of Natural Medicine.* Rocklin, CA: Prima Publishing, 1991.

Nachtigall, Lila, and Heilman, Joan Rattner. *Estrogen,* revised. New York: HarperCollins, 1991.

Northrup, Christiane. *Women's Bodies, Women's Wisdom.* New York: Bantam Books, 1994.

Notelovitz, Morris, and Tonnessen, Diana. *Menopause and Midlife Health.* New York: St. Martin's Press, 1994.

Ojeda, Linda. *Menopause Without Medicine.* Alameda, CA: Hunter House, 1992.

Ornstein, Robert, and Sobel, David. *Healthy Pleasures*. Reading, MA: Addison-Wesley, 1989.

Perry, Susan, and O'Hanlan, Katherine. *Natural Menopause*. Reading, MA: Addison-Wesley, 1992.

Quillon, Patrick. *Beating Cancer with Nutrition*. Tulsa: The Nutrition Times Press, Inc., 1994.

Rinzler, Carol Ann. *Estrogen and Breast Cancer*. New York: Macmillan, 1994.

Roth, Geneen. *Why Weight? A Guide to Compulsive Eating*. New York: New American Library, 1989.

Scott, Susan and Julian. *Natural Medicine for Women*. New York: Avon, 1991.

Seaman, Barbara, and Seaman, Gideon. *Women and the Crisis in Sex Hormones*. New York: Bantam, 1981.

Sheehy, Gail. *Menopause: The Silent Passage*. New York: Pocket Books, 1993.

Stein, Diane. *The Natural Remedy Book for Women,* Freedom, CA: The Crossing Press, 1992.

Van Stratten, Michael. *The Complete Natural Health Consultant*. New York: Prentice-Hall Press, 1987.

Weed, Susun. *Menopausal Years: The Wise Woman Way*. Woodstock, NY: Ashtree Publishing, 1992.

Weil, Andrew. *Natural Health, Natural Medicine*. Boston: Houghton Mifflin, 1990.

Weiner, Michael and Janet. *Herbs That Heal*. Mill Valley, CA: Quantum Books, 1994 [A-to-Z therapeutic index of herbs].

Werbach, Melvin. *Healing Through Nutrition*. New York: HarperCollins, 1993.

Worwood, Valerie Ann. *The Complete Book of Essential Oils and Aromatherapy*. San Rafael, CA: New World Library, 1991.

Special Reports, Journals, and Professional Articles

The Nutrition Detective Workbook: Assessing and Maximizing Your Nutritional Fitness, by Dr. Susan E. Brown, is a 100-page workbook for evaluating and maximizing your nutrient status. It helps you analyze your diet as well as detect signs and symptoms of nutrient inadequacy; lists wholesome food sources of some twenty key nutrients so you can work toward getting the required amounts in your diet. Dr.

Brown has also published *Estrogen Therapy for Osteoporosis and Heart Disease: Is It Worth It?* and *Is the Right Food Wrong for You?: A Self-Help Program to Detect and Overcome Food Allergies,* also by Dr. Brown, is a workbook. Both are available from the Nutrition Education and Consulting Service, 1200 East Genesee Street, Suite 310, Syracuse, NY 13210; 315-471-0264. Dr. Brown also provides a three-day diet analysis with personalized report, and a bi-monthly newsletter. For a sample of the newsletter send a SASE.

Adlercreutz, Herman. ''Western Diet and Western Diseases: Some Hormonal and Biochemical Mechanisms and Associations.'' *Scandinavian Journal of Clinical Laboratory Investigations,* 1990, 50, Supplement 201, p. 3 [discusses phytoestrogens and lignans].

Avorn, J., et al. ''Reduction of Bacteruria and Pyuria After Ingestion of Cranberry Juice.'' *JAMA,* March 9, 1994, p. 751.

Barradas, M., et al. ''The Effects of Olive Oil Supplementation on Human Platelet Function, Serum Cholesterol-Related Variables, and Plasma Fibrinogen Concentration: A Pilot Study.'' *Nutrition Research,* 1990, 10, p. 103.

Bauer, D. C., et al. ''Skin Thickness, Estrogen Use, and Bone Mass in Older Women.'' *Menopause: The Journal of the North American Menopause Society,* 1994, 1(3), p. 131.

Harvard Woman's Health Watch, Dept. WHW-MI93, P.O. Box 380, Boston, MA 02117-0380, has published issues on hormone replacement therapy, mammography, depression, aging and exercise, osteoporosis, breast cancer, and calcium.

The Holistic Health Directory, published annually by *New Age Journal,* contains comprehensive, state-by-state listings of practitioners under specific treatment categories. To order, call 800-782-7006.

Menopause: The Journal of the North American Menopause Society. Available from Raven Press, Department 1B, 1185 Avenue of the Americas, New York, NY 10036.

''Natural Anxiolytics—Kava and L.72 Anti-Anxiety Formula.'' *The American Journal of Natural Medicine,* October 1994, 1(2), p. 10.

''Nutritional Modulation of Women's and Men's Sex Hormone-Related Health Problems.'' *Applying New Essentials in Nutritional*

Medicine. Material from seminar by Dr. Jeffrey Bland, February 5, 1995 [discusses plant estrogens].

"St. John's Wort vs. Tricyclic Antidepressants." *The American Journal of Natural Medicine,* April 1995, 2(3), p. 8.

Borho, B. "Therapy of the Menopausal Syndrome with Mulimen— Results of a Multicentric Post-Marketing Survey." *Biological Therapy,* 1992, 10(2), p. 226 [discusses a combination homeopathic remedy].

Brody, J. E. "New Therapy for Menopause Reduces Risks." *The New York Times,* November 18, 1994.

Bitler, W. J. "Hormone Replacement Therapy in Patients with Estrogen-Sensitive Malignancies." *The Female Patient,* March 1995, p. 43 [a review of reviews].

Cardoff, Jennifer. "The Pill Over 40—Safe at Last?" *Mirabella,* September 1991.

Chambers, D. G. "Contraception in Women Over 35: Risks and Benefits." *The Canadian Journal of CME,* August 1994, p. 21.

Cobleigh, M. A., et al. "Estrogen Replacement Therapy in Breast Cancer Survivors." *JAMA,* August 17, 1994, p. 540.

Colditz, G. A., et al. "The Use of Estrogens and Progestins and the Risk of Breast Cancer in Postmenopausal Women." *The New England Journal of Medicine,* June 15, 1995.

Collins, A., and Landgren, B. "Influence of Lifestyle Factors on Women's Health at Menopause." *Menopause,* 1994, 1(3), p. 170.

Dentali, S. "Hormones and Yams: What's the Connection?" *The American Herb Association,* 1994, 10(4), p. 4.

Falck, Frank Jr., et al. "Pesticides and Polychlorinated Biphenyl Residues in Human Breast Lipids and Their Relation to Breast Cancer." *Archives of Environmental Health,* March/April 1992, p. 143.

Follingstad, A. H. "Estriol, the Forgotten Estrogen?" *JAMA,* January 2, 1978, 239(1), p. 29.

Fowler, B. "Fluoride Watch." *Natural Health,* November/December 1994, p. 14 [letter citing studies that show fluoride increases risk of hip fractures, osteoporosis, cavities, and mottled teeth].

Gaby, A. R. "Literature Review and Commentary." *The Townsend Letter for Doctors,* August/September 1994, p. 850 [on hormones].

Gelety, T. J. "Hormone Replacement Therapy and Cardiovascular Disease." *The University of Arizona Ob/Gyn Update,* Winter 1994, 2(4).

Grove, K. A., and Londeree, B. E. "Bone Density in Postmenopausal Women: High Impact vs. Low Impact Exercise." *Medicine and Science in Sports and Exercise,* 1992, p. 1190.

Hargrove, J. T., et al. "Menopausal Hormone Replacement Therapy with Continuous Daily Oral Micronized Estradiol and Progesterone." *Obstetrics & Gynecology,* April 1989, p. 606.

Hudson, Tori. "Breast Cancer News" *The Townsend Letter for Doctors,* December 1994, p. 1440 [electricity and risk, detection, beta-carotene].

———. "A Pilot Study Using Botanical Medicines in the Treatment of Menopause Symptoms." *The Townsend Letter for Doctors,* December 1994, p. 1372.

Jancin, Bruce. "Exercise Study May Point to Hormones as the Breast Cancer Culprit." *Family Practice News,* November 1, 1994, p. 5.

Joelsson, I. "Remifimin—An Alternative for the Treatment of Menopausal Disorder." *Menopause,* 1994, 1(3), p. 173 [black cohosh].

Kinzler, K., et al. "Cancer Genes: What We Know Today." *Patient Care,* April 30, 1995, p. 13.

Kuritzky, L. "Hormone Replacement Therapy: Sorting the Risks and Benefits." *Hospital Practice,* May 15, 1995, p. 24.

Miksicek, R. J. "Commonly Occurring Plant Flavonoids Have Estrogenic Activity." *Molecular Pharmacology,* 1993, 44, p. 37.

Mishell, D. R. "Is Routine Use of Estrogen Indicated in Postmenopausal Women?" *The Journal of Family Practice,* 1989, 29 (4), p. 406.

Munnings, Frances. "Calcium and Exercise Important for Bones." *The Physician and Sportsmedicine.* February 1993, p. 56.

Murase, Y., et al. "Clinically Cured Cases by Per Os Gamma-oryzanol of Menopausal Disturbances or Menopausal-like Disturbances." *Sanfujuka no Jissal,* 1963, 12(2), p. 147.

Perlmutter, Cathy. "Triumph over Menopause." *Prevention,* August 1994, p. 78.

Prior, J. C. "Progesterone as a Bone-Trophic Hormone." *Endocrine Reviews,* May 1990, 11(2), p. 386.

Reichenberg-Ullman, J. "Menopause Naturally." *Natural Health.* March/April 1992, p. 75.

Reilly, Paul. "Medicago sativa extracts." *Journal of Natural Medicine,* 1(1), p. 62 [alfalfa contains plant estrogens].

Sanchez-Guerrero, J., et al. "Postmenopausal Estrogen Therapy and the Risk for Developing Systemic Lupus Erythematosus." *Annals of Internal Medicine,* March 15, 1995, p. 430.

Sarrel, P. M. "Estrogen Changes During Menopause." *The Female Patient.* February 1995 Supplement, p. 6.

Smith, C. J. "Non-Hormonal Control of Vaso-Motor Flushing in Menopausal Patients." *Chicago Medicine,* March 7, 1964 [bioflavonoids and vitamin C relieve hot flashes].

Somer, Elizabeth. "Fish Oil Gains Credibility." *The Nutrition Report,* 1990, p. 50.

Vliet, E. L. "New Insights on Hormones and Mood." *Menopause Management,* June/July 1993, p. 14.

Weiss, R. "Estrogen and the Environment." *The Washington Post,* January 25, 1994.

Williams, D. G. "The Forgotten Hormone." *Alternatives for the Health Conscious Individual.* Mountain Home Publishing, December 1991, 4(6), p. 41 [progesterone].

Wolff, Mary S., et al. "Blood Levels of Organochlorine Residues and Risk of Breast Cancer." *Journal of the National Cancer Institute,* April 21, 1993, p. 648.

Writing Group for the PEPI Trial, Valery T. Miller, principal investigator and writer. "Effects of Estrogen or Estrogen/Progestin Regimens on Heart Disease Risk Factors in Postmenopausal Women." *JAMA,* January 18, 1995, p. 199.

About the Authors

Dr. Paula Maas is a physician board certified in Family Practice as well as Homeopathy. For over twenty years she has worked in the healing arts, integrating the most effective therapies from her eclectic study and practice. In 1988 she founded and directed the MEND Clinic in Tucson, Arizona. Multidisciplinary approaches at the MEND Clinic have included experts in osteopathy, naturopathy, psychotherapy, acupuncture, herbal therapy, homeopathy, and a variety of manual medicine disciplines. Dr. Maas has a special interest in diagnosing elusive disorders involving hormonal, environmental, nutritional, psychological, and structural origins. Dr. Maas has developed a series of unique movements that combine her background in osteopathy, tai chi, yoga, and dance, which she teaches by video and audiotape and in private sessions. She has lectured for many professional and lay groups and has given workshops with Dr. Andrew Weil and Dr. Bernie Siegel. She has written many educational handouts and has completed the book *The Natural Health Guide to Headache Relief,* forthcoming from Pocket Books. Dr. Maas is also the president of the United States Health Information Network, "USHIN," a nonprofit organization whose mission is to coordinate health information over the internet and which you may access at www.ushin.org.

Dr. Susan E. Brown, Ph.D., medical anthropologist and certified clinical nutritionist, directs the Osteoporosis Education Project and the Nutrition Education and Consulting Service in Syracuse, N.Y. Within the Osteoporosis Education Project she lectures widely on osteoporosis prevention and reversal, and teaches the use of a holistic, natural program for the regeneration of bone health. The Nutrition Education and Consulting Service (NECS) provides consulting, education, research, and lecture services for health professionals and the interested public. Dr. Brown has consulted widely on socioeconomic, cultural, education, and health issues; authored numerous academic and popular articles; and has served as assistant professor, Fulbright scholar, professor, and guest lecturer in various universities. She is a member of Sigma-Xi, the honorary Scientific Research Organization of North America.

Nancy Bruning is a writer specializing in health, fitness, and the environment. She is the author or coauthor of over a dozen other books, including *Breast Implants: Everything You Need to Know* (Hunter House, 1995), *Coping with Chemotherapy* (Ballantine, 1993), *Healing Homeopathic Remedies* (Dell, 1996), *The Natural Health Guide to Antioxidants* (Bantam, 1994), *The Real Vitamin and Mineral Book* (Avery, 1990). She also writes articles for national magazines and patient-education brochures. Nancy Bruning as a native New Yorker who currently lives in San Francisco.

Index

66, 107, 125, 138, 188, 213,
214, 226, 230, 235, 254, 257,
287, 294
Estrace, 108
Estradiol, 9–10, 18, 108, 114, 232,
288
Estriol, 18, 114, 195, 288
Estrogen, 5, 7, 9, 17–19, 232–234,
263–264, 280, 282 (*see also*
Hormone replacement therapy)
Estrone, 18, 108, 114, 232, 288
Etidronate, 260
Eucalyptus, 182, 189, 231
Excess hair, 174, 177
Exercise, 38, 39–43, 124, 143, 191–
192, 200, 213, 220, 243, 256,
270–271, 285–286
Extracts, 70, 71
Eyebright, 164

Fallopian tubes, 5
False unicorn root, 194, 198, 238
Fat consumption, 28–29, 283, 284
Fatigue, 10, 167–174, 209
Fennel, 161, 207, 215, 245
Fenugreek, 295
Fertilization, 5, 7
Feverfew, 179–180, 214
Fiber, 26, 155, 285
Fibrinogin, 107
Fight or flight response, 45
Fish oil, 66, 188, 287
Flax seed oil, 66, 138, 255
Fluorine, 267, 268, 274
Folic acid, 62, 148
Follicles, 5
Follicle-stimulating hormone (FSH),
5, 7, 186
Food allergies and sensitivities, 38,
39, 179, 220, 229, 244, 308–
309
Food and Drug Administration
(FDA), 68, 100, 104, 107, 201
Food and nutrition, 24–39

for aches and pains, 123
for anxiety, 131
for bone strength, 268–270
for breast cancer, 284–285
for breast lumps and tenderness,
137
cholesterol, 254–255
for confusion, concentration, and
forgetfulness, 140
for cramping, 143
for depression, 148
for digestive problems, 155–156
for dry mouth and bad breath,
166
for fatigue and low energy, 169
for heavy periods, 186
for hot flashes, 191
for insomnia, 199–200
for irregular menstrual periods,
206
for menstrual cramps and PMS,
212–213
for skin, 224–225
for urinary tract and bladder
infections, 228–229
Food diary, 37
Food sources, of vitamins and
minerals, 61–64
Forgetfulness, 140–142
Fosamax, 260
Foxglove, 68
Frankincense, 227
Freedman, Rita, 3
Free radicals, 12, 25, 29, 59, 250,
252, 285

Gaby, Alan, 281
Gamma-oryzanol, 66, 184, 193, 257
Garlic, 65–66, 169, 228, 238, 255,
287, 294
Gelsemium, 134, 152, 181
Genistein, 116, 117
Gentian, 157
Geranium, 152, 172, 189, 215, 227